Modeling Paradigms and Analysis of Disease Transmission Models

DIMACS
Series in Discrete Mathematics
and Theoretical Computer Science

Volume 75

Modeling Paradigms and Analysis of Disease Transmission Models

Abba B. Gumel
Suzanne Lenhart
Editors

Center for Discrete Mathematics
and Theoretical Computer Science
A consortium of Rutgers University, Princeton University,
AT&T Labs–Research, Alcatel-Lucent Bell Laboratories,
Cancer Institute of New Jersey (CINJ), NEC Laboratories America,
and Telcordia Technologies
(with partners at Avaya Labs, HP Labs, IBM Research, Microsoft
Research, Georgia Institute of Technology, Rensselaer Polytechnic
Institute, and Stevens Institute of Technology)

American Mathematical Society
Providence, Rhode Island

This DIMACS volume presents selected papers from the U.S.–Africa Advanced Study Institute on Mathematical Modeling of Infectious Diseases in Africa, held at the African Institute for Mathematical Sciences, Muizenberg, South Africa, from June 11–22, 2007, and the DIMACS Workshop of the same name, hosted by the South Africa Centre for Epidemiological Modeling and Analysis, Stellenbosch, South Africa, from June 25–27, 2007.

2000 *Mathematics Subject Classification.* Primary 34D05, 34D20, 34D23, 92B05, 92–01, 92–02, 92–06, 92D25, 92D30.

Library of Congress Cataloging-in-Publication Data

Modeling paradigms and analysis of disease transmission models / Abba B. Gumel, Suzanne Lenhart, editors.

p. cm. — (DIMACS series in discrete mathematics and theoretical computer science ; v. 75)

Includes bibliographical references.

ISBN 978-0-8218-4384-0 (alk. paper)

1. Epidemiology—Mathematical models. 2. Communicable diseases—Transmission—Mathematical models. 3. Public health—Mathematical models. I. Gumel, Abba B., 1966– II. Lenhart, Suzanne.

RA652.2M3M63 2010
614.4015118—dc22

2010016461

♾ The paper used in this book is acid-free and falls within the guidelines
established to ensure permanence and durability.
Visit the AMS home page at `http://www.ams.org/`

10 9 8 7 6 5 4 3 2 1 15 14 13 12 11 10

Contents

Foreword

In recent years, mathematical modeling of infectious diseases has had an increasing influence on the theory and practice of disease management and control with such diseases as HIV/AIDS, foot-and-mouth disease, and H1N1 virus, and this is increasingly the case with diseases of Africa. In order to understand and prevent the spread of infectious diseases endemic to or emanating from Africa, it is vitally important to train a cadre of workers who are both knowledgeable about modeling and about disease contexts and data gathering in Africa. The success of recent joint US-African modeling studies points to the major advantages of such collaborations while at the same time pointing to the vital need for more trained researchers from both sides. To address the issue of training researchers knowledgeable about African diseases and expert in mathematical modeling of disease, DIMACS, in collaboration with the South African DST/NRF Centre of Excellence in Epidemiological Modeling and Analysis (SACEMA) and the African Institute for Mathematical Sciences (AIMS), held a two-week advanced study institute (ASI) on mathematical modeling and infectious diseases in Africa, culminating in a subsequent 3-day "capstone" workshop at which ASI students and researchers from both the US and Africa interacted and established collaborations. The ASI and workshop gave rise to this volume, though it is by no means a proceedings of those two events and, in fact, is aimed at laying out in an organized way some of the major themes of infectious disease modeling, with special emphasis on infectious diseases of Africa.

The ASI, held at AIMS in Cape Town, South Africa, on June 11-22, 2007, was aimed at training junior US and African participants (graduate students and postdoctoral fellows) in mathematical epidemiology and the control of emerging and re-emerging diseases. The capstone workshop, held at Stellenbosch University, Stellenbosch, South Africa, on June 25-27, 2007, was a culmination of the ASI, enabling ASI students to participate fully in a workshop involving active US and African researchers and aimed at furthering research on the modeling of diseases in Africa. The ASI emphasized basic mathematical techniques used in modeling and reviewed key diseases of Africa. It then introduced the basic ideas of epidemiological modeling, including classical epidemic models such as SIR, SIS, and SEIR; structured modeling; deterministic vs. stochastic models; and uncertainty and sensitivity analysis. It went on to more advanced topics such as meta-population modeling; continuous vs. discrete-time stochastic models; models with vertical transmission; spatial and individual-based models; age structure; and optimal allocation of disease control resources such as vaccine and antiviral doses.

Speakers at the capstone workshop discussed the design and evaluation of cost-effective and sustainable strategies for combating disease spread in Africa, with emphasis on modern statistical tools for surveillance, network methods to elucidate patterns of spread, and evolutionary aspects of endemic African diseases. Challenges from and opportunities arising from increasing availability of data from African studies were discussed. A second theme involved the potential consequences of emerging and re-emerging diseases, in the context of shortage of resources. Speakers addressed drug resistance to tuberculosis, challenges from HIV and malaria, and alternative interventions for pandemic flu, including vaccination, targeted antiviral prophylaxis, and quarantines. Finally, a special session introduced the rapidly-emerging topic of "economic epidemiology," with its emphasis on health economics and the economic aspects of disease burden.

These activities were part of the DIMACS Special Focus on Computational and Mathematical Epidemiology. One specific special focus workshop was instrumental in leading us to develop this DIMACS activity. This was a workshop on "Evolutionary Aspects of Vaccine Use," organized at DIMACS in June 2005, and stemming from the work of the DIMACS working group on Methodologies for Comparing Vaccination Strategies. The special problems of vaccination strategies in Africa that arose in this workshop were one of the primary motivations that led Abba Gumel, one of the editors of this volume, to propose that DIMACS sponsor a workshop that would directly focus on mathematical modeling of infectious diseases in Africa.

A second activity that led to the DIMACS African activities was the summer research conference on "Modeling Dynamics of Human Diseases: Emerging Paradigms and Challenges," held at Snowbird in Utah July 17-21, 2005. One notable feature of the conference was the recognition of the central role of developing nations in the emergence of novel pathogens, and the need to involve researchers from these nations in addressing problems of the spread of disease. This recognition was central in motivating meeting participant Simon Levin, a major leader of the DIMACS Special Focus, to suggest that we pursue ways to more directly engage US researchers and students with African researchers and students.

In turn, the DIMACS African activities that led to this volume have led to a major US-African-Canadian Bio-Mathematics Initiative that includes ASIs and workshops in Uganda, Kenya, and Madagascar, modeled after those in South Africa.

DIMACS thanks Professors Gumel and Levin for their efforts in promoting the ASI and workshop on Mathematical Modeling and Infectious Diseases in Africa. Special thanks go to the Directors of SACEMA and AIMS, John Hargrove and Fritz Hahne, respectively, for their scientific, administrative, and financial support. Brenda Latka of DIMACS played a major role in helping to administer the ASI and workshop and Latka, Wayne Getz, Gumel, Hahne, Hargrove, Levin, Edward Lungu, and Alex Welte helped to organize it. Others who played an important role in developing the concept and scope of the ASI and workshop were Dominic Clemence, Ronald Mickens, Asamoah Nkwanta, and Abdul-Aziz Yakubu. DIMACS is extremely grateful to all of these people for their involvement and support in its African initiatives. Finally, DIMACS thanks Gumel and Suzanne Lenhart for their efforts in putting this volume together.

DIMACS gratefully acknowledges the generous support that makes its programs possible. Special thanks go to the National Science Foundation, under grant 0629720 to Rutgers University, which made the ASI and workshop that led to this book possible. Thanks also go to the DIMACS partners at Rutgers, Princeton, AT&T Labs - Research, Alcatel-Lucent Bell Labs, NEC Laboratories America, and Telcordia Technologies, and affiliate partners Avaya Labs, Georgia Institute of Technology, HP Labs, IBM Research, Microsoft Research, Rensselaer Polytechnic Institute, and Stevens Institute of Technology.

Fred S. Roberts
DIMACS Director

Preface

This volume is a product of two activities under the auspices of DIMACS Special Focus on Computational and Mathematical Epidemiology, namely the U.S.-Africa Advanced Study Institute (ASI) on Mathematical Modeling of Infectious Diseases in Africa, which took place at the African Institute for Mathematical Sciences (AIMS), Muizenberg, South Africa, June 11-22, 2007, and the DIMACS Workshop on Mathematical Modeling of Infectious Diseases in Africa, hosted by the South Africa Centre for Epidemiological Modeling and Analysis (SACEMA), Stellenbosch, South Africa, on June 25-27, 2007. About 50 graduate students, from across Africa and the USA, attended the ASI, and a total of about 80 people attended the workshop.

The volume consists of two types of papers: tutorial papers and research papers. While the tutorial papers introduce the basic and general principles, concepts, challenges and types of disease modeling, the research papers focus on advanced topics associated with the mathematical modeling (and analysis) of diseases relevant to Africa.

The tutorial-type papers cover topics such as basic principles and framework for modeling diseases, classical (Kermack-McKendrick type) epidemic models, modeling challenges, basic methods of analysis, epidemiological thresholds, uncertainty and sensitivity analysis and the interpretation of the analytical and simulation results obtained. In addition to the aforementioned basic topics, the volume also contains papers on more advanced topics. These include papers on optimal control techniques in disease modeling, design and analysis of discrete-time models, the role of stochasticity in disease modeling, economic aspects of disease modeling and control (including the use of greedy algorithms to obtain optimal solutions) and some advanced dynamical systems techniques for qualitatively analyzing relatively large disease transmission models. Some of these papers address the problem of the transmission dynamics and control of some diseases that inflict major socio-economic and public health burden in Africa, notably HIV and HIV-TB co-infection.

The Editors are very grateful to all those who contributed papers to the volume (S. Shrestha, J. O. Lloyd-Smith, E. M. Lungu, M. Kgosimore, F. Nyabadza, R. Miller Neilan, S. Lenhart, A.-A Yakubu, W. Ding, J. Dushoff, M. S. Sánchez, B. G. Williams, W. Getz, S. D. Hove-Musekwa, V. Runyowa, Z. Mukandavire, O. Sharomi, A. B. Gumel and F. Roberts). In addition to the great scholarly contributions of the authors, this volume would not have been possible without the support of the sponsors of the ASI and the workshop in Stellenbosch, namely AIMS, DIMACS, The U.S. National Science Foundation and SACEMA.

The Editors are immensely grateful to Fred Roberts, who made the whole U.S.-Africa program possible. We are thankful to the DIMACS staff (notably,

Margaret Barry Cozzens, Gene Fiorini, Brenda Latka, Christine Spassione and Ricardo Collado) and Ms. Christine Thivierge (Editorial Assistant, AMS) for their support. Finally, we are very grateful to the many anonymous reviewers who helped in reviewing the contributed papers. The Editors are also very thankful to Simon Levin for writing the Prologue to this volume.

Abba Gumel and Suzanne Lenhart
January 23, 2010

Prologue

In recent years, computational biology has become one of the hottest areas in science, spawning new journals, new scientific societies, new departments, and new training programs for undergraduates and graduates. The challenges of genomics and systems biology have attracted leading scientists from other disciplines—in particular physics, computer science and mathematics—who have been motivated to bring their skills to bear on some of the most important and fundamental problems facing humanity. Indeed, the excitement of the advances in genomics, and in certain branches of systems biology, has to some made these applications synonymous with the field of "computational biology." It therefore often comes as a surprise when people learn that computational biology is a very old field, tracing back more than a century, and with roots firmly planted in population genetics and in epidemiology.

The mathematical description of the dynamics of infectious diseases is one of the oldest and most successful branches of quantitative science, tracing back at least a century to the landmark malaria models of the Nobel Laureate, Sir Ronald Ross. It has remained a vibrant area of research since Ross, a subdiscipline with a rigorous theoretical foundation, a highly developed mathematical and statistical framework, and strong contact with data and with management. The concepts of theoretical epidemiology have played fundamental roles in understanding disease dynamics, and in the optimal application of vaccination and other management strategies. This volume continues that tradition, with papers by some of the leading researchers of the subject.

Infectious diseases kill millions of people worldwide every year, and sicken billions of others. Africa has always been a cauldron of devastating diseases, and malaria remains one of the world's greatest killers. Despite the heroic efforts of Ross and others, malaria remains at the top of the world's public health agenda, developing resistance to wonder drugs and frustrating public health workers. Charitable foundations, like the Gates Foundation, have thus placed the elimination or control of malaria and other diseases, especially in Africa, at the tops of their agendas; but money alone cannot solve the problems. We need new approaches, new insights, and new methodologies. The quantitative study of infectious diseases has made remarkable advances in the years since Ross, and powerful new mathematical, statistical and computational tools are available; but much more needs to be done.

It is thus urgent that quantitative biologists increase their efforts to attack the problems of infectious diseases in the African subcontinent, and that has led DIMACS to sponsor a variety of ongoing efforts to address the scientific challenges and to train African scientists in the modern methods of the theory of infectious diseases. This volume is one product of that effort, and will help to strengthen the foundations and the partnerships that have been initiated. It is a mixture of pedagogy and research, building from the foundations of the subject to recent mathematical advances, including especially the application of modern control theory. Most impressively, through a mixture of contributions from U.S., Canadian and African scientists, it is testimony to the vision of Fred Roberts in sponsoring these activities, and to the success of his efforts.

Simon Levin
Princeton University
October 14, 2009

DIMACS Series in Discrete Mathematics
and Theoretical Computer Science
Volume 75, 2010

Introduction to Mathematical Modeling of Infectious Diseases

Sourya Shrestha[1] and James O. Lloyd-Smith[2,3]

1. Introduction

Despite major advances in science and public health, infectious diseases continue to cause significant morbidity and mortality in human populations worldwide, with disproportionate impact in developing countries. A recent survey estimated that infectious diseases are responsible for more than half of human deaths in sub-Saharan Africa, and sub-lethal effects of disease impose heavy burdens on quality of life and economic development (Lopez et al., 2002). Impacts of infectious disease extend beyond human populations, exacting tolls on domestic animal, wildlife and plant populations. The combination of complex ecology, rapid evolution in response to changing circumstances, and the on-going emergence of novel pathogens, ensures that infectious diseases will continue to pose serious challenges for the foreseeable future.

Thus there is strong motivation to pursue the scientific study of infectious diseases, and mathematical models make a unique contribution to this endeavor. Infectious diseases can exhibit complex nonlinear dynamics, and mathematical models enable clear and rigorous analysis of the underlying mechanisms. Models provide a crucial link between individual-level 'clinical' knowledge of disease properties and population-scale patterns of incidence and prevalence, and help to establish the relative importance of different processes to focus research and management effort. Models can provide a testing ground to investigate the possible efficacy of alternative disease control policies, in settings where direct experimentation is often ethically or logistically impossible. Finally, the process of formulating and analyzing models has the salutary effect of focusing research questions and forcing clear enunciation of assumptions and hypotheses.

This chapter is a summary of lectures given by JL-S at the DIMACS Advanced Studies Institute at AIMS in 2007. We are grateful to Ottar Bjørnstad and Matt Ferrari for sharing materials that helped with the preparation of these lectures. We are also very grateful to the students and other instructors at the institute, whose questions and comments helped to improve the presentation of this material. JL-S was funded by a Center for Infectious Disease Dynamics Fellowship at Penn State University, and by the RAPIDD program of the Science & Technology Directorate, US Department of Homeland Security, and the Fogarty International Center, National Institutes of Health.

In this article we seek to provide a concise introduction to the concepts and basic methods of infectious disease modelling. We begin by briefly reviewing some key concepts and terminology for the study of infectious disease dynamics, then introduce some classical models and broad decisions faced in model design. We discuss formulation of the transmission term that sits at the heart of infectious disease models, and approaches to incorporating population heterogeneity and structure. We conclude with a survey of approaches to parameter estimation, model fitting, and sensitivity and uncertainty analysis. Our treatment is far from comprehensive and for details we refer the reader to books by Anderson & May (1991), Diekmann & Heesterbeek (2000) or Keeling & Rohani (2007).

2. Basic concepts in infectious disease dynamics

2.1. Pathogens. It is conventional among disease modellers to categorize disease-causing organisms into two broad groups based on their size and life cycle. (i) **Microparasites** are very small organisms that multiply, often to reach very large population sizes, within individual hosts. This category includes viruses (such as influenza or HIV), bacteria (such as *Bordetella pertussis* that causes whooping cough and *Bacillus anthracis* that causes anthrax), protozoa (such as *Trypanosoma* species that cause sleeping sickness and *Plasmodium* species that cause malaria), and pathogenic fungi (such as *Candida* species that cause thrush and *Tinea pedis* that causes Athlete's foot). Microparasitic infections range from acute to chronic, lasting days to years, and cause effects ranging from asymptomatic infection to rapid death. Host individuals that survive infection often have some degree of immunity to re-infection, though the duration of this protection varies greatly among pathogens. Microparasites have a short generation time relative to their host, and undergo many generations in the course of a single infection. Hence microparasites can evolve rapidly, with important applied consequences for development of drug resistance, evasion of host immune responses, and adaptation to changing environmental circumstances.

(ii) **Macroparasites** are larger multicellular organisms, which multiply outside of the host. Macroparasites can be further divided into endoparasites that enter the host's body, such as roundworms and flukes, and ectoparasites that dwell on the surface of the host, such as ticks and mites. Macroparasites typically have longer generation times than microparasites, and their life cycles tend to be complex often comprising stages both within and outside the host and specialized infective stages. Macroparasitic infections are often chronic and sub-lethal, and the host immune response often serves to contain or limit the infection rather than eliminate it.

From a disease modelling standpoint, there are several important distinctions between macroparasites and microparasites. Typically, microparasite models classify hosts according to infection status (e.g. susceptible vs infected), while macroparasite models explicitly quantify the parasite burden within each host. The burden of macroparasites, which accumulates as a result of multiple infection events of the same host individual, is assumed to affect transmission rates from that host and morbidity or mortality of the host. In contrast, parasite burden and multiple infection events are typically assumed to be unimportant for microparasites (i.e. once infected, further exposures do not matter) – though exceptions exist for models addressing multi-strain dynamics or other particular questions.

2.2. Host immune response. Immunology is a vast and fast-moving field, and we certainly do not aim to summarize it here. Instead we present a few deliberately simplified concepts that motivate the formulation of basic disease models. A more in-depth treatment with a focus on dynamical aspects can be found in Perelson & Weisbuch (1997). The host immune response can be broadly divided into two parts. The **innate immune response** is an intrinsic, mostly non-specific response to any foreign intruder, which provides a first line of defense particularly for pathogens that the host has not encountered before. The **acquired** or **adaptive immune response** is a pathogen-specific defense based on recognition of characteristic molecular 'signatures' of pathogens that have been encountered before. The acquired immune response is the basis for the practice of vaccination, which is based on exposing the host to molecules from the parasite to prime the immune system for subsequent exposures.

A greatly simplified timecourse of the immune response to an acute microparasitic infection is as follows. Following infection with a bacterial pathogen, the innate immune response is activated immediately as macrophages recognize molecules in the bacterial wall as foreign particles. Macrophages begin killing the bacteria, and they also produce chemical signals or chemokines that recruit neutrophils and other innate effectors to the site of infection to aid in killing the bacteria. The adaptive part of the immune response begins several days after the beginning of the infection, stimulated by other chemokines and antigens (molecular motifs from the parasite) which stimulate antigen-specific B cells. These stimulated B cells multiply to produce plasma B cells that in turn produce antibodies (large molecules that bind the corresponding antigen with high affinity). These antibodies bind to the antigens on the bacteria, and cytotoxic T cells recognize the bound antibodies and kill the bacteria, eventually eliminating the infection. Apart from producing plasma cells, the stimulated B cells also produce long-lived memory B cells. This helps the immune system to react swiftly and effectively if the host is later exposed to the same antigen, so re-infection by the same bacterial strain is less likely. Depending on the efficacy of the memory response, that host may be said to be 'immune' to that bacterial pathogen. The duration and efficacy of immunity can vary greatly from one pathogen to another, from essentially no lasting immunity in the case of gonorrhea to lifelong protective immunity in the case of measles.

Immunology has mostly been a stand-alone field, but recent advances in immunology as well as epidemiology and disease ecology have generated both the need and the interest to study the immune system in conjunction with epidemiological aspects of disease dynamics. The interaction between pathogens and the host immune system is likely to affect various characteristics of an infection, such as how much pathogen the host will be carrying during the infection or how long the infection will last. These characteristics in turn will influence epidemiological properties of the disease, including transmissibility. These complexities are beyond the scope of this chapter, so we will direct readers to a sampling of recent papers that address the interaction between immunology and epidemiology. (Schmid-Hempel, 2008; Antia et al., 2005; Mideo et al., 2008; King et al., 2009)

2.3. Clinical course of disease. Once a pathogen becomes established in a host, the infection goes through different phases as it runs its course. Understanding the details of the course of infection is crucial when modelling disease spread. One is typically concerned about the time it takes for a newly infected host to become

TABLE 1. Incubation, latent and infectious periods (in days) for a variety of viral and bacterial infections. Adapted from Anderson and May (1991).

Infectious disease	**Incubation period**	**Latent period**	**Infectious period**
Measles	8 - 13	6 - 9	6 - 7
Mumps	12 - 16	12 - 18	4 - 8
Pertussis	6 - 10	21 - 23	7 - 10
Rubella	14 - 21	7 - 14	11 - 12
Diphtheria	2 - 5	14 - 21	2 - 5
Chicken pox	13 - 17	8 - 12	10 - 11
Hepatitis B	30 - 80	13 - 17	19 - 22
Poliomyelitis	7 - 12	1 - 3	14 - 20
Influenza	1 - 3	1 - 3	2 - 3
Smallpox	10 - 15	8 - 11	2 - 3
Scarlet fever	2 - 3	1 - 2	14 - 21

infectious and begin transmitting, the time it takes for the onset of symptoms, and the duration of infectiousness. These details correspond to basic parameters in epidemic models, and their values will determine basic properties of the resulting epidemic curves, some of which we shall discuss in the later sections. For now we introduce some of the frequently-used terminologies:

Incubation period: the time from infection to the onset of symptoms.
Latent period: the time from infection to the onset of transmissibility. This is also called the pre-patent period for macroparasites.
Infectious period: the time during which individual can transmit disease.
Generation time (or serial interval): the time period between infection of one host and infection of other secondary cases caused by that host.

Table 1 shows the range of values for these periods for some important microparasites. Note that the incubation and latent periods are not always equal, so the onset of transmission can come before or after the onset of symptoms for some pathogens. This has important consequences for the ability to control these disease (Fraser et al., 2004).

2.4. Transmission. Transmission of infection between individuals is the central process of infectious disease dynamics – indeed it is the reason why these disease are 'infectious' – so it is essential to consider transmission carefully in designing an epidemic model. There are many different modes of transmission (see Table 2), and models must account for the relevant modes and how they affect the disease spread. Often one has to confront questions such as:

- What is the host contact structure relevant to this mode of transmission? For example, sexually transmitted diseases (STDs) clearly follow different contact structures from respiratory pathogens.
- Are there important heterogeneities among hosts that will impact transmission?
- What disease control measures are relevant for this mode of transmission?

The answers to these questions gives us a good platform to develop accurate models of disease dynamics. We will return to the topic of different transmission models and their consequences in section 4.1.

2.5. Epidemiological terms and population-level patterns. Infectious disease epidemiology is the study of the spread of disease at the population level. Here are a few basic terms that are used in epidemiological descriptions of infectious diseases:

Incidence: the number of new infections per unit time.

Prevalence: the proportion of population that is infected at a particular time.

Attack rate: the proportion of susceptible individuals in a given setting that become infected during a given interval.

Force of infection: the per capita rate of infection per unit time (i.e. the hazard rate of infection experienced by each susceptible individual).

Seroprevalence: the proportion of population carrying antibodies indicating past exposure to pathogen.

The population-level patterns of disease spread can be broadly categorized as follows (see Fig 1 for schematic depictions):

Endemic infections: infections which do not exhibit wide temporal fluctuations in incidence or prevalence in a defined place. For microparasites, the term 'endemic' can also be used to indicate an infection that can persist locally without the need for reintroduction from outside host communities. Stable endemicity is where the incidence of infection or disease shows no secular trend for increase or decrease.

Simple epidemic: an outbreak of infection entailing a rapid increase in incidence followed by decline and (possibly temporary) disappearance of the pathogen. This epidemic pattern is typical of the microparasitic infections with high transmission rates, short generation times, and long-lasting host immunity. An epidemic usually begins with an exponential rise in the number of cases and a subsequent decline as the population of susceptible hosts is exhausted (or control measures are imposed).

Recurrent epidemics: a population-level pattern in which simple epidemics occur sporadically due to repeated introduction of the pathogen. Following each epidemic there may be a 'refractory period' in which the susceptible population is diminished so that another epidemic cannot occur. After

TABLE 2. Different modes of transmission

Modes	Diseases
Direct (droplet, aerosol, fomite)	influenza, measles, SARS
Sexual transmission	HIV, gonorrhea, HSV-2, chlamydia
Vector-borne (mosquitoes, tsetse flies, sandflies)	malaria, trypanosomiasis, leishmaniasis
Free-living infectious stages and environmental reservoirs	helminths, anthrax
Waterborne, food-borne, fecal-oral	cholera, polio, Salmonella

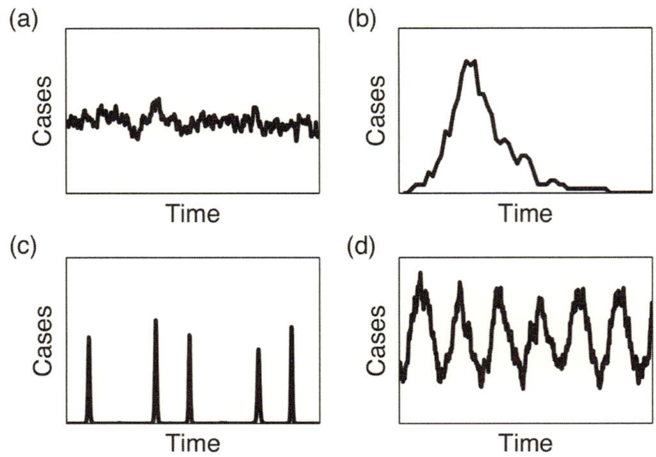

FIGURE 1. Population level patterns. (a) Endemic infection; (b) Simple epidemic; (c) Recurrent epidemic; and (d) Seasonal endemism.

sufficient time the susceptible population will be replenished (by births, immigration, or loss of acquired immunity) and subsequent introduction of the pathogen can lead to another epidemic.

Seasonal endemism: a situation in which the pathogen circulates persistently within a given population, but incidence rates vary seasonally due to changing contact rates or environmental factors. Such systems may exhibit annual epidemics of varying intensity, or marked multi-annual cycles arising from the interaction of seasonal factors with longer-period cycles of susceptible depletion and replenishment.

3. Introduction to infectious disease modelling

3.1. SIR-type compartment models for microparasite infections. The most common approach to understanding the dynamics of microparasite infections is the family of compartmental models. These models divide the population into compartments, where all individuals in a given compartment share some common attributes — where the choice of these attributes will depend on the questions that you are trying to answer and the complexity of the dynamics that you are modelling. For microparasites, these models are often referred to as SIR-type models, where S, I, and R represent compartments of Susceptible, Infectious, and Removed (or Recovered) populations, respectively. These are represented by state variables $S(t)$, $I(t)$ and $R(t)$ that track how the numbers of individuals in each compartment change with time. The set of equations below describe how the quantities in each of the compartments are changing in a standard SIR model with frequency-dependent transmission.

$$\begin{aligned}
\frac{dS}{dt} &= -\frac{\beta\, S\, I}{N} \\
\frac{dI}{dt} &= \frac{\beta\, S\, I}{N} - \gamma\, I \\
\frac{dR}{dt} &= \gamma\, I
\end{aligned} \tag{1}$$

Here, β is the transmission coefficient, which relates the current prevalence of infectiousness to the force of infection, and γ is the per capita rate of recovery for infected individuals. Susceptible individuals become infected upon successful transmission of the pathogen when two individuals from the S and I compartments interact (see section 4.1 for more details). Infectious individuals are removed from the infectious state at the given recovery rate. In this very simple model, recovered individuals remain in the R compartment indefinitely.

The set of differential equations given by (1) can be solved approximately. Because $S+I+R = N$ is a constant, we can write $\frac{dR}{dt} = \gamma(N-S-R)$. Introducing $\hat{\beta} = \frac{\beta}{N}$, we find $\frac{dS}{dR} = \frac{\frac{dS}{dt}}{\frac{dR}{dt}} = -\frac{\hat{\beta}}{\gamma} S$. Now S can be expressed in terms of R as $S = S_0\, e^{-\frac{\hat{\beta}}{\gamma} R}$, where S_0 is the initial condition, i.e. $S(t=0)$. Hence, the differential equation for R can be written in terms of R alone, $\frac{dR}{dt} = \gamma(N - S_0\, e^{-\frac{\hat{\beta}}{\gamma} R} - R)$. The approximate solution to this, due to Kermack & McKendrick, is:

$$\begin{aligned}
R &= \frac{\gamma^2}{S_0\, \hat{\beta}^2} \left[\frac{\hat{\beta}}{\gamma} S_0 - 1 + q \tanh\left(\frac{1}{2} q\, \gamma\, t - \phi \right) \right], \\
&\text{where } \phi = \tanh^{-1}\left(\frac{\hat{\beta}}{\gamma} S_0 - 1 \right) / q, \\
&\text{and } q = \left[\left(\frac{\hat{\beta}}{\gamma} S_0 - 1 \right)^2 + 2\, S_0\, I_0 \frac{\hat{\beta}^2}{\gamma^2} \right]^{1/2}.
\end{aligned} \tag{2}$$

The total size of an epidemic is approximately $\frac{2\gamma}{S_0 \hat{\beta}} \left(S_0 - \frac{\gamma}{\hat{\beta}} \right)$ (Bailey, 1955).

The SIR model can be altered or customized to suit the biological and social details of the disease system being modelled, or the question that one wants answered. A number of these alterations are shown in figure 2, including very common models (e.g. SEIR, SIS) and models that we have designed for particular problems (e.g. SICR).

3.2. Basic reproductive number, R_0. A central concept in the analysis of infectious disease dynamics is the basic reproductive number, or R_0. R_0 is defined as the expected number of new infections caused by a typical infectious individual in a wholly susceptible population. It is a threshold parameter that determines whether a disease starting from a typical infectious individual can cause an epidemic. In most cases, the same threshold also determines whether a disease can persist at the population scale (i.e. is there an 'endemic equilibrium' for the model or is

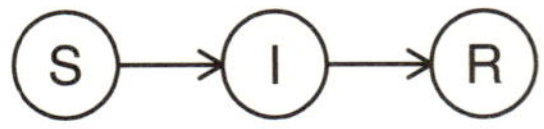

(i) Standard **SIR** model described by equation 1.

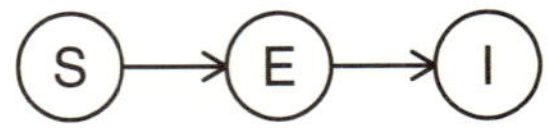

(ii) **SEI** model, where E stands for exposed but not yet infectious.

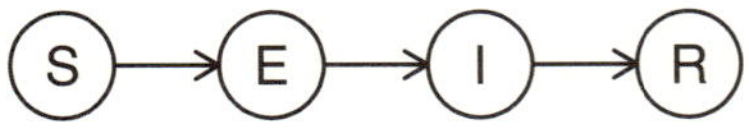

(iii) **SEIR** model with exposed and recovered classes.

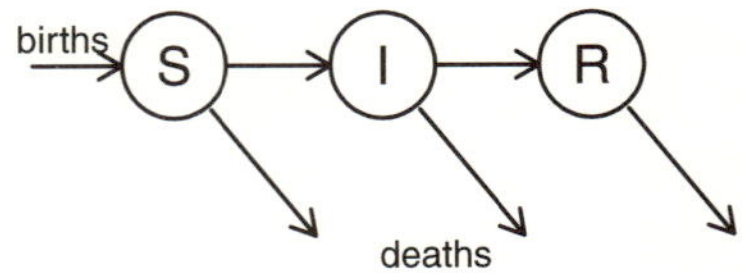

(iv) **SIR** model with birth and death processes included.

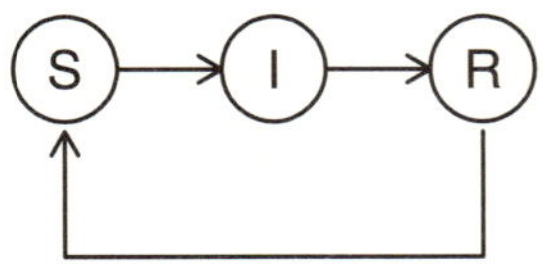

(v) **SIRS** model; recovered hosts become susceptible via loss of immunity.

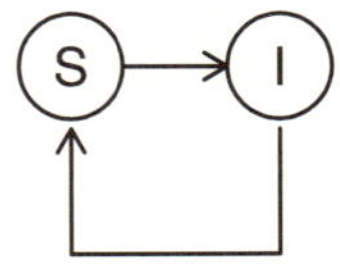

(vi) **SIS** model; infected hosts return directly to the susceptible class.

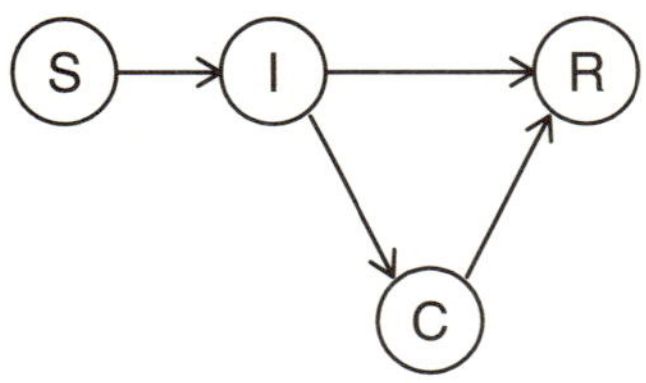

(vii) **SICR** model allows for some infectious hosts to pass through a chronic shedding phase, denoted by class C.

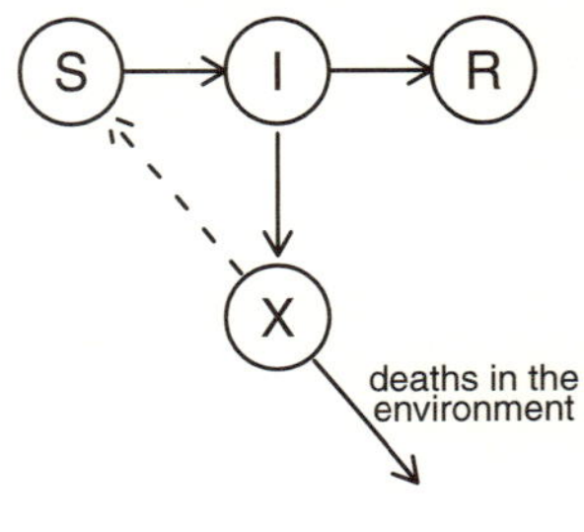

(viii) **SIR** model with class X, an environmental reservoir of the pathogen, which can contribute to new infections.

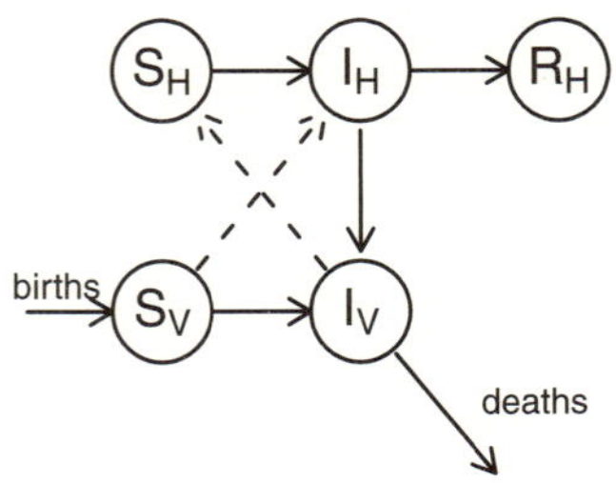

(ix) For vector-borne diseases, one tracks epidemic dynamics in both host and vector populations, where transmission occurs via vector bites.

FIGURE 2. Various adaptations of the SIR-type family of compartmental models.

the 'disease-free equilibrium' globally asymptotically stable?). If $R_0 \leq 1$, then on average an infectious individual will spread the disease to less than one individual, and the disease will not be able to spread and cause a major epidemic (though note that it can 'stutter along' for some time before it goes extinct). By contrast, if $R_0 > 1$, then a typical infectious individual will spread the disease to more than one other individual on average, and hence the disease can take off and result in an epidemic (though note that $R_0 > 1$ does not guarantee that an epidemic will occur, due to stochastic effects that we discuss below). If an epidemic does occur, then the value of R_0 gives important information about the initial growth rate of the epidemic, the prevalence at the peak of an epidemic, and the proportion of the population ultimately infected by a simple epidemic. In an endemic setting, R_0 gives insight into the endemic equilibrium prevalence and the mean age of infection.

For a simple SIR model, R_0 can be calculated in a fairly intuitive manner: it is the product of the per capita rate of infecting others, and the mean duration of infection. Under frequency-dependent transmission, the per capita rate of infecting others is $\beta S/N$ (which reduces to β if the population is wholly susceptible), and the duration of the infection is simply the reciprocal of the recovery rate, so $R_0 = \beta/\gamma$.

Generally, R_0 is taken in the context of a wholly susceptible population. To talk about a population that is not wholly susceptible, we define $R_{\text{effective}}$, which is the expected number of cases caused by a typical infectious individual in a population that is not wholly susceptible. In the simplest case, $R_{\text{effective}} = R_0 \times S/N$. This formulation will help us calculate the endemic level of disease in the population, since at equilibrium $R_{\text{effective}} = 1$ (by definition, because at equilibrium each infected case replaces itself), so the endemic equilibrium level of disease in the population is $1/R_0$. This simple formulation of $R_{\text{effective}}$ also allows us to understand the concept of **herd immunity**. If there is a sufficiently low proportion of the population that is susceptible to the disease, then $R_{\text{effective}}$ will be below 1 and the infection will be unable to circulate persistently in the population. The critical proportion of the population that needs to be immune is determined simply: since $R_{\text{effective}} = R_0 \times S/N$, then for $R_{\text{effective}} < 1$ we need $S/N < 1/R_0$. Hence, we need a proportion $1 - 1/R_0$ of the population to be immune, and the remainder of the population may be individually susceptible but is protected by herd immunity. This sets a target level for vaccination campaigns to stop disease circulation. $R_{\text{effective}}$ is sometimes also used to denote the reproductive number when other control measures have been put in place (e.g. drug treatment or case isolation). In these cases, one can use R_0 and $R_{\text{effective}}$ to determine the threshold coverage (proportion of the population that is subject to the control measure) and efficacy (proportional reduction in transmission) needed to stop disease circulation.

3.3. Models for macroparasite infection. As noted above, the basic model for macroparasite infection differs fundamentally from SIR-type models for microparasites, because for macroparasites the intensity of the infection needs to be taken into consideration. The number of disease-causing macroparasites within a host affects the way in which the disease gets transmitted. Given below is a basic model for a directly-transmitted macroparasite (Anderson & May, 1991).

$$
\begin{aligned}
\frac{dM}{dt} &= d_1\beta\, L(t-\tau_1) - (\mu+\mu_1)\, M \\
\frac{dL}{dt} &= s\, d_2\, \lambda\, N\, M(t-\tau_2) - \mu_2\, L - \beta\, N\, L
\end{aligned} \tag{3}
$$

where $N(t)$ represents the size of the host population, $M(t)$ represents the mean number of sexually mature worms in the host population, and $L(t)$ represents the number of infective larvae in the habitat. The parameter β is the infection rate; λ is the per capita fecundity rate of the parasites; μ, μ_1 and μ_2 are the death rates of the hosts, adult worms within the hosts, and larvae in the environment, respectively; d_1 and d_2 are the proportions of ingested larvae that survive to adulthood, and eggs shed that survive to become infective larvae, respectively; τ_1 is the time delay for parasite maturation to the reproductive stage; τ_2 is the time delay for maturation from egg to infective larva; and s is the proportion of offspring that are female. We will not go into greater depth on macroparasite modelling, but note that this model is a truly simplified depiction of macroparasite dynamics, and that even simple models typically account for complexities such as the density dependence of parasite fecundity and mortality, and the well-known pattern of parasite aggregation within host individuals.

3.4. R_0 and $R_{\text{effective}}$ for macroparasites. For macroparasites, R_0 is the average number of female offspring (or just offspring in the case of hermaphroditic species) produced throughout the lifetime of a mature female parasite, which themselves achieve reproductive maturity, in the absence of density-dependent constraints on the parasite establishment, survival or reproduction. $R_{\text{effective}}$ is the average number of female offspring produced in a host population within which density dependent constraints limit parasite population growth.

Note the distinction in usage of $R_{\text{effective}}$ across classes of parasites. For microparasites, $R_{\text{effective}}$ is the reproductive number in the presence of competition for hosts at the population scale (i.e. due to herd immunity), whereas for macroparasites, $R_{\text{effective}}$ is the reproductive number in the presence of competition at the within-host scale (i.e. due to density dependence within the host). For both cases, $R_{\text{effective}} = 1$ under the conditions of stable endemic infection.

3.5. Modelling decisions. Even after choosing an appropriate compartmental structure, there are many more decisions faced in the course of designing a model for a particular system and problem. Different modelling approaches are suited to different kinds of analysis, and important assumptions are often implicit in model designs. Here we review a few key dimensions of model design.

3.5.1. *Deterministic versus stochastic models.* One basic assumption made in compartmental models based on ordinary differential equations is that the course of the dynamics is **deterministic**. That is, given a model structure, parameter values and initial conditions, the model output is absolutely determined with no variation. This deterministic framework does not capture the effects of chance, or of variability in the parameters and processes involved in the model. Sometimes this is an acceptable approximation, and deterministic models do have the advantage that they are well studied and often easier to analyze. The results, when attained are definite and easy to intrepret.

In certain situations, however, it is important to consider the influence of chance events by using a **stochastic** model which incorporates variability in dynamic outcomes by modelling some processes in a probabilistic manner. One such situation is when some crucial processes in the model involve small populations or rare events. In these situations, substantial variations in population-level outcome can arise because individual-level events are discrete and uncertain. For example, an infection may have $R_0 = 1.5$ but each infected host will transmit the infection to an integer number of other hosts (0,1,2,3,...). If there is only one infected host in a population, then it matters a great deal whether he/she transmits to 0 or 1 or 2 other hosts, because the infection is very vulnerable to going extinct in that host population. (If there are 1000 infected hosts, then this individual-level uncertainty is less important because the population average outcome will dominate.) This uncertainty arising from the discreteness of individual-level events is called 'demographic stochasticity'. A second source of variation in dynamic outcomes is 'environmental stochasticity', which arises from fluctuations in the environment. Note that this includes factors in the natural environment, such as the weather, but also any other factors or processes that are not explicitly included in the model.

There are many different approaches to stochastic modelling. **Monte Carlo simulations** are models that use computers' pseudo-random number generators to determine the occurrence of events according to appropriate probability distributions. **Branching processes** and **birth-death processes** are simple analytic approaches to modelling invasion in relatively large susceptible populations. These models allow for flexibility in the distribution of secondary infections, and can be solved explicitly for quantities such as the probability of extinction, but they do not account for depletion of the susceptible population. **Chain binomials** or **Reed-Frost models** are used to model stochastic epidemics in finite populations. For each generation of transmission, these models enable us to calculate the number of newly infected individuals as a binomial random draw from the remaining susceptibles. **Diffusion processes** can be used to model infectious disease spread in large populations. Here the number of infectious individuals is modeled as a random walk around the equilibrium value, giving rise to a so-called 'quasi-stationary distribution' which is the long-term steady state distribution of values, conditioned on non-extinction.

3.5.2. *Continuous-time versus discrete-time models.* A fundamental decision in formulating a dynamic model is how to treat time. The models we have described using differential equations are continuous-time models, i.e. the time variable can take any real value. The key advantage of continuous-time models is that they are well-suited for mathematical analysis. They also allow for full flexibility in quantities like residence times and other durations. However, there are several factors that may favour the use of discrete-time models, in which the time variable changes by fixed increments. Data are typically reported in discrete time intervals, and it can be convenient to design the model to match the data. Discrete-time models can also match natural time scales of the system, such as the generation time or length of a season. Some people find discrete-time models more intuitive, and simulation code is easy to write as a basic 'for' loop. It can also be argued that for most epidemic models, especially the ones that are more complicated, it is not possible to obtain analytical results for any models; then continuous-time models have to be solved numerically, which involves discretizing time anyways.

While most discrete-time models can be compared to continuous-time models in the limit of small time steps, there are properties of discrete-time models that differ fundamentally from continuous-time models. The possibility of chaotic dynamics is one property of some discrete-time models that does not translate into continuous-time models. Whether chaotic dynamics are biologically meaningful is a topic of open debate. As ever, whichever formulation is used, one should be judicious in interpreting model results and always wary of artefacts (i.e. model behaviors that arise from quirks of the model design rather than from the basic biological processes under study). One common guideline to guard against artefactual results from discrete-time models is to repeat your model simulations with time-steps that are twice as long and half as long. If most of your work uses a time-step of 1 day, then check whether the model gives wildly different results using time-steps of 2 days or half a day. If it does, then examine the results closely to ensure that your choice of time-step – which is to some degree arbitrary – is not unduly influencing your results.

3.5.3. *Residence time distributions.* A related topic concerns the probability distributions of so-called 'residence times' that are implied by the model. The residence time refers to the duration that individuals in the model spend in a given compartment. In continuous-time models, a constant per capita rate of leaving a compartment gives rise to an exponentially distributed residence time, e.g. in equation 1, the constant recovery rate implies that the duration that individuals remain infectious is exponentially distributed. Analogously, in discrete-time models with constant probabilities per time step of leaving a compartment, the residence time is geometrically distributed.

For example, the constant recovery rate in equation 1 implies that the distribution of infectious periods in the population is exponential (and hence the most common infectious period duration approaches zero!), whereas data from real infections invariably show that such infectious period distributions are peaked at non-zero values. Numerous studies over the years have shown that modelling the incubation and infectious period distributions inaccurately can introduce undesirable biases into model results (Keeling & Grenfell, 1998; Lloyd, 2001; Wearing et al., 2005). Fortunately there is a useful trick to adapt the ordinary differential equation framework to reflect more realistic residence time distributions. This is known informally as the 'box-car' model. In this box-car model, a particular compartment is broken into a chain of sub-compartments, e.g. the E compartment could be broken into $E_1, E_2, \ldots, E_n$, as shown in figure 3. This changes the distribution of residence times from exponential in the usual framework to the gamma distribution, which can adopt a range of shapes depending on the number of sub-compartments included in the box-car model (Wearing et al., 2005).

3.5.4. *Continuous versus discrete state variables.* State variables are continuous in the models described by differential equations, in the sense that the state variables (such as the number of infected individuals) can take any positive real value. While these models have the advantage of being tractable mathematically, their precise biological interpretation is often vague. Sometimes the state variables are defined as densities, so non-integer values are acceptable. In other cases the state variables are meant to describe numbers of individuals, with the hope that the numbers in most compartments are sufficiently high that 'fractional individuals' do not exert an important influence on dynamics. This assumption can lead to serious

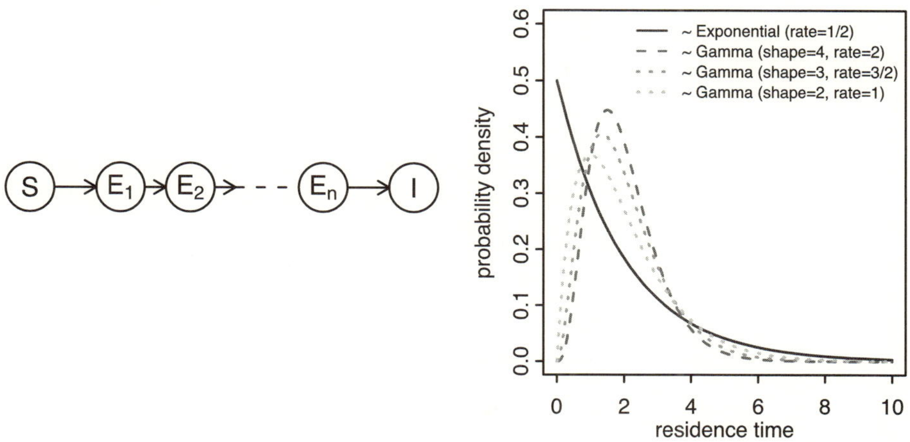

FIGURE 3. In a 'box-car' model, individuals move through a chain of sub-compartments to generate a more realistic distribution of residence times, e.g. for the Exposed compartment. If the rate of moving between sub-compartments is constant, then the total residence time in the Exposed compartment is gamma distributed. The gamma distribution can assume a range of forms depending its 'shape' parameter, which corresponds to the number of sub-compartments in the box-car model. By varying the 'rate' parameter for movement between sub-compartments, one can ensure that all of the distributions have the same mean (in the example shown, this is 2 time units). Note that the exponential distribution is actually a special case of the gamma distribution – in the example shown it is gamma (shape=1, rate=1/2).

problems, however, as famously exemplified by the "atto-fox" problem identified by Mollison (1991), wherein infinitesimal fractions of infected foxes allowed rabies to persist between epidemics in a differential equation model. It is thus crucial to recognize situations when key state variables may approach very low values during your system's dynamics, and to design your model accordingly. One convenient work-around is to impose a so-called quasi-extinction threshold, which asserts that a continuous-valued state variable in a deterministic model goes extinct if its value passes below some arbitrary lower bound. Discrete state variables, which count individuals in integer units, arise naturally in many stochastic models. These models are sometimes less amenable to mathematical analysis, but they are also safe from yielding artefactual results.

3.5.5. *Models for population structure and heterogeneities.* Simple compartmental models make two other important assumptions. These models assume that each individual in a compartment is identical to any other (i.e. that the populations are homogeneous), and that all individuals in the modeled population mix randomly and completely. It is increasingly recognized that for almost all real-world populations, neither of these assumptions is valid, so they need to be considered carefully when formulating a disease model. 'Population structure' refers to non-random

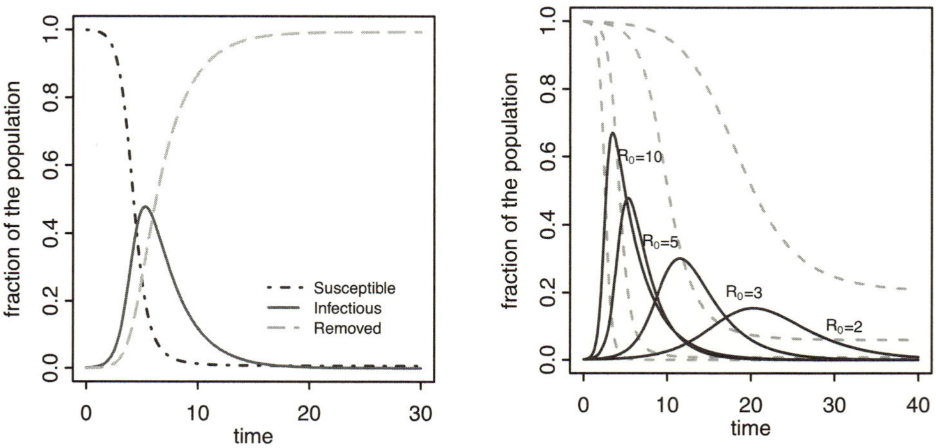

FIGURE 4. Epidemic curves for SIR model with frequency-dependent transmission. (Left) Typical population level epidemic pattern. The parameter values used here are $\beta = 2$ and $\gamma = 0.4$, which gives $R_0 = 5$. (Right) Epidemic curves for different values of R_0.

patterns of mixing in a population, due to factors such as spatial separation or social contact patterns. 'Population heterogeneity' refers to situations where basic properties such as infectiousness or contact rate vary among individuals in a population. There are numerous frameworks for modeling population structure and heterogeneity with varying degrees of complexity; these will be discussed in section 5.

3.6. Basic analysis of SIR-type compartmental model. The SIR family of models has been studied in great detail, and many analytic results can be derived from simple ordinary differential equation formulations. Here we summarize a few expressions that can be derived from the basic models, to give a sense of what is possible. For details we refer the reader to the classic treatment of these analyses given by Anderson & May (1991). For the simple deterministic SIR model without host demographics, diseases with $R_0 > 1$ will initiate an epidemic, which eventually burns itself out because the pool of susceptible individuals is depleted. Figure 4 shows graphs of epidemic curves generated by the SIR model with frequency-dependent transmission described by equation 1. In this case, the **exponential growth rate** at the outset of an epidemic is given by $r = (R_0 - 1)/D$, where D is the mean duration of infectiousness. The fraction of hosts infected when the epidemic reaches its peak, or **peak prevalence**, is given by $I_{\max} = 1-(1+\ln R_0)/R_0$. The **final proportion susceptible** in the host population, after the epidemic has run its course and burned out, is given by $f = \exp(-R_0(1-f)) \approx \exp(R_0)$.

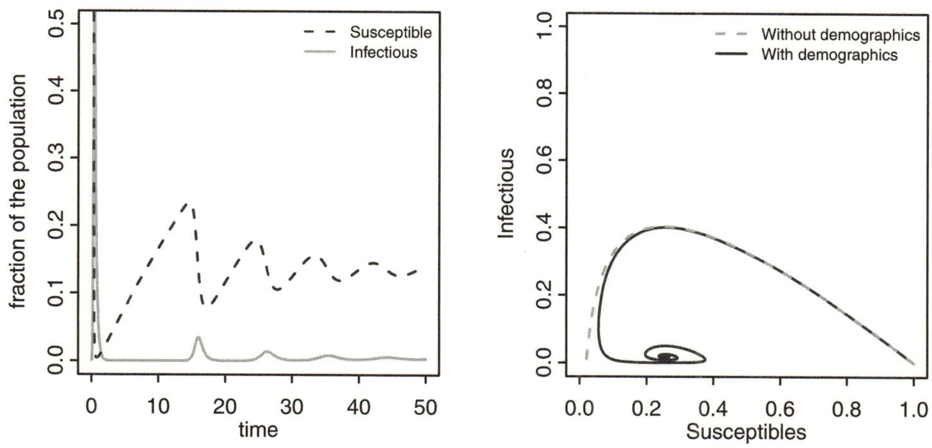

FIGURE 5. (Left) Typical population level epidemic pattern for SIR model with demographics. Introduction of demographics allows persistence and introduces periodicity due to repeated cyclic epidemics. (Right) S-I phase plane with phase diagram for both SIR models, with and without demographics.

Introduction of host demographics changes the model as shown in equation 4, and can fundamentally change the dynamics exhibited by the system.

$$\begin{aligned}\frac{dS}{dt} &= \mu N - \frac{\beta S I}{N} - \mu S\\ \frac{dI}{dt} &= \frac{\beta S I}{N} - \gamma I - \mu I \\ \frac{dR}{dt} &= \gamma I - \mu R\end{aligned} \tag{4}$$

Here we have introduced host births and deaths, which both occur at per capita rate μ so the population size remains constant. Depending on parameter values, this model can now exhibit endemic persistence, and can give rise to periodicity in incidence that was not present in the simpler model without demographics (Figure 5). The period of the cycles can be calculated roughly, $T \approx 2\pi (A\,D)^{1/2}$, where A is the mean age of infection, and D is the mean disease generation interval Anderson & May (1991). The reproductive number, $R_0 = \beta/(\gamma+\mu)$. Intuitively, this is because the average duration an individual host will remain infected will be shortened to $1/(\gamma+\mu)$ from $1/\gamma$, which was the case in the simpler model described by (1). One can find a more thorough and general mathematical treatment in van den Driesche & Watmough (2002).

3.7. Roles and types of data. Mathematical modelling of infectious disease dynamics is a scientific endeavor aimed at improving our understanding of real biological systems, so it is desirable to relate our models to reality by incorporating data whenever possible. Broadly speaking, there are two primary uses of data: to construct and parameterize models, and to validate model output.

When considering what data are needed to construct a model, one can delineate three rough categories. The first category includes data describing the progression of infection at the scale of individual hosts, including parameters describing clinical progression of the infection such as the infectious period, the latency period and the duration and efficacy of immunity once it is attained. For some pathogens, these data are readily available from the medical or veterinary literature, although fine points (such as how infectiousness varies through time) may be unknown. For many pathogens, particularly those circulating in wildlife hosts or newly emerged in human populations, even these basic data aren't available.

The second category of data entails information about the host population in the absence of disease, such as the size and structure of the host population, basic demographic characteristics such as rates of birth, death, and migration, and rates of contacts between people in a community and between communities. These types of data are very useful in designing epidemic models, particularly with regard to population structure and contact patterns.

The third category of data describes epidemiological patterns of disease circulation in the host population. These data can take the form of time series of estimated incidence or prevalence, or point estimates of quantities such as prevalence or seroprevalence. The data may be structured by host age or spatial location. Occasionally the data will be very detailed, such as contact tracing reports of transmission chains, or household studies that track generations of transmission among household members.

Epidemiological data can be used either to construct or to validate a model. If there are significant unknowns remaining after other classes of data have been used, then fitting the model to epidemiological data is an excellent way to estimate values for remaining free parameters. The most fundamental quantity is the transmissibility of the pathogen (i.e. R_0), which is rarely directly observable but can sometimes be estimated indirectly from other quantities (see section 7.1). Other aspects of transmissibility such as its seasonality or density dependence can also be estimated. If it is possible to construct and parameterize the model without using all the data that are available, then there is an opportunity to validate the model by making appropriate predictions and comparing them to data that were not used in model construction. If the model predictions are relatively close to these 'out-of-sample' data, then there are grounds for much greater confidence that the model is an accurate depiction of the system dynamics. This is particularly true (though rare in practice) if the model is able to predict responses to perturbations that were not included in the training data.

It is important to note that individual, population and epidemiological data are widely available, in the scientific literature and elsewhere. The websites for The World Health Organization (WHO), and The Center for Disease Control (CDC) are excellent places to search for epidemiological data. Two recent books full of data on important global health problems can be downloaded for free from the following websites: `http://www.dcp2.org/pubs/GBD` and `http://www.dcp2.org/pubs/DCP`.

4. Incidence function and population threshold

4.1. Incidence rate. The incidence rate is the rate at which new infections arise in a host population. Since the production of new infectious individuals drives the dynamics of infectious disease spread, the formulation of the incidence term is of central importance to epidemic modelling. Formulation of the incidence rate will reflect the biological and social processes inherent in disease transmission, as well as the assumptions made by the modeler. It is typically formulated as a product of (i) the number of susceptible individuals in the population, S, and (ii) the force of infection experienced by each susceptible, λ. The force of infection, in turn, constitutes of a number of other factors, depending on the transmission mechanism of the disease and the structure of the host population. In the most basic terms, the force of infection can be expressed as $\lambda = c(N)\,p\,I/N$, where $c(N)$ is the per capita rate of contacting other hosts (with an arbitrary dependence on the population size, N); p is the probability of transmission given that contact with an infectious host has occurred; and I/N is the probability that a randomly chosen host is infectious. Hence, the incidence rate can be expressed as:

$$f(S, I) = c(N)\,p\,\frac{S\,I}{N} \tag{5}$$

The contact rate $c(N)$ is commonly modeled in two different ways. Under **density-dependent transmission**, the contact rate is assumed to depend linearly on the host population size, i.e. $c(N) = k\,N$. Then the incidence rate is $f(S, I) = k\,N\,p\,S\,I/N = \beta_{\mathrm{DD}}\,S\,I$, where $\beta_{\mathrm{DD}} = k\,p$. In contrast, under **frequency-dependent transmission** the contact rate is assumed to be constant with respect to the host population, i.e. $c(N) = c_0$. In this case, the incidence rate is $f(S, I) = c_0\,p\,S\,I/N = \beta_{\mathrm{FD}}\,S\,I/N$, where $\beta_{\mathrm{FD}} = c_0\,p$. The frequency-dependent model is sometimes also called the standard incidence. The density-dependent model used to be called "mass action", in reference to the model from chemistry which was the original inspiration for early disease models, but since the mid 1990s the terminology has become confused with some authors calling the frequency-dependent model "mass action" (McCallum et al., 2001).

There is an ongoing debate about which transmission model is a more realistic representation of disease spread in human and natural populations. Classically, it was assumed that the transmission rate increases with population size, because contacts increase with crowding. For that reason, the density-dependent model was dominant until the 1980s. However, it has since been argued that many modes of contact (e.g. sexual contact) are governed more by social norms than by density, favoring use of frequency-dependent transmission (Hethcote & Van Ark, 1987). In recent years, evidence has been accumulating from many human and animal studies that even for infections transmitted by casual contact there is little evidence for clear density dependence in transmission rates (Bjørnstad et al., 2002; Begon et al., 1999).

Putting aside the debate, it is always worthwhile to think carefully about the natural history of the disease-host interaction — with particular attention to the mechanism of transmission — in formulating the incidence term. As a general rule frequency-dependent transmission is more appropriate in a large well-mixed population, whereas density-dependent transmission probably applies in smaller populations where individuals' contact budgets may not be saturated. A more realistic general model may be one which links these two regimes via a simple saturating function (Antonovics et al., 1995). It is important to realize the shortcomings and limitations of all these simple transmission models, and to think about the underlying population structure and mechanisms of mixing at the temporal and spatial scales which apply for the pathogen being considered. In many circumstances an explicit population structure is appropriate to capture the relevant mechanisms (see section 5). We refer the reader to McCallum et al. (2001) for further discussion regarding the choice of the transmission model and related issues.

4.2. Population thresholds in epidemic dynamics.

4.2.1. *Population threshold for invasion.* The basic reproduction number, R_0, has been the central concept in epidemic dynamics since the early 1980s, thanks largely to the work by Anderson and May (Heesterbeek, 2002). Long before this, people studying epidemic dynamics have focused on population thresholds. In their classic study, Kermack & McKendrick (1927) focused on the **population threshold for invasion**, which is defined as the host population size below which the parasite cannot invade. This is readily derived from the density-dependent transmission model, in which $R_0 = \beta\, N\, D$ where β is the rate of transmission, N is the size of the host population, and, D is the average duration of an infection. Because R_0 is positively related to N, an increase in the host population size increases R_0 and reduces the probability of extinction of a pathogen in a host population. In particular, since a pathogen can only successfully invade when $R_0 > 1$, this implies that there is a threshold population size N_T, such that the pathogen has a positive probability of successful invasion only if the host population $N > N_T$. This N_T can be thought of as the population threshold for invasion. Note that this phenomenon is not observed in the model with frequency-dependent transmission, where $R_0 = \beta\, D$ and since R_0 is not a function of N there is no population threshold for invasion.

Apart from looking at the population threshold in a fully susceptible host population, one can also examine a similar threshold for a population that is only partially susceptible. As introduced in section 3.2, $R_{\text{effective}} = R_0\, S/N$, where S and N are the susceptible and total host populations, respectively. An epidemic is possible in a population if $R_{\text{effective}} > 1$. This translates into a threshold condition on the fraction of the population that is susceptible, i.e., the pathogen can invade only if $S/N > 1/R_0$. This susceptibility threshold for disease invasion is applicable to either density-dependent or frequency-dependent transmission models. Conversely, the pathogen fails to survive in a host population when $S/N \leq 1/R_0$, and this is the basis for herd immunity as described above.

Despite its conceptual simplicity, real-world evidence for invasion thresholds is hard to find, for two major reasons (Lloyd-Smith et al., 2005a). First, while we can gather various kinds of epidemiological data for a successful disease invasions, it is very difficult to gather data for unsuccessful pathogen invasion. Failure of a disease invasion implies that the disease did not spread, and such an event usually does not get noticed. Thus there is an inherent bias in the observation process. Second, even with perfect observation, demographic stochasticity leads to substantial variation in outbreak sizes which can obscure the distinction between populations below and above the invasion threshold. Consider the stochastic simulation results shown in figure 6, which show the distribution of outbreak sizes following introduction of a single infected individual into populations of various sizes, with various values of R_0. Higher population sizes and higher values of R_0 lead to relatively clear bimodal distributions, where success versus failure of invasion can be clearly delineated. In contrast, small N or $R_0 \approx 1$ lead to distributions with density throughout the range of possible outbreak sizes. For example, compare the outbreak size distributions

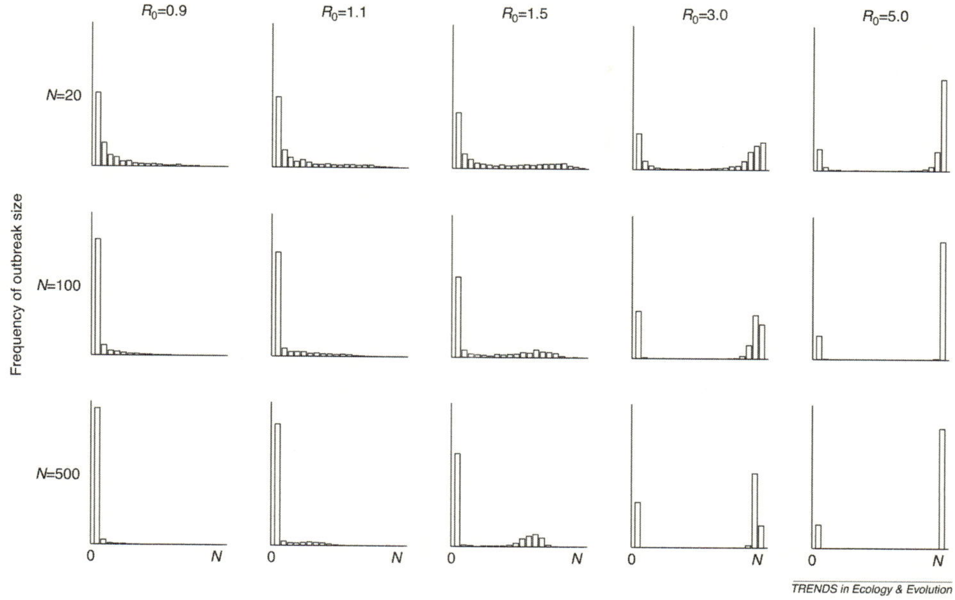

FIGURE 6. Histograms showing the distribution of total outbreak size for simulated stochastic outbreaks in populations of three sizes under five values of R_0. Figure reproduced from Lloyd-Smith et al (2005).

for populations of 100 hosts, and R_0 values of 0.9 and 1.1. Here the two values of R_0 are on the two sides of the threshold of $R_0 = 1$, so in principle outbreaks are possible for one and not for the other. Yet limited chains of transmission can still occur for $R_0 < 1$, while epidemics can still die out by chance when $R_0 > 1$, and the resulting distributions of outbreak size look very similar. Considering these intrinsic challenges in light of the substantial logistical problems in completely observing the outcome of many replicate disease introductions, we can see why clear empirical demonstrations of threshold population sizes for disease invasion are so rare.

4.2.2. *Population threshold for persistence.* A disease that successfully invades a host population is not necessarily guaranteed to persist long-term. There are two broad mechanisms whereby an established disease can fail to persist, or fade out. **Endemic fadeout** can occur when a disease is prevalent in the host population at a relatively low endemic level, but then the transmission chain is broken (i.e. the number of infected hosts goes to zero) due to a stochastic fluctuation. **Epidemic fadeout** occurs following a major epidemic, when the pool of susceptible individuals is depleted and the pathogen runs out of new individuals to infect. Epidemic fadeout typically occurs for highly infectious pathogens which exhibit strongly overcompensatory dynamics with very dramatic outbreaks and hence deep post-epidemic troughs in the susceptible population. Fig 7 illustrates endemic and epidemic fadeouts for a stochastic SIR model.

Measles is the classic example of a pathogen for which epidemic fadeouts are relevant, although the phenomenon certainly applies to other acute immunizing infections. In his seminal work, Bartlett (1957) observed that measles frequently

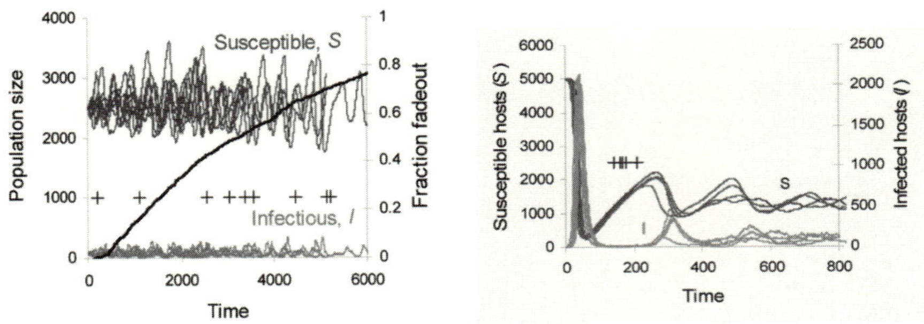

FIGURE 7. Endemic (left) and epidemic (right) fadeouts for a stochastic SIR model with frequency-dependent transmission and $R_0 = 4$. The graphs plot the number of susceptibles (in dark grey) and number of infecteds (in light grey) in 10 simulations. + signs show times when the disease fades out in particular simulations. The bold black line in the left graph indicates the fraction of 1000 simulations that had faded out as a function of time. Figure reproduced from Lloyd-Smith et al. (2005a).

disappeared from smaller towns in Britain, but circulated persistently in larger cities (note that this work was conducted before the measles vaccine was available). By analyzing the likelihood of fadeouts as a function of the population of the towns or cities, Bartlett concluded that there was a **critical community size** required for long-term persistence of the virus in a given population. This phenomenon has since been corroborated and analyzed in great detail (Anderson & May, 1991; Keeling & Grenfell, 1997; Bjørnstad et al., 2002; Grenfell et al., 2002). It is important to note, though, that the critical community size is not simply a fixed population size, but arises from a complex interaction between population size, demographic rates, and epidemiological properties of the disease (Lloyd-Smith et al., 2005a). Endemic fadeouts have proved more difficult to identify in empirical data, but Nåsell (2005) has developed important theory for defining and estimating such a threshold.

5. Population structure, heterogeneity and mixing

The simple models we have discussed so far have assumed that each individual host in a chosen compartment is exactly the same as all the others, neglecting variation in host genetics and condition, patterns of interaction with other individuals, and spatial location among many other factors. These assumptions are bound to have significant bearing on the results we obtain from the model. In this section, we will attempt to lay out several ways in which we can relax these assumptions, and discuss the consequences of such extensions. We can roughly group these methods into two very broad categories—methods that focus on population heterogeneity and those that focus on population structure. **Heterogeneity** refers to differences among individuals or groups in a given population, for instance due to different occupations or levels of nutrition. By **population structure** we mean the deviations in the mixing patterns of the population from the standard random mixing assumption in the SIR model. These deviations could be due to spatial proximity (you may be likely to interact with another host living nearby, but much less likely with someone in a different continent) or social factors (you are more likely to mingle co-workers than with strangers, regardless of where you live). This nomenclature is somewhat arbitrary and can be somewhat confusing — for instance models that include heterogeneity in host age are called 'age-structured', while models where parameters vary through space may be called 'spatially heterogeneous'.

5.1. Models for population structure. The most simple models for population structure, implicit in differential equations of the simple SIR-type models, are **random mixing** or **mean-field** models. In these models, every individual in the population is assumed to have equal probability of contacting any other individual. As we have discovered, they are mathematically tractable in the simple mass-action formulations analogous to mixing of small particles in chemistry models. The number of contacts that result in transmission simplifies to the product of the number of susceptible and number of infected individuals, and hence the incidence rate, $f(S, I) = \beta S I$. Sometimes, this form is modified to $\beta S^a I^b$ by including exponents as a phenomenological representation of non-random mixing. The dynamical properties of the resulting system is also more rich (Lui et al., 1987), and one needs to be cognizant of unintended consequences while adopting this technique. See Koelle et al. (2005) for an example of application of this technique to model cholera dynamics.

Multi-group, **multi-patch** or **metapopulation** models incorporate differences in host mixing behavior in a more mechanistic way, by dividing the host population into multiple groups based on the spatial location (or some other attribute that is expected to differentiate host mixing, such as social groups). The transmission function resulting from this mixing can be modeled in a couple of different ways. The most common approach is to construct a matrix that specifies the rate of transmission between individuals of any two chosen groups — often called the 'who acquires infection from whom' or WAIFW matrix. For a multi-group model with n groups, one constructs a $n \times n$ matrix whose component β_{ij} gives the transmission rate from an individual in group i to group j. β_{ii} is taken to be the transmission rate between two individual hosts within group i. Hence, the force of infection on a susceptible host in group j is:

$$\sum_i \beta_{ij} \frac{I_i}{N_i}.$$

See Anderson & May (1991) or Keeling & Grenfell (1997) for examples of the construction and use of WAIFW matrices. Here the authors subdivide the host population into groups based on their age — age being an important criterion for mixing in relation to measles epidemic.

An alternative approach to modelling transmission in multi-group models is to assume that transmission occurs only within groups (often using a random mixing assumption within the group), but to explicitly model movements of individual hosts between groups. The advantage of this approach is that the stochasticity involved in between-group movements can be captured, which is important if the groups are small or movement events are rare (see section 5.3.1).

Metapopulation models are particularly useful to study spatial patterns. To explore spatial dynamics of raccoon rabies epidemic in Connecticut, for example, Smith et al. (2002) divide the host population into 169 spatial groups corresponding to townships. By constructing a transmission matrix, the authors model both transmission between adjacent townships and longer-distance translocations of infected hosts, and as a result are able to quantify the roles of human habitats and rivers in the spatial spread of the disease.

For some disease systems (or research questions), it is important to consider the fine structure in interactions among hosts, or to capture the reality of persistent relationships between host individuals. As an example, for STDs, the number and identity of sexual partners for each infected host — which tend to vary substantially from one individual to another — will play a fundamental role in the spread of the disease. **Network models**, based on a branch of mathematics called graph theory, are well-suited to address problems where the details or 'memory' in the host contact structure are important. A network, or a 'graph', is a collection of nodes and edges, where nodes represent individual hosts and edges between two nodes represent contact between those hosts. When appropriate, an edge can have a weight and a direction to represent the intensity of the contact and the direction of the contact. This information is captured in an adjacency matrix, A, where values of a component, A_{ij}, denote the strength of contact between hosts i and j. By tracing the edges starting from a node, referred to as the index case, one can find which other hosts can be infected in the network. This type of contact tracing can be useful for assessing the risk of and to an individual host and for designing control strategies. There are several basic mathematical tools that have been developed to study different properties of these networks. These include the degree distribution, which the distribution of number of edges per node, and the clustering coefficient, which for a given node is the number of neighboring nodes that also share edges between themselves. Finally, it is important to realize that, despite their complexity, many network models make the very strong assumption that the contact structure is static, which can have the effect of artificially limited disease spread. There is increasing interest in dynamics network models which allow for changes in the network structure over time. We refer readers to Newman (2002), Keeling & Eames (2005) and Bansal et al. (2007) for reviews of network models in epidemiology.

Individual-based models or **microsimulation models** go even further in capturing the differences between individuals. Every individual in the model carries its own attributes, such as age, sex, location, contact behavior, or any other property that is deemed important. This extremely flexible framework allows one to represent arbitrarily complex systems and ask detailed questions. But this additional complexity comes at a high price. The dynamics of the model are simulated stochastically, often requiring major computational facilities. Results from model simulations can be difficult to reproduce and understand, and lack the clear cause-and-effect relationships of simpler models. Also, for each parameter that the modeler incorporates, he/she will then need to figure out what values they take, and how it interacts with others in the model. Often there are not sufficiently detailed data to estimate all these parameters, and sensitivity analyses can be burdensome. STDSIM is a famous example of this type of model used to study transmission and control of STDs including HIV in East Africa.

5.2. Models for heterogeneity. Incorporation of population heterogeneity into epidemic models has been a major topic of research for decades, motivated by both the clear influence of heterogeneity on patterns of disease spread and the potential to take advantage of population differences to design targeted control measures. The topic is treated in depth elsewhere (Anderson & May, 1991; Keeling & Rohani, 2007; Lloyd-Smith et al., 2006; Diekmann & Heesterbeek, 2000; Becker & Marschner, 1990); here we will briefly summarize a few key concepts.

5.2.1. *Group-level heterogeneity.* The most common approach to modelling heterogeneity is to divide the population into several sub-groups, which have some differences in parameter values but are themselves homogeneous. The model can then be analyzed using well-developed methods related to the metapopulation approaches described above. Again we can generalize R_0 for a multi-group population by defining R_{ij} as the expected number of new infections caused in group j due to the infected individuals in group i. Under the assumption that group membership is static, $R_{ij} = D_i \beta_{ij}$ where D_i is the expected infectious period, spent entirely in group i, and β_{ij} is the transmission rate from group i to group j. The value of R_0

If we assume that hosts can move from one group to another but transmission can occur only locally, then we can define D_{ij} to be the expected time spent in group j, while still infectious, by an individual infected in group i, and β_j to be the transmission rate within group j, so that $R_{ij} = D_{ij} \beta_j$. This helps us construct a $n \times n$ matrix of reproductive numbers for an n-group model. If the movement rules are Markovian, then the process can be defined by an absorbing Markov chain, with overall transition matrix:

$$\begin{bmatrix} P_{n\times n} & m \\ 0 & 1 \end{bmatrix},$$

where p_{ij} is the per-timestep probability that an individual moves from group i to group j, and m_j is the probability that an infected individual will recover or die while in group j. The expected residence times D_{ij} are then given by the fundamental matrix $\mathbf{D} = (\mathbf{I} - \mathbf{P})^{-1}$, and so $R_{ij} = D_{ij} \beta_j$. These arguments are generalized, and further conclusions are derived about the invasion dynamics of a disease in a heterogeneous population with movement among groups, in Schreiber & Lloyd-Smith (in press).

5.2.2. *Individual heterogeneity and superspreaders.* Individuals differ from one another in many ways, but from the perspective of a disease modeler, the most important heterogeneities are those that affect disease transmission. There are many accounts, for many diseases, of 'superspreader' individuals who are responsible for much more transmission than is typical for the disease (Lloyd-Smith et al., 2005b). For sexually-transmitted and vector-borne infections, this phenomenon has been attributed to the long-recognized fact that contact rates (i.e. contacts with sexual partners or bites by vectors) differ greatly across individuals. Indeed, Woolhouse et al. (1997) analyzed contact rate data for a suite of sexually-transmitted and vector-borne infections, and proposed that they are described by a 20/80 rule which states that 20% of hosts are responsible for 80% of the net transmission potential. This approach cannot be applied for many directly-transmitted infections, however, because it is not possible to quantify contact rates (e.g. for influenza or SARS or any other infections transmitted in casual contact, contacts are not discrete and identifiable events). Furthermore, for all infections, many other factors contribute to a host's infectiousness – including properties of the host, pathogen and environment – so we expect the degree of infectiousness to be distributed continuously in a population, and not identifiable *a priori.* For all of these reasons, the conventional group-based approach to modelling population heterogeneity is not well-suited to the challenge of capturing individual variation in infectiousness.

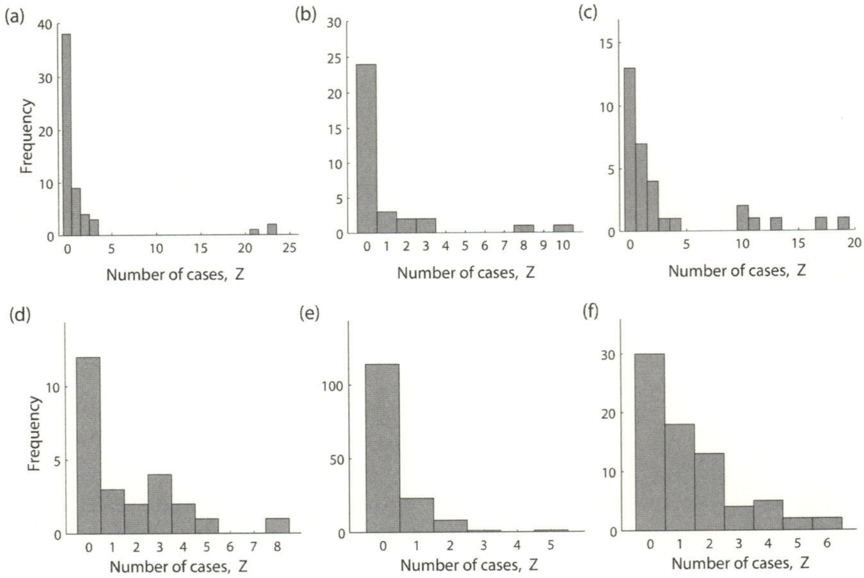

FIGURE 8. Data from contact tracing studies highlight the substantial individual-level heterogeneity in infectiousness. The variability in the number of secondary cases caused by a single infected individual is shown for various infectious diseases: (a) SARS in Singapore; (b) SARS in Beijing; (c) Smallpox; (d) Variola minor; (e) Monkeypox; and (f) Pneumonic plague.

One approach to this challenge was presented by Lloyd-Smith et al. (2005b), who proposed an extension of the idea of the basic reproductive number, R_0, to a population distribution. They defined the individual reproductive number, ν, as the expected number of infections caused by a particular infectious individual in a susceptible population. This quantity is allowed to vary among individuals in the population according to any continuous distribution with a mean of R_0. The actual number of cases caused by a particular individual, Z, is determined by this expectation filtered by demographic stochasticity in the transmission process, and under simple assumptions is given by $Z \sim \text{Poisson}(\nu)$. Lloyd-Smith et al. propose a flexible model wherein ν follows a gamma distribution, so that Z follows a negative binomial distribution. By comparing this model with data from real outbreaks on the distribution of the number of secondary cases resulting from single infected individuals (Figure 8), they were able to estimate the distribution of ν for several infections. The 20/80 rule did not hold as a generality, but for all diseases there was a substantial degree of individual heterogeneity, and it was shown that the standard models assuming homogeneous infectiousness are statistically inconsistent with many of the available data sets. Their analysis went on to analyze the stochastic dynamics of disease outbreaks using the branching process framework introduced in section 3.5.1, showing that increased heterogeneity leads to a higher probability that a disease outbreak will go extinct, but that those outbreaks that do succeed will grow faster in their early stages.

A second approach to modelling superspreading events was suggested by James et al. (2006). In this model infections occur in two ways: 'normal' infections can be caused by all individuals according to a branching process with Z following a Poisson distribution, and superspreading events occur as a Poisson process with rate ρ. Each superspreading event is assumed to cause a number of infections that is Poisson distributed with mean λ. The authors show that this model can fit some data sets about as well as the model proposed by Lloyd-Smith et al. (2005b). Closer examination of epidemiological reports indicates that reality probably falls somewhere between the two models, with heterogeneity in infectiousness arising sometimes from individual differences in transmission rate, and sometimes from events that occur unpredictably.

5.3. The importance of mechanism. In formulating an epidemic model, it is essential to think carefully about the mechanisms of contact underlying transmission for the system at hand. Sometimes these considerations can lead to greater complexity in your model, but for particular scenarios it is often possible to reduce this complexity by working in various limits. As a rule, one needs to consider the timescales of the relevant processes, such as mixing, recovery and transmission, to determine what limits are applicable. In situations where these timescales have similar magnitudes, it is often important to use mechanistic models to capture the dynamics accurately.

5.3.1. *Contact between groups.* For populations structured into groups, transmission occurs within groups and large-scale spread arises when infected individuals move between groups. As described in section 5.1, this situation can be modelled by explicitly tracking the movement of individuals or by introducing a 'between-group' transmission rate that implicitly describes both movements and transmission in other groups. Keeling & Rohani (2002) show that, when movements between groups are rapid, these two approaches give similar results. Subsequent work by Cross et al. (2005), however, shows that this similarity breaks down as the movements between groups become less frequent. In particular, Cross et al. examine how the timescales of host movement and disease recovery interact to determine invasion success in structured populations. They show that it is essential to consider the discrete and stochastic nature of movement for systems where group sizes are small and between-group moves occur on the same (or slower) timescales as disease recovery. That is, if the expected number of between-group moves by a host during its infectious period is 1 or lower, then a widespread disease outbreak is unlikely even if the local $R_0 \gg 1$ (Figure 9). Thus we expect acute and chronic diseases to exhibit different invasion dynamics in a structured population, even if they have the same R_0.

So we see that R_0 can fail to properly predict the invasion threshold for a structured population. For a metapopulation, it is then appropriate to develop a similar threshold quantity. Ball et al. (1997) introduce a quantity R_*, which is defined to be the expected number of groups infected by the first infected group, and present elegant analyses of this quantity in systems with large numbers of groups and without tracking host movements. Analytical expressions for R_0 or R_* are hard to find for systems with mechanistic movement, finite group sizes and finite numbers of groups, so Cross et al. (2005) tested the applicability of the R_* concept to their model by computing 'empirical' values, $\hat{R}_0$ and $\hat{R}_*$, from their simulation results. Figure 10 shows how the two quantities compare in their ability to predict

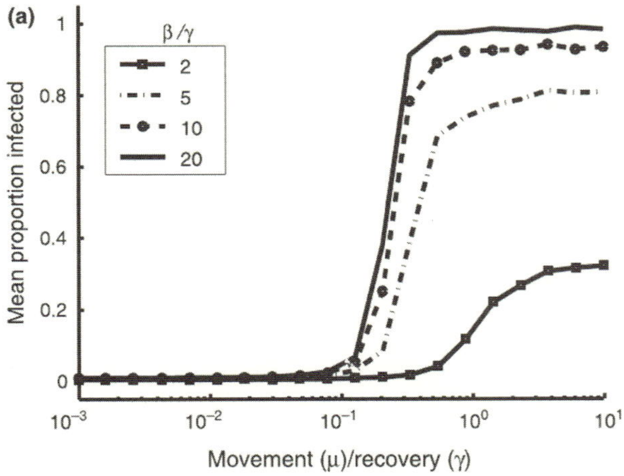

FIGURE 9. The interaction of movement rate (μ) and recovery rate (γ) determines the mean proportion of a structured population that becomes infected in an outbreak. The reproductive number within a group is given by β/γ. These results are the average of 1000 stochastic simulations of disease invasions initiated by a single infected individual introduced into a toroidal 11×11 array of groups, where each group began with 10 hosts. Figure reproduced from Cross et al. (2005).

invasion in a structured population. A system can have $\hat{R}_0 \gg 1$ and not experience a major outbreak, because movements between groups are too infrequent, but if $\hat{R}_*$ is greater than about 2 then a major outbreak is very likely. Clearly R_* is a better predictor of invasion.

We have summarized one study of the complexities arising in group-structured populations, but there is an extensive literature addressing these issues. We refer the reader to papers by Ball et al. (1997) and Ball & Neal (2002) for further details on mixing at different levels, and to Cross et al. (2004, 2005, 2007) for further analysis on disease invasion in structured populations.

5.3.2. *Pair formation and STD transmission.* Sexually-transmitted diseases are often modeled using ordinary differential equations with a frequency-dependent incidence rate. Following the presentation introduced in section 4.1, the incidence rate, $f(S, I)$ is given by the following function:

$$f(S,I) = c_{\mathrm{FD}}\, p_{\mathrm{FD}} \left(\frac{S}{N}\right) I, \tag{6}$$

where c_{FD} is the rate of acquiring new partners, p_{FD} is the probability of transmission in S-I partnership, S/N is the probability that a partner is susceptible, and I is the abundance of infected hosts. But the derivation of the incidence rate given earlier was based upon random mixing in a population, whereas most sexual transmission takes place within monogamous pairs of varying duration. Lloyd-Smith et al. (2004) examined the underlying dynamics of pair formation and dissolution to

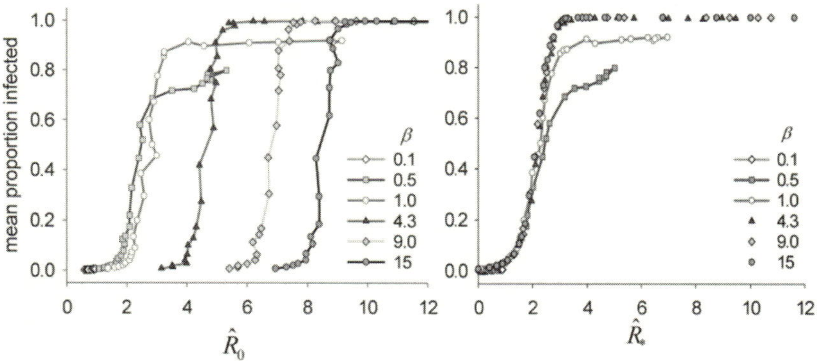

FIGURE 10. Comparing the ability of $\hat{R}_0$ and $\hat{R}_*$ to predict invasion success in a structured population. Details as in Figure 9, with $\gamma = 0.1$. Figure reproduced from Cross et al. (2005).

understand how this basic mechanism related to the common frequency-dependent formulation of incidence for these diseases.

Consider a population of host individuals that can be either susceptible, X_{S} or infected, X_{I}. These individuals form pairs P_{SS}, P_{SI},and P_{II} where the subscripts indicate the infection status of the individuals in the pair. Pairs form at per capita rate k and dissolve at per-pair rate l. For generality, and to incorporate the observation that infected individuals often exhibit different contact behavior Lloyd-Smith et al. (2004), we let k_S and k_I be the pairing rates for susceptible and infected hosts, and l_{SS}, l_{SI}, l_{IS},and l_{II} be the dissolution rates for pairs with different compositions. We introduce m_{SS}, m_{SI}, m_{IS}, and m_{SS} as the mixing rates between individuals of different categories.

Now we introduce a strong assumption that pair formation and dissolution dynamics are fast compared to the disease dynamics (i.e. transmission and recovery). Under this assumption we can separate the timescales of pairing and disease, and assume that the pairing dynamics are at a quasi-steady-state relative to the disease dynamics. This means that disease status is constant on the timescales relevant to pairing dynamics, so the dynamics of the pairing system are described by:

$$
\begin{aligned}
\frac{dX_{\mathrm{S}}}{dt} &= -k_{\mathrm{S}}\, X_{\mathrm{S}} + 2l_{\mathrm{SS}}\, P_{\mathrm{SS}} + l_{\mathrm{SI}}\, P_{\mathrm{SI}} \\
\frac{dX_{\mathrm{I}}}{dt} &= -k_{\mathrm{I}}\, X_{\mathrm{I}} + 2l_{\mathrm{II}}\, P_{\mathrm{II}} + l_{\mathrm{SI}}\, P_{\mathrm{SI}} \\
\frac{dP_{\mathrm{SS}}}{dt} &= \frac{1}{2}k_{\mathrm{S}}\, m_{\mathrm{SS}}\, X_{\mathrm{S}} - l_{\mathrm{SS}}\, P_{\mathrm{SS}} \\
\frac{dP_{\mathrm{SI}}}{dt} &= \frac{1}{2}k_{\mathrm{S}}\, m_{\mathrm{SI}}\, X_{\mathrm{S}} + \frac{1}{2}k_{\mathrm{I}}\, m_{\mathrm{IS}}\, X_{\mathrm{I}} - l_{\mathrm{SI}}\, P_{\mathrm{SI}} \\
\frac{dP_{\mathrm{II}}}{dt} &= \frac{1}{2}k_{\mathrm{I}}\, m_{\mathrm{II}}\, X_{\mathrm{I}} - l_{\mathrm{II}}\, P_{\mathrm{II}}
\end{aligned}
\tag{7}
$$

The disease dynamics take place on a much slower timescale. Transmission can only occur in discordant S-I pairs, so we are interested in the quasi-steady-state abundance P^*_{SI}. If transmission occurs within such pairs at rate β_{pair}, then the incidence rate for the whole population is $\beta_{\text{pair}}\, P^*_{\text{SI}}$. The disease dynamics are then captured by the following equations:

$$
\begin{aligned}
\frac{dS}{dt} &= \lambda - \beta\text{pair}\, P^*_{\text{SI}} + \sigma\, I - \mu\, S \\
\frac{dI}{dt} &= \beta\text{pair}\, P^*_{\text{SI}} - (\sigma + \mu)\, I
\end{aligned} \tag{8}
$$

where λ is the recruitment rate of new susceptibles, σ is the rate of recovery to the susceptible class, and μ is the rate of leaving the population (by death, emigration, or entering a permanent relationship). Then to understand the incidence term we must solve the system for P^*_{SI}. Lloyd-Smith et al. (2004) show that it is straightforward to calculate P^*_{SI} under the assumption that partners are chosen at random (although the choice is weighted by the abundance and pairing rates of unpaired S and I individuals), by solving for the steady state of equation 7.

In the simplest case where infection status does not affect pairing behavior, we can take a single pairing rate k and a single break-up rate l and the incidence rate is

$$f(S, I) = \beta_{\text{pair}}\, P^*_{\text{SI}} = \beta_{\text{pair}} \left(\frac{k}{k+l}\right) \frac{SI}{N}. \tag{9}$$

Noting the similarity to equation 6, we recall that c_{FD} is the per capita rate of acquiring new partners, so

$$c_{\text{FD}} = \frac{1}{1/l + 1/k},$$

and p_{FD} is the probability of transmission in S-I partnership, so

$$p_{\text{FD}} = 1 - \exp(-\beta_{\text{pair}}/l) \approx \beta\text{pair}/l, \qquad \text{since } \beta_{\text{pair}} \ll 1.$$

Thus we find that

$$c_{\text{FD}}\, p_{\text{FD}} \left(\frac{S}{I}\right) I \approx \beta_{\text{pair}} \left(\frac{k}{k+l}\right) \frac{SI}{N}$$

i.e., we have derived the frequency-dependent incidence rate from a mechanistic pair-formation model. This means that this standard formulation of STD incidence can represent pair-based transmission, but several strong assumptions were required – most notably the timescale approximation that pairing dynamics are much faster than disease dynamics. (Conversely, we know that STD dynamics are driven by pair-based transmission, which means that models using frequency-dependent incidence are implicitly making this timescale approximation.)

To assess the validity of this approximation, Lloyd-Smith et al. (2004) compared epidemics simulated using frequency-dependent transmission with those simulated using the full pair-formation/epidemic system, for parameters corresponding to different types of STD. For transient and highly transmissible diseases such as gonorrhea, frequency-dependent incidence is a good depiction of pair-based transmission only for populations that change sexual partners very frequently (i.e. mean partnership duration 1 day). For chronic and less-transmissible diseases such as HIV, frequency dependence is a reasonable model for populations with mean partnership duration of several months. For populations outside these ranges, mechanistic models that track pairing dynamics should be used. Note also that generalized forms of frequency-dependent incidence can be derived for situations where pairing behavior depends on infection status.

6. Disease Control

6.1. Approaches to disease control. The primary goal of disease control measures is to reduce morbidity and mortality due to disease. Sometimes the control measures are focused on protecting vulnerable populations, such as elderly people for influenza, or endangered populations of wildlife. Most often, however, the aim is to reduce the disease burden in the whole population, by reducing transmission of the infection.

In section 3.2, we established that the effective reproductive rate for transmission within a population can be expressed as $R_{\text{effective}} = cpD(S/N)$, where, c is the contact rate, p is the probability of transmission given contact, D is the duration of infection, and S/N is the proportion of the population that is susceptible. Examination of this expression allows us to classify control measures according to which component of $R_{\text{effective}}$ they address. The contact rate, c, can be reduced by measures such as quarantine, case isolation, promotion of abstinence, and reduction of mass gatherings (e.g. in theaters or schools). In animal populations, there is also the option of culling hosts which reduces the population density and hence the contact rate. The probability of transmission, p, can be reduced by promoting the use of condoms and safe sex practices, increasing barrier precautions such as masks, gloves, gowns etc., by male circumcision (which now is known to reduce female to male transmission of HIV (Williams et al., 2006)), and by prophylactic treatment. The duration of infectiousness, D, can be reduced by treatment, by contact tracing and case isolation, by improved diagnostics (which enable faster identification of cases) and again by culling of infected hosts. Finally, one can reduce the proportion of susceptibles, S/N in the population by carrying out different types of vaccination programs. Mass vaccination is the simplest program, and involves trying to vaccinate the entire population experiencing or threatened by an infectious disease. Ring vaccination involves vaccinating individuals epidemiologically linked to suspected cases, e.g. by tracing contacts of the cases and vaccinating them. Spatially targeted vaccination targets neighborhoods of affected cities and is particularly effective at containing transmission localized to specific geographical area. Other sub-groups in a population can also be targeted if they are thought to be epidemiologically important.

Another aim of some control measures is to reduce transmission between groups (i.e. to reduce R_* rather than R_0). Such measures include movement restrictions and ring vaccination for human hosts, and fencing and ring culling for animals. For vector-borne diseases, further measures are available in addition to the approaches listed above. Bednets and insect repellents are used to reduce biting rates. Many measures aim to reduce the vector population, including the application of larvicides or insecticides, removal of standing water, and use of biological control methods such as larval predators or fungal pathogens.

6.2. Basic theory of disease control. The fundamental question that arises in disease control is "what amount of control is needed to stop sustained transmission of the pathogen?" The question is posed most simply in terms of vaccination, i.e. "what fraction of the population do we need to vaccinate?", but can apply equally to other modes of control. The question is readily answered with reference to the R_0 and $R_{\text{effective}}$ concepts introduced above. Since $R_{\text{effective}} = R_0 \times S/N$, we need $S/N < 1/R_0$ to achieve $R_{\text{effective}} < 1$. Therefore the critical vaccination

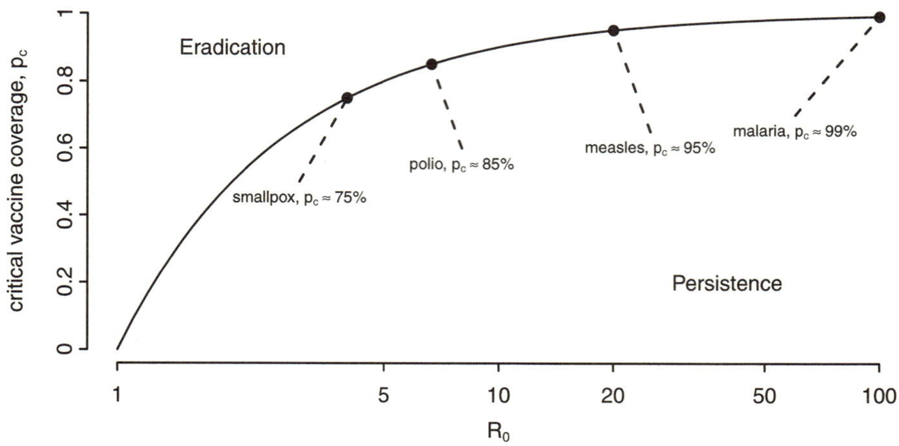

FIGURE 11. Critical vaccination coverage for various diseases, which is determined by R_0.

coverage to eradicate a disease is $p_c = 1 - 1/R_0$. Figure 11 shows this critical vaccination coverage, p_c for various infectious diseases. Note that the disease can be eradicated without vaccinating the entire population, due to herd immunity (Anderson & May, 1985b,a). However, as R_0 increases, eradication by vaccination becomes very challenging due to logistical problems in achieving high coverage levels. It is also important to remember that this calculation makes numerous strong assumptions, including mass untargeted vaccination in a randomly mixing homogeneous population, and that vaccination occurs at birth and is 100% effective. The critical vaccination coverage should thus be treated as a rough guideline, and more detailed mechanistic models are needed to calculate more refined targets.

Based on the considerations of section 5, it is clear that heterogeneity or population structure will influence the efficacy of control measures. For instance, in a classic study May & Anderson (1984) considered vaccination strategies in a patchy population, with host patches of different sizes (e.g. a city and surrounding villages). They assumed that transmission was density dependent so it varied strongly among patches. They showed that, if vaccination was applied uniformly (i.e. the same fraction vaccinated on each patch), spatial heterogeneity increased the critical vaccination coverage relative to the expectation for a homogeneous and well-mixed population. However, if information about the heterogeneity is used to design a targeted campaign, then the disease can be eradicated with a lower overall coverage. Under the assumption of density dependent transmission, the optimal strategy is the one that leaves the same number of individuals susceptible on each patch. In an important follow-up study, Hethcote & Van Ark (1987) showed that weaker density dependence in transmission greatly reduced the magnitude of these effects, but the qualitative result still held.

Eames & Keeling (2003) studied the efficacy of contact tracing in a network epidemic model, considering the critical 'efficiency' of contact tracing (i.e. the proportion of contacts of an infected individual that need to be traced and treated) required to stop transmission. They found that for a model with non-random mixing the critical tracing efficiency was $\approx 1 - 1/R_0$, as predicted for models based on random mixing, provided the network had a negligible degree of clustering. For clustered networks, they found that a lower tracing efficiency was sufficient to contain an epidemic.

Other studies have emphasized the importance of individual heterogeneity for control efforts. Woolhouse et al. (1997) highlighted the marked heterogeneity in contact rates for STDs and vector-borne diseases, and showed how control measures targeting the hosts with highest contact rates could disproportionately help to reduce transmission. Lloyd-Smith et al. (2005b) broadened this point to directly-transmitted diseases, showing that the existence of individual variation in infectiousness – and superspreaders – presented an opportunity for potent targeted control, but also emphasized the challenges in identifying highly-infectious individuals *a priori*. This study also introduced the distinction between two idealized classes of control measures: **population-wide** control measures that are partially effective, such as wearing masks or reducing time in public areas, and **individual-specific** measures that are wholly effective, such as case isolation. (Note that these two extremes are also relevant to contemporary issues in vaccination, since there is interest in the impacts of partially-effective vaccines for diseases like HIV or malaria. Such vaccines can act by protecting all individuals partially, or by protecting a proportion of individuals fully.) For a given reduction in R_0, individual-specific control measures are likely to stop a disease outbreak (because they lead to increased heterogeneity among individuals; see section 5.2.2).

6.3. Success stories. A number of major success stories demonstrate the potential efficacy of disease control measures. The greatest example is the global eradication of smallpox, via a worldwide effort led by the World Health Organization, which culminated with the last naturally occurring case in Somalia in 1977. The epidemiology, control and eradication of smallpox is described in a fascinating book (available online) written by the leaders of the effort (Fenner et al., 1988). Smallpox was a terrible disease, and has been estimated to have killed 300-500 million humans during the 20th century alone. However, it had certain characteristics that made it vulnerable to eradication. It was not too highly transmissible ($R_0 \approx 3.5 - 6$), requiring a critical vaccine coverage of about 70-85% (Gani & Leach, 2001). It had a relatively long incubation period ($\approx$ 21 days) giving sufficient time for control if an outbreak is detected in its early stages (Ferguson et al., 2003). Smallpox had conspicuous symptoms and few subclinical cases, leading to easy case finding. Crucially, smallpox was a disease of humans only, so there was no animal reservoir from which the infection could re-emerge (although there is concern that monkeypox, which is a zoonotic infection, may fill the niche left vacant by smallpox eradication). Despite these beneficial characteristics, however, the eradication effort struggled in its final phases to stop transmission in the last hot-spots of smallpox transmission. Interestingly, the success of local eradication efforts depended on both vaccination coverage and population density – i.e. factors beyond the predictions of the basic theory of control – and involved intensive contact tracing and ring vaccination. In recent years there has been renewed interest in the dynamics of smallpox transmission, due to concern about its possible use as a bioterror agent (Ferguson et al., 2003).

Another significant success story is the containment of SARS in 2002-2003 (Anderson et al., 2004). SARS is the best case study of an emerging viral pathogen, which had potential for pandemic spread ($R_0 \approx 3$) but was arrested by global efforts.

This outbreak has been extensively modelled (Bauch et al., 2005), with particular focus on quarantine and case isolation measures (since there were no drugs or vaccines available to fight this new disease). There was also considerable focus on hospital-based control measures, since 18 – 63% of SARS cases were reported in health care workers (Lloyd-Smith et al., 2003).

A more controversial example is the containment of the foot and mouth disease epizootic in Britain in 2001. The effort was successful in eliminating the infection, but the massive targeted culling program which led to the success has remained controversial. This outbreak is an important example of epidemic models playing a clear role in guiding policy, with two early modelling studies being quite influential (Ferguson et al., 2001; Keeling et al., 2001). Further studies have weighed prophylactic and reactive vaccination strategies, as well as the impact of heterogeneities in the landscape (Keeling et al., 2003; Tildesley et al., 2006).

6.4. Challenges. Disease control efforts are also confronted by many challenges, with causes ranging from fundamental biology to human behaviour. An important example of a biological challenge is drug resistance. Rapid evolutionary rates of pathogens, coupled with strong selection pressure imposed by drug treatments, often result in evolution of drug-resistant pathogen strains. Drug resistance poses grave public health threats worldwide, from methicillin-resistant *Staphylococcus aureus* (MRSA) to chloroquine-resistant malaria. Anti-retroviral resistance is a major concern in the effort to treat HIV and AIDS victims all over the world. Epidemic modellers can play a useful role in integrating information from clinical, experimental and epidemiological data to understand the spread of drug-resistant pathogens. It is important to recognize, though, that some crucial aspects of the basic biology of drug resistance are complex or incompletely understood, such as the relationship between drug dose regimens and evolutionary selection on the pathogen strains (Lipsitch & Samore, 2002) and the relative transmissibility of resistant strains. Models should be designed to reflect (or better still, address) these uncertainties.

Human behaviour can pose a challenge to disease control through vaccine scares, when the belief spreads in a population that a particular vaccine has more adverse effects than benefits. It is true that vaccination typically carries a slight risk, but these risks are much less than those arising from infection with the pathogen. Vaccine scares can arise from an overestimation of the risk of vaccines, or an underestimation of the risk of infection (e.g. for diseases like measles, which have have been eliminated from developed countries for long enough that people may have forgotten that infection can cause serious side effects or death). It is also possible that vaccine refusal arises from selfish behaviour, since if enough of a population is vaccinated then an unvaccinated individual can get all the benefits of herd immunity while avoiding the small risk of vaccination. The individual benefits from refusing vaccine, but the costs of lower coverage are shared among the group – this is a classic ‘tragedy of the commons’ situation, and accordingly there have been efforts to apply game theory to vaccination behaviour (Bauch & Earn, 2004). Drops in vaccine coverage resulting from vaccine scares have had severe public health consequences. Vaccine scares in the late 1970s for whooping cough in the UK led to slump in immunization, resulting in several major epidemics affecting millions of children (Rohani et al., 1999). The decline in MMR (measles-mumps-rubella) vaccine coverage through the late 1990s and early 2000s in Britain led to increased outbreak size (Jansen et al., 2003). A vaccine scare in Nigeria in 2004 led to increased circulation of polio virus, which was then re-seeded in several other countries by infected travellers, dealing a serious blow to the current campaign to eradicate polio worldwide (Minor, 2004).

7. Parameter estimation, model fitting, and sensitivity analysis

7.1. Estimating R_0. Given its central role in infectious disease dynamics, R_0 is the one parameter we would most like to estimate for any disease. We have already seen that in its simplest form, $R_0 = \beta/\gamma = c\,p\,D$, where, c is the contact rate, p is the probability of transmission given contact, D is the duration of infectiousness, β is the transmission rate, and γ is the recovery rate. It is tempting to think that if we can estimate these parameters at the individual level, then we would be able to estimate R_0. Unfortunately, estimation of these parameters at the individual level is often difficult. The contact rate is particularly challenging, because for many infectious diseases 'contacts' are not defined precisely. This ambiguity also complicates estimation of p. Furthermore, estimates based on R_0 expressions are highly model-dependent, so any assumptions made in model construction will influence the resulting estimate. Finally, it is important to note that in general parameters, c, p and D are not independent of each other. So, the expectation, $\mathrm{E}(c\,p\,D) \neq \mathrm{E}(c)\,\mathrm{E}(p)\,\mathrm{E}(D)$, and any correlations among the constituent parameters would need to be accounted for.

Fortunately, there are many techniques available to estimate R_0 from epidemic data (Dietz, 1993; Anderson & May, 1991). Simple analysis of the SIR model yields two useful approaches. First, during the initial phase of an epidemic the growth rate in the number of cases is roughly exponential. If the exponential growth rate is r, then $R_0 = 1 + rD$. Equivalently, if t_d is the doubling time of the number of infected individuals, then

$$R_0 = 1 + \frac{D \ln 2}{t_d}.$$

On the other hand, if s_0 and s_∞ are the susceptible proportions before the epidemic and after it runs to completion, respectively, then

$$R_0 = \frac{\ln(s_0) - \ln(s_\infty)}{(s_0 - s_\infty)}.$$

All of these estimates are based on simple differential equation models, and hence assume exponentially distributed infectious periods (see section 3.5.3). Wallinga & Lipsitch (2007) provide a general analysis of how the distribution of the serial interval influences the relationship between r and R_0. They find that $R_0 = \frac{1}{M(-r)}$, where $M(z)$ is the moment generating function for the distribution of the serial interval. This allows one to calculate R_0 from r for any arbitrary distribution of the serial interval. Furthermore, they prove that the upper bound on R_0 is $R_0 = e^{rT}$, where T is the mean serial interval.

If the case data are collected in discrete intervals, estimation from continuous-time models is moe difficult. Ferrari et al. (2005) derive an approach based on chain binomial models that provides a maximum-likelihood estimator for R_0 and the associated uncertainty. Note that, like the previous approach based on s_∞, this approach requires that the epidemic runs to its natural completion. The reproductive number can also be estimated based on data from the self-limiting outbreaks that occur when $R_0 < 1$. Branching process models allow analysis of the distribution of outbreak sizes to make inference about the effective reproductive number (Farrington & Whitaker, 2003).

It is also possible to estimate R_0 from epidemiological data in endemic settings. Anderson & May (1991) present simple expressions based on the mean age at first infection, A, and the mean lifespan in a population L. The precise results depend on the age-dependent rate of mortality in the population, $\mu(a)$, where they treat two idealized cases. In "Type I" mortality, all individuals live to age L, so that:

$$\mu(a) = 0 \qquad \text{for} \quad a < L$$
$$\mu(a) = \infty \qquad \text{for} \quad a > L.$$

In "Type II" mortality, individuals are subject to a constant death rate:

$$\mu(a) = \mu = \text{constant} = 1/L.$$

For a population with Type I mortality, $R_0 \approx L/A$. For Type II mortality, the relationship is exact, $R_0 = L/A$. These simple estimates are based on a number of strong assumptions, including random mixing, the absence of heterogeneities or age dependence in the force of infection, and a constant population size. For more advanced treatments, see later chapters of Anderson & May (1991), or Dietz (1993).

R_0 can also be estimated from data on the seroprevalence as a function of age ("age-seroprevalence curves"), by calculating the age-dependent force of infection and making assumptions on the WAIFW matrix for the age-structured population. We refer the readers to Farrington et al. (2001) for a comprehensive review in this topic.

7.2. Parameter estimation. In this and the next section, we give a very cursory overview of various approaches to the estimation of parameter values and their associated uncertainties. Our aim is to introduce the reader to the general principles, and perhaps provide enough basic concepts and vocabulary to enable independent forays into the literature to search for greater detail. In a few instances we have followed the presentation of material by Bolker (2008), and we encourage readers to refer to this excellent book for a more in-depth treatment of these issues (and tips on how to implement estimation algorithms in R).

7.2.1. *Method of moments.* Many problems in parameter estimation can be reduced to the problem of estimating the parameters of a relevant probability distribution to describe the data. For most standard probability distributions, the parameters can be expressed in terms of the moments of the distribution, such as the mean and the variance. The most simple method of estimating your parameter is using these moments directly. For example, consider an exponential distribution whose probability density function, $f(x) = \lambda \exp(-\lambda x)$. If μ is the mean of the distribution, then the exponential rate parameter can be expressed as $\lambda = 1/\mu$. One can calculate the sample moments from the data, and substitute them in the expression, i.e. in our example, $\lambda \approx 1/\bar{\mu}$, where $\bar{\mu}$ is the estimate for μ derived from the data. This approach provides a quick and simple way of getting rough a estimate for your parameter, but the estimates are sometimes biased.

7.2.2. *Maximum likelihood.* For a more formal approach to fitting single distributions, one can use the method of maximum likelihood. Maximum likelihood estimates have certain desirable statistical properties when the data points are independent and identically distributed ("iid") and as the number of data points gets large (the "asymptotic limit"). In particular, maximum likelihood estimates are asymptotically unbiased, asymptotically efficient (i.e. no other asymptotically unbiased estimator has lower uncertainty), and asymptotically normal (i.e. the sampling distribution of the maximum likelihood estimate is normal). These properties, in addition to other useful properties of maximum likelihood estimates (see section 7.5), contribute to the great popularity of this approach for relatively simple estimation problems.

The **likelihood** is the probability of observing the data given the model (which includes the parameter values for the model). If Y is the data set, such that $Y = \{Y_1, Y_2, \ldots, Y_n\}$ and θ is the set of model parameters, then the likelihood is $\mathcal{L} = \Pr(Y|\theta)$, where the model (e.g. the probability distribution we are fitting) will determine the form the probability. The basic idea of the maximum likelihood estimation method is to find the parameter set that maximizes the likelihood of observing the data that you have.

As a simple example, consider the binomial distribution. The binomial distribution describes the number of successes out of N independent trials, if each trial has a probability p of success. In a disease context, this could be the number of individuals infected in a day, out of total susceptible population of N. If the per capita probability of infection is p, then the probability that k out of N are infected is

$$\Pr(k|p, N) = \binom{N}{k} p^k (1-p)^{N-k}$$

Now imagine that we have n independent observations of this process, each with the same initial number of susceptible individuals, N. If the number of individuals infected on the ith observation is k_i, then the likelihood is

$$\mathcal{L} = \prod_{i=1}^{n} \binom{N}{k_i} p^{k_i} (1-p)^{N-k_i}$$

Note that we have applied the principle that the joint probability of several independent events is the product of the probabilities of the single events.

It is conventional to work with the log-likelihood, $L = \log(\mathcal{L})$ for two reasons: (1) it turns the product into a sum, and (2) the probabilities are often very small numbers (usually $\ll 1$), and working with a product of small numbers causes numerical problems in computation. The log-likelihood for the binomial example is:

$$L = \sum_{i=1}^{n} \left(\log \binom{N}{k_i} + k_i \log p + (N - k_i) \log(1-p) \right)$$

For our example, the parameter N is known and we want to find the parameter p that maximizes L. For this simple example, it can actually be calculated analytically (see Bolker (2008)), and yields an intuitive answer:

$$\hat{p} = \frac{\sum_{i=1}^{n} k_i}{nN}$$

Other common probability distributions also have maximum likelihood estimators for their parameters that have simple, intuitive forms. For instance, the maximum likelihood estimators for the means of the Poisson, normal, exponential, gamma, and the negative binomial distributions are all equal to the mean of the data.

For most problems, though, this optimization cannot be solved analytically, so we optimize numerically. It is conventional to do this by minimizing the negative log-likelihood (NLL). For more complex distributions, this can be a multidimensional optimization problem as we may be trying to estimate values for several parameters at once. The optimization can be handled using basic commands in various scientific computing environments (e.g. `fminsearch` and related commands in Matlab, and `optim` in R).

In addition to finding the the optimal parameter value(s) via the maximum likelihood estimate, it is very useful to examine the values of the likelihood for other nearby values of the parameter(s). For a univariate estimation problem this is called the likelihood curve, and gives information about the uncertainty in your estimate (see section 7.4) as well as an indication of any pathological behaviour of your model. For a multivariate problem, this will be a likelihood surface, and it gives information about correlations between parameter estimates as well as their uncertainty.

7.2.3. *Bayesian approaches.* The maximum likelihood approach is an example of frequentist statistics. In frequentist statistics, parameters are assumed to have fixed values that we are trying to estimate as precisely as possible. In Bayesian statistics, in contrast, parameters are treated as random variables, with probabilities assigned to particular values of a parameter to reflect the degree of evidence for that value. Bayesian estimation of distribution parameters is also based on the likelihood, but there are two major differences from MLE (Bolker, 2008):

(1) The likelihood is combined with a **prior probability distribution**, which represents information from other sources regarding the values of the parameters. These elements are combined to yield a **posterior probability distribution**, which represents our best estimate of the probability that the parameter takes certain values.
(2) The Bayesian parameter estimates are usually given as the mean of the posterior distribution rather than its mode (as in maximum likelihood estimation), because the mean encapsulates more information about the shape of the distribution.

In the setting of parameter estimation, if we have a data set Y and model parameters θ, then Bayes' theorem states that the posterior distribution on θ is

$$\Pr(\theta|Y) = \frac{\Pr(Y|\theta)\Pr(\theta)}{\Pr(Y)},$$

where $\Pr(Y|\theta)$ is the likelihood (as in the previous section), $\Pr(\theta)$ is the prior distribution, which we define, and $\Pr(Y)$ is the probability of observing the data.

The choice of the prior distribution is somewhat subjective, and there are diverse opinions as to how it should be done. The prior distribution be viewed as a useful tool to incorporate background knowledge regarding the parameter, in which case an 'informative prior' can be chosen that places higher density on parameter values that reflect your knowledge. The prior distribution can also be viewed as a necessary evil required to use the tools of Bayesian inference, in which case a 'flat prior' can be chosen that does not include much information about particular values (e.g. a uniform distribution over a plausible range of values). In this case a prior can also be chosen to simplify the computation.

Another challenge in applying Bayesian methods is how to handle the $\Pr(Y)$ term. For very simple situations, the probability of observing a particular data set can be calculated formally, but in most real-world situations this term is somewhat mysterious. There are two important facts to remember about the $\Pr(Y)$ term. The first is that it's a constant for any given data set. This fact is very useful for some numerical techniques which work with the ratio of posterior probabilities, so the $\Pr(Y)$ terms factor out. The second fact is that the posterior probability distribution must be normalized, so it can be re-written:

$$\Pr(\theta|Y) = \frac{\Pr(Y|\theta)\Pr(\theta)}{\int \Pr(Y|\theta)\Pr(\theta)\,d\theta}.$$

For simple problems this integral can be calculated numerically, but for higher dimensional problems we need other tricks. The important insight to derive from this expression is that the posterior distribution is proportional to the product of the likelihood and the prior. It follows that the more 'informative' the prior, the more it will influence the shape of the posterior distribution.

This technique can readily be generalized to estimation of multiple parameters. For example, for a negative binomial distribution with parameters m and k, we can estimate the joint posterior distribution:

$$\Pr(m,k|Y) = \frac{\Pr(Y|m,k)\Pr(m,k)}{\int\int \Pr(Y|m,k)\Pr(m,k)\,dm\,dk}.$$

Then to learn about parameters individually, you can examine the marginal posterior distributions, e.g.

$$\Pr(k|Y) = \int \Pr(m,k|Y)\,m\,dm$$

or take the mean values, e.g.

$$\bar{k} = \int \Pr(k|Y)\,k\,dk.$$

7.3. Fitting more complex models. The approaches described above are readily applied to the problem of fitting a probability distribution to a set of iid data points, but often we will want to estimate parameters from more complex models — sometimes even from our whole dynamic model. The challenge here is to define the likelihood for the model. Because the likelihood is based on probabilities, it requires that we think about the stochastic components of the processes that generated the data — including both the underlying mechanisms and the observation process. This is not a simple problem, in general, but there are two main approaches:

(1) Consider whether the basic mechanisms of the model corresponds to a clearly defined stochastic process.
(2) Do a rough fit of the model to the data, and examine the residuals to look for systematic patterns that corresponds to basic distributions.

We can apply some rules of thumb to choosing a likelihood model, drawn from the excellent discussion of this problem by Hilborn & Mangel (1997). When the quantities in the data are proportions, consider a binomial distribution; if the quantities are rare events, consider a Poisson distribution, or a negative binomial if there seems to be over-dispersion; if the quantities are sums of many contributions, consider a normal distribution, and if they are products of multiplicative probabilities, consider a log-normal distribution. Always examine the residuals from any model you fit to the data, and be alert for patterns that indicate that the likelihood model is inappropriate. Also remember that these are not definitive rules but rather guidelines.

In epidemic models, one example of a clear stochastic mechanism enabling use of a simple likelihood is the situation where the number of susceptible and infectious individuals are known at each point in time. In this case, the likelihood describing the number of new infections in a given interval is binomial. Let $S(t)$ be the number of susceptible individuals, and $\lambda = \beta I(t)/N(t)$ be the force of infection. Then the probability that each susceptible becomes infected in time Δt is $p(t) = 1 - \exp(-\lambda(t)\Delta t)$, and the number of new infections generated in $(t, t + \Delta t) \sim \text{Binomial}\,(S(t), p(t))$. A more sophisticated example of a mechanistic approach to defining the likelihood for an epidemic model is presented by Eichner & Dietz (2003).

If the model is too complex to infer the appropriate likelihood function, one can resort a simpler method. Many studies are published based on simpler fitting procedures, most frequently the method of least squares, or its close relative the χ^2 goodness-of-fit. This approach is based on minimizing the statistic

$$G = \sum_i (O_i - E_i)^2/E_i,$$

where O_i is the observed value at point i from the the real data, and E_i is the expected value at point i from the model output. While this approach does not have the theoretical foundation or powerful ancillary tools associated with the maximum likelihood or Bayesian approaches (though note that least-squares fitting is closely related to maximum likelihood for a normally distributed likelihood (Hilborn & Mangel, 1997)), it will typically yield a decent fit to the data.

7.4. Estimating uncertainties. In any estimation problem, it is essential to obtain some measure of uncertainty that describes the precision and reliability of the point estimate. In frequentist approaches this is often presented as a **confidence interval**, which is defined as an estimated range of values that will contain the unknown parameter with a given probability. In Bayesian approaches, the uncertainty is often presented as a **credible interval**, defined as the region in the center of the posterior distribution containing a given proportion of the density.

7.4.1. *Likelihood profiles.* Likelihood curves and surfaces map out not only the best fit but also the "badness-of-fit" of different parameter values to the data. We can analyze the curvature of these surfaces — or actually, of surfaces of the negative log-likelihood (NLL) — to find confidence intervals for our parameter estimates. For a one-parameter problem, the confidence interval can be calculated directly from the likelihood curve. For higher-dimensional problems, it is often necessary to reduce the dimensionality to focus on the contribution of one parameter to the overall likelihood of the model. The correct approach to this problem is via "likelihood profiles". Likelihood profiles are generated by choosing a range of values for the focal parameter, and for each value maximizing the likelihood with respect to all other parameters. The multiple parameter problem has now been reduced to a one-dimensional profile likelihood curve, which can then be analyzed by the same method that is used for a one-parameter problem to estimate a confidence interval for that parameter value.

The difference in NLL values between the maximum likelihood estimate and other points on a likelihood profile is asymptotically χ^2-distributed with one degree of freedom. To find the $(1-\alpha)\%$ confidence limits on our estimate, we find the parameter values corresponding to NLL values of $\mathbf{NNL}_{\text{MLE}} + \chi_1^2(1-\alpha)/2$, where $\chi_1^2(x)$ is the xth quantile of the cumulative distribution function of the χ^2 distribution with one degree of freedom. For a 95% confidence interval, the increment is $\chi_1^2(0.95)/2$ or 1.92 log-likelihood units. These methods can be generalized to higher dimensions, e.g. to calculate joint confidence regions for two parameters by generating the profile likelihood surface across a fixed grid of values for the parameters. See Bolker (2008) for more details.

7.4.2. *Quadratic approximations.* The likelihood profile approach works very well when you have a small number of parameters, but becomes computationally impractical for models with many parameters, since for an n-parameter model, you have to optimize $n-1$ parameters for each point on your likelihood profile. Luckily, classical likelihood theory tells us that we can learn about the variance of our estimate by considering the second derivative of the likelihood curve — essentially by using a quadratic approximation to the region around the minimum. Here we follow the excellent presentation by Bolker (2008) to summarize this approach.

As mentioned above, maximum likelihood estimates have the property of asymptotically normality. For large enough samples, the sampling distribution for the parameter estimate is approximately normal with standard deviation $\left(\frac{d^2L}{dp^2}\right)^{-1/2}$, where recall that $L = \log \mathcal{L}$. The width of the interval that gives a $(1-\alpha)$ confidence interval is then $N(\alpha)\left(\frac{d^2L}{dp^2}\right)^{-1/2}$, where $N(\alpha)$ is the appropriate quantile from the standard normal distribution. The second derivative with respect to parameter p at a given value p_0 can be computed numerically using the basic formula:

$$\left.\frac{d^2f}{dp^2}\right|_{p=p_0} \approx \frac{f(p_0+2\triangle p) - 2f(p_0+\triangle p) + f(p_0)}{(\triangle p)^2}.$$

For models with several parameters, the same idea applies, but we need to work with the matrix of the second derivatives (the Hessian). For example, if we are estimating the negative binomial parameters m and k:

$$\begin{pmatrix} \frac{\partial^2 L}{\partial m^2} & \frac{\partial^2 L}{\partial m \partial k} \\ \frac{\partial^2 L}{\partial m \partial k} & \frac{\partial^2 L}{\partial k^2} \end{pmatrix}$$

If we evaluate the Hessian at the maximum likelihood estimate and invert it, we obtain the variance-covariance matrix for the parameters:

$$V = \begin{pmatrix} \sigma_m^2 & \sigma_{mk} \\ \sigma_{mk} & \sigma_k^2 \end{pmatrix}$$

Here the diagonal terms can be used to estimate confidence intervals on single parameters, as above, and the off-diagonal terms reflect any correlation between the parameter estimates.

7.4.3. *Bootstrapping.* Bootstrapping is a completely different approach to estimating uncertainties. It is completely non-parametric, meaning that it does not depend on any assumptions about the probability distributions that underlie your data and instead relies on heavy computation to examine the statistical properties of the data set directly. The basic idea is to simulate new data sets by randomly re-sampling with replacement from the observed data. One can then calculate the parameter of interest for each of these simulated data sets, and the distribution of these estimates gives an indication of the uncertainty in your true estimate.

7.5. Model selection. To this point we have focused entirely on how to fit parameters of a single model to the observed data. It is often informative to ask whether the model we are using is the best one, or more generally, to select the best model from a set of candidate models using some objective criterion. The field of model selection and multi-model inference addresses the challenge of comparing models and weighting their outputs in the context of data. It is treated comprehensively by Burnham & Anderson (2002). There are many approaches to model selection, but all have two properties in common: (i) models that fit the data better are preferred; and (ii) parsimonious models are preferred (i.e. there is a penalty for having more parameters).

A classical approach to model selection is the likelihood ratio test. It provides a pair-wise comparison between two models when one model is nested within the other. Model A is said to be nested within model B if it corresponds to some special case of model B where one or more parameters have particular values. For example, $f(x) = ax^2 + c$ is nested in $g(x) = ax^2 + bx + c$ for the value of $b = 0$. An epidemiological example might be whether an additional parameter is justified to describe the possible effect of male circumcision on male-to-female transmission of HIV. For any such pair of models for which likelihood function can be defined, the likelihood ratio test test computes a statistic that compares the log-likelihoods calculated from the two models, and determines whether the additional complexity is justified by the data.

The Akaike information criterion (AIC) provides a more flexible framework for model selection, that does not require models to be nested and can compare many models at once. It is important to note that the AIC can be applied only to models which have been fit by the method of maximum likelihood. The AIC statistic takes the value $\text{AIC} = -2L + 2K$, where, L is the log-likelihood of the maximum likelihood estimate and K is the number of free parameters in the model. For small sample sizes, i.e. when the number of data points N is such that $N/K < 40$, a corrected AIC should be used. Here,

$$\text{AIC}_\text{c} = \text{AIC} + \frac{2K(K+1)}{N-K-1}.$$

In fact the AIC_c converges to the AIC statistic as the sample size grows, so it is always safer to use the AIC_c.

Many models can be compared by simply comparing their AIC values, and the model with the lowest AIC value is generally preferred. Only the relative values of the AIC matter, so they are often reduced to differences from the lowest value obtained, AIC_min:

$$\Delta\text{AIC}_i = \text{AIC}_i - \text{AIC}_\text{min}.$$

As a rule of thumb, models with AIC < 2 units apart have roughly equivalent support, models with AIC between 4 and 7 units apart are clearly distinguishable, and models with AIC > 10 units apart are definitely different.

The ΔAIC values can also be used to calculate the Akaike weight associated with each model i,

$$w_i = \frac{e^{\Delta \mathrm{AIC}_i/2}}{\sum_j e^{\Delta \mathrm{AIC}_j/2}}.$$

These weights are often interpreted as the probability that a given model is the best of the candidate models considered, but this is not formally accurate (Burnham & Anderson, 2002). The weights can be used for model averaging, i.e. to generate an "average" output from several models that is weighted by the support for each model from the data.

7.6. Sensitivity and Uncertainty Analysis. After constructing a model, choosing parameter values, and generating some simulated epidemics, it is important to keep a critical eye on your model output via sensitivity and uncertainty analyses. Model outputs contain uncertainties from two main sources: parameter values and model structure. Parameter values are inevitably uncertain, either because of statistical uncertainties in the estimation process, or because there are no data from which to make an estimate so you have hypothesized a plausible range of values. Model structure is also a source of uncertainty, because there are many possible models that could be built to describe a given system, and all of them make simplifying assumptions while trying to capture the important mechanisms.

Uncertainty analysis aims to assess the variability in model outputs that arises from uncertainty in model inputs. This will determine how much confidence one should place in any quantitative projections that are generated by the model. **Sensitivity analysis** aims to determine which parameters or changes in model structure are most important in determining the model output. It quantifies the influence of each parameter or modelled process on the particular outputs you have obtained. By revealing the relative importance of different mechanisms in the model, sensitivity analysis also tells us which components of the system are good targets for possible disease control measures, or where further efforts to collect data and information should be focused.

A formal definition of **sensitivity** of an outcome λ to the parameter value θ is $S = \frac{\partial \lambda}{\partial \theta}$. By holding all other parameters constant, the partial derivative gives us exactly the rate of change of the outcome, λ, with respect to change in the chosen parameter value θ. However different parameters often have different units or scales of measurement, making sensitivity values difficult to compare. To address this we define **elasticity**, which is the proportional response of an outcome to a proportional perturbation to a parameter. The elasticity of the outcome λ to the value of parameter θ is $E = \frac{\theta}{\lambda}\frac{\partial \lambda}{\partial \theta} = \frac{\partial \log \lambda}{\partial \log \theta}$.

For complex models these quantities typically cannot be calculated analytically, but there are various methods to investigate the influence of parameter values on the model outputs. At the *ad hoc* extreme, it is fairly common to explore a model's range of behaviours by examining different sets of parameters chosen to represent a range of 'scenarios'. This is certainly preferable to no exploration of parameter space, but is not a formal sensitivity analysis. More formally, it is common to examine the sensitivity or elasticity of an output to one or two parameters by running simulations for a range of values of the parameters of interest, while all other parameters are held constant. However, in nonlinear models there can be complex interactions among parameter values, so it is desirable to consider the influence of each parameter in the context of all plausible values of the other parameters. For a model with more than a few parameters, it becomes computationally intensive to investigate all parameters in a full-factorial manner, so more efficient approaches to sampling parameter space have been devised. A popular approach for epidemic models is **Latin Hypercube Sampling**, which is introduced clearly in an influential paper by Blower & Dowlatabadi (1994). Results from this approach are often presented in terms of partial rank correlation coefficients, which describe the influence of each parameter on a given model output in a non-parametric manner.

Structural sensitivity analysis, on the other hand, describes how changes in the design of a model influence its output. There are many subjective decisions, and many assumptions, involved in constructing a model — but too few modelling studies take the time to test explicitly how aspects of their model structure affect their findings. This is probably because it is not a well-defined problem (because there are an infinite number of possible model structures), and there are not established methods for these analyses. Testing for structural sensitivity is an important endeavor, though, because we do not want our assumptions to bias the output of our modelling studies. As a modeller, it is often clear which structural assumptions are most tenuous or have greatest potential to influence the results, and it is good practice to test whether your conclusions are robust to these. The ultimate structural sensitivity analysis occurs when several independent groups of researchers work on the same problem, as has been the case for some recent outbreaks such as H5N1 influenza, SARS, and foot and mouth disease in Britain.

References

R. M. Anderson, C. Fraser, A. C. Ghani, C. A. Donnelly, S. Riley, N. M. Ferguson, G. M. Leung, T. H. Lam, & A. J. Hedley (2004). 'Epidemiology, transmission dynamics and control of SARS: The 2002-2003 epidemic.' *Philosophical Transactions of the Royal Society of London Series B-Biological Sciences* **359**:1091–1105.

R. M. Anderson & R. M. May (1985a). 'Herd immunity to helminth infection and implications for parasite control.' *Nature* **315**:493–496.

R. M. Anderson & R. M. May (1985b). 'Vaccination and herd immunity to infectious diseases.' *Nature* **318**:323–329.

R. M. Anderson & R. M. C. May (1991). *Infectious Diseases of Humans: Dynamics and Control.* Oxford University Press.

R. Antia, V. V. Ganusov, & R. Ahmed (2005). 'The role of models in understanding CD8+ T-cell memory.' *Nat. Rev. Immunol.* **5**(2):101–111.

J. Antonovics, Y. Iwasa, & M. P. Hassell (1995). 'A generalized model of parasitoid, veneral, and vector-based transmission processes.' *American Naturalist* **145**:661–675.

N. T. J. Bailey (1955). 'Some problems in the statistical analysis of epidemic data.' *Journal of the Royal Statistical Society. Series B* **17**:35–68.

F. Ball, D. Mollison, & G. Scalia-Tomba (1997). 'Epidemics with two levels of mixing.' *Ann. Appl. Probab.* **7**:46–89.

F. Ball & P. Neal (2002). 'A general model for stochastic SIR epidemics with two levels of mixing.' *Mathematical Biosciences* **180**:73–102.

S. Bansal, B. T. Grenfell, & L. A. Meyers (2007). 'When individual behaviour matters: homogeneous and network models in epidemiology.' *Journal of the Royal Society Interface* **4**:879–891.

M. S. Bartlett (1957). 'Measles periodicity and community size.' *Journal of the Royal Statistical Society. Series A (General)* **120**:48–70.

C. T. Bauch & D. J. D. Earn (2004). 'Vaccination and the theory of games.' *Proceedings of the National Academy of Sciences of the United States of America* **101**:13391–13394.

C. T. Bauch, J. O. Lloyd-Smith, M. Coffee, & A. P. Galvani (2005). 'Dynamically modeling SARS and respiratory EIDs: past, present, future.' *Epidemiology* **16**:791–801.

N. Becker & I. Marschner (1990). 'The effect of heterogeneity on the spread of disease.' In P. Picard, J. P. Gabriel, & C. Lefevre (eds.), *Stochastic Processes in Epidemic Theory*, vol. 86 of *Lecture Notes in Biomathematics*, pp. 90–103. Springer-Verlag, New York.

M. Begon, S. M. Hazel, D. Baxby, K. Brown, R. Cavanagh, J. Chantrey, T. Jones, & M. Bennett (1999). 'Transmission dynamics of a zoonotic pathogen within and between wildlife host species.' *Proceedings of the Royal Society of London Series B-Biological Sciences* **266**:1939—1945.

O. N. Bjørnstad, B. F. Finkendtädt, & B. T. Grenfell (2002). 'Dynamics of measles epidemics: Estimating scaling of transmission rates using a time series SIR model.' *Ecological Monographs* **72**:169–184.

S. M. Blower & H. Dowlatabadi (1994). 'Sensitivity and uncertainty analysis of complex models of disease transmission: an HIV model, as an example.' *International Statistical Review* **62**:229–243.

B. M. Bolker (2008). *Ecological models and data in R.* Princeton University Press.

K. P. Burnham & D. R. Anderson (2002). *Model Selection and Multimodel Inference: A Practical Information-Theoretic Approach.* Springer.

P. C. Cross, P. L. F. Johnson, J. O. Lloyd-Smith, & W. M. Getz (2007). 'Utility of R_0 as a predictor of disease invasion in structured populations.' *Journal of the Royal Society Interface* **4**:315–324.

P. C. Cross, J. O. Lloyd-Smith, J. Bowers, C. Hay, M. Hofmeyr, & W. M. Getz (2004). 'Integrating association data and disease dynamics in a social ungulate: bovine tuberculosis in african buffalo in kruger national park.' *Annales Zoologici Fennici* **41**:879–892.

P. C. Cross, J. O. Lloyd-Smith, P. L. F. Johnson, & W. M. Getz (2005). 'Duelling timescales of host movement and disease recovery determine invasion of disease in structured populations.' *Ecology Letters* **8**(6):587–595.

O. Diekmann & J. A. P. Heesterbeek (2000). *Mathematical Epidemiology of Infectious Diseases: Model Building, Analysis, and Interpretation.* Wiley, Chichester.

K. Dietz (1993). 'The estimation of the basic reproduction number for infectious diseases.' *Statistical methods in medical research* **2**:23–41.

K. T. D. Eames & M. J. Keeling (2003). 'Contact tracing and disease control.' *Proceedings of the Royal Society, London, Series B* **270**:2565–2571.

M. Eichner & K. Dietz (2003). 'Transmission potential of Smallpox: Estimates based on detailed data from an outbreak.' *American Journal of Epidemiology* **158**:110–117.

C. P. Farrington, M. N. Kanaan, & N. J. Gay (2001). 'Estimation of the basic reproduction number for infectious diseases from age-stratified serological survey data.' *Journal of Royal Statistical Society* **50**:251–292.

C. P. Farrington & H. J. Whitaker (2003). 'Estimation of effective reproduction numbers for infectious diseases using serological survey data.' *Biostatistics* **4**:621–632.

F. Fenner, D. Henderson, I. Arita, Z. Jezek, & I. Ladnyi (1988). *Smallpox and Its Eradication.* World Health Organization, Geneva.

N. M. Ferguson, C. A. Donnelly, & R. Anderson (2001). 'The Foot-and-Mouth epidemic in Great Britian: Pattern of spread and impact of intervensions.' *Science* **292**:1155—1160.

N. M. Ferguson, M. J. Keeling, W. J. Edmunds, R. Gani, B. T. Grenfell, R. M. Anderson, & S. Leach (2003). 'Planning for Smallpox outbreaks.' *Nature* **425**:681–685.

M. J. Ferrari, O. N. Bjørnstad, & A. P. Dobson (2005). 'Estimation and inference of R_0 of an infectious pathogen by removal method.' *Mathematical Biosciences* **198**:14–26.

C. Fraser, S. Riley, R. M. Anderson, & N. M. Ferguson (2004). 'Factors that make an infectious disease outbreak controlable.' *Proceedings of the National Academy of Sciences of the United States of America* **101**:6146—6151.

R. Gani & S. Leach (2001). 'Transmission potential of smallpox in contemporary populations.' *Nature* **414**:748–751.

B. T. Grenfell, O. N. Bjørnstad, & B. F. Finkendtädt (2002). 'Dynamics of measles epidemics. ii. scaling noise, determinism and predictability with the times series SIR model.' *Ecological Monographs* **72**:185—2002.

J. A. P. Heesterbeek (2002). 'A brief history of R_0 and a recipe for its calculation.' *Acta Biotheoretica* **50**:189–204.

H. W. Hethcote & J. W. Van Ark (1987). 'Epidemiological models for heterogenous populations: Proportionate mixing, parameter estimation, and immunization programs.' *Mathematical Biosciences* **84**:85–118.

R. Hilborn & M. Mangel (1997). *The ecological detective: confronting models with data.* Princeton University Press.

A. James, J. W. Pitchford, & M. J. Plank (2006). 'An event-based model of superspreading in epidemics.' *Proceedings of the Royal Society of London Series B-Biological Sciences* **274**:741–747.

V. A. A. Jansen, N. Stollenwerk, H. J. Jensen, M. E. Ramsay, W. J. Edmunds, & C. J. Rhodes (2003). 'Measles outbreaks in a population with declining vaccine uptake.' *Science* **301**.

M. J. Keeling & K. T. D. Eames (2005). 'Networks and epidemic models.' *J. R. Soc. Interface* **2**(4):295–307.

M. J. Keeling & B. T. Grenfell (1997). 'Disease extinction and community size: Modeling the persistence of measles.' *Science* **275**:65–67.

M. J. Keeling & B. T. Grenfell (1998). 'Effect of variability in infection period on the persistence and spatial spread of infectious diseases.' *Mathematical Biosciences* **147**:207–226.

M. J. Keeling & P. Rohani (2002). 'Estimating spatial coupling in epidemiological systems: a mechanistic approach.' *Ecology Letters* **5**:20–29.

M. J. Keeling & P. Rohani (2007). *Modeling infectious diseases in humans and animals.* Princeton University Press.

M. J. Keeling, M. E. J. Woolhouse, R. M. May, & B. T. Grenfell (2003). 'Modelling vaccination strategies against foot-and-mouth disease.' *Nature* **421**:136–142.

M. J. Keeling, M. E. J. Woolhouse, D. J. Shaw, L. Matthews, M. Chase-Topping, D. T. Haydon, S. J. Cornell, J. Kappey, J. Wilesmith, & B. T. Grenfell (2001). 'Dynamics of the 2001 UK Foot and Mouth epidemic: Stochastic dispersal in a heterogeneous landscape.' *Science* **294**:813—817.

W. O. Kermack & A. G. McKendrick (1927). 'A contribution to the mathematical theory of epidemics.' *Proceedings of the Royal Society of London, Series A* **115**:700–721.

A. A. King, S. Shrestha, E. T. Harvell, & O. N. Bjørnstad (2009). 'Evolution of acute infections and the invasion-persistence trade-off.' *The American Naturalist* **173**:446—455.

K. Koelle, X. Rodo, M. Pascual, M. Yunus, & G. Mostafa (2005). 'Refractory periods and climate forcing in cholera dynamics.' *Nature* **436**(7051):696–700.

M. Lipsitch & M. H. Samore (2002). 'Antimicrobial use and anitmicrobial resistance: a population perspective.' *Trends in Microbiology* **8**:347–354.

A. L. Lloyd (2001). 'Destabilization of epidemic models with the inclusion of realistic distributions of infectious periods.' *Proceedings of the Royal Society of London Series B-Biological Sciences* **268**:985–993.

J. O. Lloyd-Smith, P. C. Cross, C. J. Briggs, M. Daugherty, W. M. Getz, J. Latto, M. S. Sanchez, A. B. Smith, & A. Swei (2005a). 'Should we expect population thresholds for wildlife disease?' *Trends in Ecology and Evolution* **20**(9):511–519.

J. O. Lloyd-Smith, A. P. Galvani, & W. M. Getz (2003). 'Curtailing transmission of severe acute respiratory syndrome within a community and its hospital.' *Proceedings of the Royal Society, London, Series B* **270**:1979–1989.

J. O. Lloyd-Smith, W. M. Getz, & H. V. Westerhoff (2004). 'Frequency-dependent incidence in models of sexually transmitted diseases: portrayal of pair-based transmission and effects of illness on contact behaviour.' *Proceedings of the Royal Society of London, Series B* **271**:625–635.

J. O. Lloyd-Smith, S. J. Schreiber, & W. M. Getz (2006). 'Moving beyond averages: individual-level variation in disease transmission.' In A. B. Gumel, C. Castillo-Chavez, R. E. Mickes, & D. P. Clemence (eds.), *Mathematical studies of human disease dynamics: emerging paradigms and challenges*, vol. 410 of *AMS Contemporary Mathematics*, pp. 235–258. American Mathematical Society.

J. O. Lloyd-Smith, S. J. Schreiber, P. E. Jopp, & W. M. Getz (2005b). 'Superspreading and the effect of individual variation on disease emergence.' *Nature* **438**:355–359.

A. D. Lopez, C. D. Mathers, M. Ezzati, D. T. Jamison, & C. J. L. Murray (eds.) (2002). *Global Burden of Disease and Risk Factors.* Oxford University Press, Oxford.

W. M. Lui, H. W. Hethcote, & S. A. Levin (1987). 'Dynamical behaviour of epidemiological models with nonlinear incidence rates.' *Journal of Mathematical Biology* **25**:359—380.

R. M. May & R. M. Anderson (1984). 'Spatial heterogeneity and the design of immunization programs.' *Mathematical Biosciences* **72**:83–111.

H. McCallum, N. Barlow, & J. Hone (2001). 'How should pathogen transmission be modelled?' *Trends in Ecology and Evolution* **16**:295–300.

N. Mideo, S. Alizon, & T. Day (2008). 'Linking within- and between-host dynamics in the evolutionary epidemiology of infectious diseases.' *Trends Ecol. Evol.* .

P. D. Minor (2004). 'Polio eradication, cessation of vaccination and re-emergence of disease.' *Nature Reviews Microbiology* **2**:473–482.

D. Mollison (1991). 'Dependence of epidemic and population velocities on basic parameters.' *Mathematical Biosciences* **107**:255–287.

I. Nåsell (2005). 'A new look at the critical community size for childhood infections.' *Theor. Popul. Biol.* **67**(3):203–216.

M. E. J. Newman (2002). 'Spread of epidemic disease on networks.' *Physical Review E* **66**.

A. S. Perelson & G. Weisbuch (1997). 'Immunology for physicists.' *Reviews in Modern Physics* **69**:1219–1268.

P. Rohani, D. J. D. Earn, & B. T. Grenfell (1999). 'Oppopsite patterns of synchrony in sympatric disease metapopulations.' *Science* **286**:968–971.

P. Schmid-Hempel (2008). 'Parasite immune evasion: a momentous molecular war.' *Trends Ecol. Evol.* **23**:318—326.

S. J. Schreiber & J. O. Lloyd-Smith (in press). 'Invasion success and extinction risk in spatially heterogeneous environments.' *The American Naturalist* .

D. L. Smith, B. Lucey, L. A. Waller, J. E. Childs, & R. L. A. (2002). 'Predicting the spatial dynamics of rabies epidemics on heterogenous landscapes.' *Proceedings of the National Academy of Sciences of the United States of America* **99**:3668–3672.

M. J. Tildesley, N. J. Savill, D. J. Shaw, R. Deardon, S. P. Brooks, M. E. J. Woolhouse, B. T. Grenfell, & M. J. Keeling (2006). 'Modelling vaccination strategies against foot-and-mouth disease.' *Nature* **440**:83–86.

P. van den Driesche & J. Watmough (2002). 'Reproduction number and subthreshold endemic equilibria for compartmental models of disease transmission.' *Mathematical Biosciences* **180**:29–48.

J. Wallinga & M. Lipsitch (2007). 'How generation intervals shape the relationship between growth rates and reproductive numbers.' *Proceedings of the Royal Society, Series B* **274**:599–604.

H. J. Wearing, P. Rohani, & M. J. Keeling (2005). 'Appropriate models for the management of infectious diseases.' *PLoS Medicine* **2**:e174.

B. G. Williams, J. O. Lloyd-Smith, E. Gouws, C. Hankins, W. M. Getz, J. Hargrove, I. de Zoysa, C. Dye, & B. Auvert (2006). 'The potential impact of male circumcision on HIV in sub-Saharan Africa.' *PLoS Medicine* **7**:e262.

M. E. J. Woolhouse, C. Dye, J. F. Etard, T. Smith, J. D. Charlwood, G. P. Garnett, P. Hagan, J. L. K. Hii, P. D. Ndhlovu, R. J. Quinnell, C. H. Watts, S. K. Chandiwana, & R. M. Anderson (1997). 'Heterogeneities in the transmission of infectious agents: Implications for the design of control programs.' *Proceedings of the National Academy of Sciences of the United States of America* **94**:338–342.

[1]Department of Ecology & Evolutionary Biology, and Center for the Study of Complex Systems, University of Michigan, Ann Arbor, MI 48109

[2]Department of Ecology & Evolutionary Biology, University of California, Los Angeles, 90095,

[3]Fogarty International Center, National Institutes of Health, Bethesda, MD 20892, USA

DIMACS Series in Discrete Mathematics
and Theoretical Computer Science
Volume **75**, 2010

Tools for Mathematical Epidemiology

E.M. Lungu, M. Kgosimore, and F. Nyabadza

1. Introduction to mathematical epidemiology

In this chapter, we introduce simple epidemic models on the spread of an infectious disease. The aim is to introduce basic ideas in epidemiological modeling to someone being initiated to this area. Epidemiological modeling has become important because humans are facing challenges from old diseases such as tuberculosis (TB), malaria, influenza and new diseases such as the human immunodeficiency (HIV) syndrome and AIDS [**9**]. Increasingly, animal or bird diseases are mutating and are infecting humans, for example, swine flu (H1N1 flu), bird flu [**8**]. The TB bacteria and the malaria parasite have developed resistance to treatment drugs thereby compounding an already complex situation. In this chapter, however, we shall consider a simple situation when a small group of people carrying an infectious disease is introduced into a large population, the members of which are liable to catch the disease. We ask the questions: (i) What happens as time goes on? (ii) Is it inevitable that all healthy individuals will catch the disease?

It is impossible to capture reality but we shall be content with an approximation of reality, meaning that we will make some assumptions in order to build a simple model. We shall assume (i) that anyone who catches the disease either dies or recovers with permanent immunity. In either case such individuals will be removed from the sub-population of susceptibles. (ii) We shall assume that there is a negligibly short incubation period so that anyone who catches the disease becomes infective immediately afterwards and (iii) lastly, we shall assume that there is homogeneous mixing between susceptibles and infectives. Our population will be divided into three classes of individuals namely, the susceptible class, S, the infective class, I, and the removed class, R. Before we translate this into an epidemic model in the form of ordinary differential equations, we need to develop the tools that will be used to understand the behavior of the disease in terms of its spread, control etc. The examples we shall use to develop the basic tools are not from epidemiology but at this stage we want to achieve simplicity in developing the tools and clarity in understanding the interpretation.

1991 *Mathematics Subject Classification.* Primary 92B05.

2. Introduction to nonlinear systems

An n th-order continuous-time system has the following form [4, 5]:

$$
\begin{array}{rcl}
\dot{x}_1(t) & = & f_1(x_1(t), x_2(t), \cdots, x_n(t)), \\
\dot{x}_2(t) & = & f_1(x_1(t), x_2(t), \cdots, x_n(t)), \\
. & . & \ldots\ldots\ldots\ldots\ldots \\
. & . & \ldots\ldots\ldots\ldots\ldots \\
\dot{x}_n(t) & = & f_n(x_1(t), x_2(t), \cdots, x_n(t))
\end{array} \tag{2.1}
$$

which can be expressed in matrix form as

$$\dot{X}(t) = f(X(t), t), \tag{2.2}$$

where $X = [x_1, x_2, ..., x_n]^T$ and $f = [f_1, f_2, ..., f_n]^T$, T denotes matrix transpose.

In general, one does not seek detailed solutions either in numerical or analytical form, but rather one seeks to characterize some aspects of system behavior. For example, one might ask whether there are equilibrium points and whether they are stable. In nonlinear systems, one might look for threshold effects. The role of analysis therefore, is to characterize in broad outline the critical aspects of the system behavior.

3. Main tools for analysis of nonlinear systems

3.1. Equilibrium Points.

DEFINITION 3.1. [4] A vector $\bar{X}$ is an equilibrium point for a dynamical system if once the state vector is equal to $\bar{X}$ it remains equal to $\bar{X}$ for all future time. That is, if

$$\dot{X}(t) = f(X(t), t)$$

then an equilibrium point is a state $\bar{X}$ satisfying

$$f(\bar{X}, t) = 0.$$

An analysis of a nonlinear dynamical system may devote considerable attention to the characterization of the equilibrium points. In the linear systems, equilibrium points are basically solutions to linear equations. The nonlinear case is different in two essential respects:

(1) First, since the equilibrium points are solutions to nonlinear equations, finding such solutions is somewhat more of an accomplishment than in the linear case.
(2) The equilibrium point distribution is potentially more complex in the nonlinear case than in the linear case.

Thus, characterization of equilibrium points is not only technically more difficult, it is a much broader question. Ultimately, interest centers not just on the existence of the equilibrium points but also on their stability properties.

4. Stability

4.1. Stability definitions. Stability properties characterize how a system behaves if its state is initiated close to, but not precisely at a given equilibrium point.

(1) If a system is initiated with the state exactly equal to an equilibrium point, then by definition it will never move.
(2) When initiated close by, however, the state may remain close by, or it may move away.

Roughly speaking, an equilibrium point is stable if whenever the system state is initiated near that point, the state remains near it, perhaps even tending towards the equilibrium point as time increases. Suppose $\bar{X}$ is an equilibrium point of a time-invariant system, that is, $\bar{X}$ is an equilibrium point of

$$\dot{X}(t) = f(X(t)).$$

For a precise definition of stability, it is convenient to introduce the notation $D(\bar{X}, \rho)$ to denote a spherical region in the state space with center at $\bar{X}$ and radius ρ.

DEFINITION 4.1. An equilibrium point $\bar{X}$ is stable if there is a $\rho_0 > 0$ for which the following is true. For every $\rho < \rho_0$, there is r, $0 < r < \rho$, such that if $X(0)$ is inside $D(\bar{X}, r)$, then $X(t)$ is inside $D(\bar{X}, \rho)$ for all $t > 0$.

DEFINITION 4.2. An equilibrium point $\bar{X}$ is asymptotically stable if whenever it is stable and in addition there is an $\bar{\rho}_0 > 0$ such that whenever the state is initiated inside $D(\bar{X}, \bar{\rho}_0)$, it tends to $\bar{X}$ as time increases.

DEFINITION 4.3. An equilibrium point $\bar{X}$ is marginally stable if it is stable but not asymptotically stable.

DEFINITION 4.4. An equilibrium point $\bar{X}$ is unstable if it is not stable. Equivalently, $\bar{X}$ is unstable if for some $\rho_0 > 0$ and any $r > 0$ there is a point in the spherical region $D(\bar{X}, r)$ such that if initiated there, the system state will eventually move outside of $D(\bar{X}, \rho_0)$.

4.2. Linearization and stability. According to the basic definitions, stability properties depend only on the nature of the system near the equilibrium point. Therefore, to conduct an analysis of the stability, it is often theoretically legitimate and mathematically convenient to replace the full nonlinear description by a simpler description that approximates the true system near the equilibrium point. Often a linear approximation is sufficient to reveal the stability properties.

The linearization of a nonlinear system is based on linearization of the nonlinear function f in its description. For the first-order system, defined by a single function $f(x)$ of a single variable, the procedure (see [**5**]) is to approximate f near $\bar{x}$ by

$$f(\bar{x} + y) \approx f(\bar{x}) + \frac{df(\bar{x})}{dx} y. \tag{4.1}$$

An n-order system is defined by n functions, each of which depends on the n variables. In this case each function is approximated by the relation

$$\begin{aligned} f_i(\bar{x}_1+y_1,\bar{x}_2+y_2,\cdots,\bar{x}_n+y_n) \approx\ & f_i(\bar{x}_1,\bar{x}_2,\cdots,\bar{x}_n)+\frac{\partial f(\bar{x}_1,\bar{x}_2,\cdots,\bar{x}_n)}{\partial x_1}y_1+ \\ & \frac{\partial f(\bar{x}_1,\bar{x}_2,\cdots,\bar{x}_n)}{\partial x_2}y_2+\frac{\partial f(\bar{x}_1,\bar{x}_2,\cdots,\bar{x}_n)}{\partial x_3}y_3+ \\ & \cdots\cdots+\frac{\partial f(\bar{x}_1,\bar{x}_2,\cdots,\bar{x}_n)}{\partial x_n}y_n. \end{aligned} \tag{4.2}$$

In matrix form

$$f(\bar{x}+y)\approx f(\bar{x})+Fy \tag{4.3}$$

where

$$F=\begin{pmatrix} \frac{\partial f_1}{\partial x_1} & \frac{\partial f_1}{\partial x_2} & \cdots & \frac{\partial f_1}{\partial x_n} \\ \frac{\partial f_2}{\partial x_1} & \frac{\partial f_2}{\partial x_2} & \cdots & \frac{\partial f_2}{\partial x_n} \\ \cdots & \cdots & \cdots & \cdots \\ \cdots & \cdots & \cdots & \cdots \\ \cdots & \cdots & \cdots & \cdots \\ \frac{\partial f_n}{\partial x_1} & \frac{\partial f_n}{\partial x_2} & \cdots & \frac{\partial f_n}{\partial x_n} \end{pmatrix}$$

The matrix F is called the Jacobian matrix of f. Now consider the matrix equation

$$\dot{x}(t)=f(x(t)). \tag{4.4}$$

Setting $x(t)=\bar{x}+y(t)$, we obtain

$$\dot{y}(t)=f(\bar{x}+y(t))\approx f(\bar{x})+Fy(t). \tag{4.5}$$

Since $\bar{x}$ is an equilibrium point of f, $f(\bar{x})=0$. Therefore, to the first order of approximation equation (4.5) becomes

$$\dot{y}(t)=Fy(t). \tag{4.6}$$

The stability properties of the original system can be inferred from the linearized system using the following results.

(1) If all eigenvalues of F are strictly in the left half-plane, then $\bar{x}$ is asymptotically stable for the nonlinear system.
(2) If at least one eigenvalue of F has a positive real part, then $\bar{x}$ is unstable for the nonlinear system.
(3) If the eigenvalues of F are all in the left half-plane, but at least one has a zero real part then $\bar{x}$ may be either stable, asymptotically stable or unstable for the nonlinear system.

EXAMPLE 4.5. Consider the system

$$\begin{aligned} \dot{x}(t) &= x(t) \\ \dot{y}(t) &= -ky(t). \end{aligned} \tag{4.7}$$

The system (4.7) has one fixed point $(0,0)$, and its solution is given by:

$$x(t) = x_0e^{-t},\ y(t)=y_0e^{-kt}. \tag{4.8}$$

If $x_0 \neq 0$, then this solution can be expressed as

$$y = y_0 e^{-kt} = bx^k,$$

where $b = y_0 x_0^{-k}$. Below, we consider several cases of this solution for various values of k.

Case: $k = 1$

For $k = 1$ the solution (4.8) becomes

$$x(t) = x_0 e^{-t}, \; y(t) = bx.$$

Clearly, $y = bx$ represents a family of straight lines with slope b. As $t \to \infty$, $x(t) \to 0$, and $y(t) \to 0$. Thus, for $k = 1$ the fixed point $(0,0)$ is an asymptotically stable proper node since the trajectories are rays that tend to $(0,0)$ as $t \to \infty$.

Case: $k = 2$

For $k = 2$ the solution (4.8) becomes

$$x(t) = x_0 e^{-t}, \; y(t) = bx^2.$$

The solution $y = bx^2$ represents a family of parabolas. As $t \to \infty$, $x(t) \to 0$, and $y(t) \to 0$. The fixed point $(0,0)$ is now an asymptotically stable improper node. It is improper because the trajectories are parabolas rather than straight lines.

Case: $k = -1$

For $k = -1$ the solution (4.8) has the form

$$x(t) = x_0 e^{-t}, \; y(t) = y_0 e^{t} \text{ or } xy = C.$$

$x(t)$ decreases with increasing time t but y increases with increasing t. The fixed point $(0,0)$ is now a saddle point (unstable).

EXAMPLE 4.6. Consider the system

$$\begin{aligned} \dot{x}(t) &= y(t) \\ \dot{y}(t) &= -\omega^2 x(t). \end{aligned} \tag{4.9}$$

This system (4.9) has one fixed point $(0,0)$. Alternatively, we can express this system as a second order differential equation with constant coefficients, that is,

$$\ddot{x}(t) = -\omega^2 x(t)$$

which reveals that the given system (4.9) represents simple harmonic motion.

The solution of (4.9) is given by

$$\begin{aligned} x(t) &= C\cos(\omega t - \alpha) \\ y(t) &= -\omega C \sin(\omega t - \alpha), \end{aligned} \tag{4.10}$$

which by simple algebraic manipulation can be put in the form

$$\frac{x^2}{C^2} + \frac{y^2}{\omega^2 C^2} = 1 \tag{4.11}$$

Equation (4.11) represents a family of ellipses with period $2\pi\omega^{-1}$. The fixed point $(0,0)$ is stable but not asymptotically stable.

We can modify the system (4.9) slightly as below:

EXAMPLE 4.7. Consider the system

$$\begin{aligned} \dot{x}(t) &= y(t) \\ \dot{y}(t) &= -2x(t) - 2y(t). \end{aligned} \tag{4.12}$$

Like (4.9), the system (4.12) has one fixed point $(0,0)$, and can be expressed as a second order differential equation of the form

$$\ddot{x}(t) + 2\dot{x} + 2x = 0.$$

The solution of the modified system is given by

$$\begin{aligned} x(t) &= Ce^{-t}\cos(t-\alpha) \\ y(t) &= -C\sqrt{2}e^{-t}\sin(t-\alpha+\frac{\pi}{4}). \end{aligned}$$

Note that the amplitude is now time dependent which decreases as $t \to \infty$, implying that the modified system represents damped harmonic motion. The fixed point $(0,0)$ is now asymptotically stable.

4.3. Examples on Linearization - Local Stability. In order to emphasize the idea of linearization and introduce the concept of bifurcation, we use the following example from predator-prey systems but which is simple enough to modify for the purpose of studying both linearization and bifurcation.

EXAMPLE 4.8. Consider the system

$$\begin{aligned} \dot{x}_1 &= k_1(1-x_2)x_1, \\ \dot{x}_2 &= -k_2(1-x_1)x_2,\ x_1,\ x_2 \geq 0,\ k_1,\ k_2 > 0. \end{aligned} \tag{4.13}$$

This system has two equilibrium points $(0,0)$ and $(1,1)$. We can linearize the system about $(0,0)$ by discarding the quadratic terms giving

$$\begin{aligned} \dot{x}_1 &= k_1x_1, \\ \dot{x}_2 &= -k_2x_2, \end{aligned} \tag{4.14}$$

or in matrix form

$$\begin{pmatrix} \dot{x}_1 \\ \dot{x}_2 \end{pmatrix} = \begin{pmatrix} k_1 & 0 \\ 0 & -k_2 \end{pmatrix} \begin{pmatrix} x_1 \\ x_2 \end{pmatrix}.$$

The eigenvalues of (4.15) are $\lambda_1 = k_1 > 0$ and $\lambda_2 = -k_2 < 0$. Because one eigenvalue is positive and the other negative, the fixed point $(0,0)$ is a saddle point.

Let us now consider the equilibrium point $(1,1)$. Because the fixed point $(1,1)$ is not the origin of the x_1x_2 coordinate system, we define new local variables so that the point $(1,1)$ is the origin of the new coordinate system. Let

$$y_1 = x_1 - 1 \text{ and } y_2 = x_2 - 1. \tag{4.15}$$

Then, substituting (4.15) in (4.13) gives

$$\begin{aligned} \dot{y}_1 &= k_1y_2(y_1+1), \\ \dot{y}_2 &= -k_2y_1(y_2+1). \end{aligned} \tag{4.16}$$

The associated linear system of equation (4.16), obtained by discarding the quadratic terms, is

$$\begin{pmatrix}\dot{y}_1\\ \dot{y}_2\end{pmatrix} = \begin{pmatrix}0 & k_1\\ -k_2 & 0\end{pmatrix}\begin{pmatrix}y_1\\ y_2\end{pmatrix}. \tag{4.17}$$

The eigenvalues of equation (4.17) are $\lambda_1 = i\sqrt{k_1k_2}$ and $\lambda_2 = -i\sqrt{k_1k_2}$. Because the eigenvalues are purely imaginary, the fixed point $(1,1)$ is a center. The equilibrium point $(1,1)$ is stable but it is not asymptotically stable.

EXAMPLE 4.9. Consider the system

$$\begin{aligned}\dot{x}_1 &= k_1(1-\epsilon x_1 - x_2)x_1,\ 0<\epsilon<<1\\ \dot{x}_2 &= -k_2(1-x_1)x_2.\end{aligned} \tag{4.18}$$

This system (4.18) is a slight modification of the system (4.13). The modification takes into account self regulation by the population x_1 through the term $-\epsilon k_1 x_1^2$. The system has three equilibrium points $(0,0)$, $(1,1-\epsilon)$ and $(\epsilon^{-1},0)$.

Consider $(0,0)$: Since $(0,0)$ is the origin of the x_1x_2 coordinate system, we can linearize the system (4.18) by discarding the quadratic terms giving

$$\begin{pmatrix}\dot{x}_1\\ \dot{x}_2\end{pmatrix} = \begin{pmatrix}k_1 & 0\\ 0 & -k_2\end{pmatrix}\begin{pmatrix}x_1\\ x_2\end{pmatrix}.$$

This is exactly the same as (4.15) in example (4.8). The extra term $-\epsilon k_1 x_1^2$ does not change the nature of the equilibrium point $(0,0)$. Thus, $(0,0)$ remains a saddle point.

Consider $(\epsilon^{-1},0)$: Let

$$y_1 = x_1 - \epsilon^{-1} \text{ and } y_2 = x_2. \tag{4.19}$$

Then, substituting (4.19) into (4.18) and discarding the quadratic terms gives

$$\begin{pmatrix}\dot{y}_1\\ \dot{y}_2\end{pmatrix} = \begin{pmatrix}-k_1 & -k_1\epsilon^{-1}\\ 0 & k_2(\epsilon^{-1}-1)\end{pmatrix}\begin{pmatrix}y_1\\ y_2\end{pmatrix}. \tag{4.20}$$

The characteristic equation of (4.20) is

$$\begin{vmatrix}-k_1-\lambda & -k_1\epsilon^{-1}\\ 0 & k_2(\epsilon^{-1}-1)-\lambda\end{vmatrix} = 0.$$

with solutions

$$\lambda_1 = -k_1 < 0 \text{ and } \lambda_2 = k_2(\epsilon^{-1}-1) > 0.$$

Therefore, the equilibrium point $(\epsilon^{-1},0)$ is another saddle point.

Consider $(1,1-\epsilon)$: Note that this equilibrium point was a center when $\epsilon = 0$. Let

$$y_1 = x_1 - 1 \text{ and } y_2 = x_2 - 1 + \epsilon. \tag{4.21}$$

Then, substituting (4.21) into (4.18) and linearizing gives

$$\begin{pmatrix}\dot{y}_1\\ \dot{y}_2\end{pmatrix} = \begin{pmatrix}-k_1\epsilon & -k_1\\ k_2(1-\epsilon) & 0\end{pmatrix}\begin{pmatrix}y_1\\ y_2\end{pmatrix}.$$

The eigenvalue equation is

$$\begin{vmatrix} -k_1\epsilon - \lambda & -k_1 \\ k_2(1-\epsilon) & -\lambda \end{vmatrix} = 0,$$

with solutions

$$\lambda_1, \lambda_2 = \frac{-k_1\epsilon \pm \sqrt{k_1^2\epsilon^2 - 4k_1k_2(1-\epsilon)}}{2}.$$

If $\epsilon << 1$ then

$$\lambda_1, \lambda_2 \approx \frac{-k_1\epsilon \pm 2i\sqrt{k_1k_2(1-\frac{\epsilon}{2})}}{2}.$$

We have two complex roots with negative real parts indicating a stable focus at $(1, 1-\epsilon)$.

So, the effect of a very small perturbation ϵx_1 is to change the center at $(1,1)$ to a stable focus (spiral point) at $(1, 1-\epsilon)$.

Note that if $-1 << \epsilon < 0$ then the eigenvalues would be

$$\lambda_1, \lambda_2 = \frac{1}{2}k_1|\epsilon| \pm i\sqrt{k_1k_2(1+\frac{1}{2}|\epsilon|)}$$

and since the real parts are now positive the focus at $(1, 1+\epsilon)$ is unstable. So we have

- $\epsilon > 0$ stable focus at $(1, 1-\epsilon)$
- $\epsilon = 0$ Center at $(1,1)$
- $\epsilon < 0$ Unstable focus at $(1, 1+|\epsilon|)$

The system has a bifurcation (splitting into two) point at $\epsilon = 0$.

5. Liapunov Functions - Global Stability

The method of Liapunov functions enables the analysis to be extended beyond only a small region near the equilibrium point. The basic idea of this technique for verifying stability is to seek an aggregated summarizing function that continually decreases towards a minimum as the system evolves.

Suppose that $\bar{X}$ is an equilibrium point of a given dynamic system. A Liapunov function for the system and the equilibrium $\bar{X}$ is a real valued function V, which is defined over a region Ω of the state space that contains $\bar{X}$ and satisfies the three requirements:

(1) V is continuous
(2) V has a unique minimum at $\bar{X}$ with respect to all other points in Ω.
(3) Along any trajectory of the system contained in Ω, the value of V never increases.

5.1. Liapunov Theorem for Continuous Case. Consider the system

$$\dot{X}(t) = f(X(t)) \tag{5.1}$$

together with a given equilibrium point $\bar{X}$. In the time continuous case the requirement that the value of a Liapunov function never increases along a trajectory is expressed in terms of the time derivative.

Suppose $X(t)$ is a trajectory. Then $V(X(t))$ represents the corresponding value of $V(X(t))$ along the trajectory. In order for V not to increase, we require that

$$\dot{V}(X(t)) \leq 0$$

for all t. This derivative can be expressed, using the chain rule for differentiation as

$$\dot{V}(X(t)) = \frac{\partial V}{\partial x_1}\dot{x}_1(t) + \frac{\partial V}{\partial x_2}\dot{x}_2(t) + \cdots + \frac{\partial V}{\partial x_n}\dot{x}_n(t). \tag{5.2}$$

Then using the original system, this becomes

$$\begin{aligned} \dot{V}(X(t)) &= \frac{\partial V}{\partial x_1}f_1(t) + \frac{\partial V}{\partial x_2}f_2(t) + \cdots + \frac{\partial V}{\partial x_n}f_n(t) \\ &= \nabla V(X(t))f(X(t)). \end{aligned} \tag{5.3}$$

Therefore, the requirement that V is non-increasing along any trajectory of the system translates into the requirement that

$$\dot{V}(X) = \nabla V(X))f(X) \leq 0 \tag{5.4}$$

for all X is Ω.

Definition 5.1. A function V defined on a region Ω of the state space and containing $\bar{X}$ is a Liapunov function if it satisfies the following three requirements

(1) V is continuous and has continuous first partial derivatives.
(2) V has a unique minimum at $\bar{X}$ with respect to all other points in Ω.
(3) The function $\dot{V}(X) = \nabla V(X)f(X)$ satisfies $\dot{V}(X) \leq 0$ for all $X(t)$ in Ω.

Theorem 5.2 (Liapunov Theorem). *If there exists a Liapunov function $V(X)$, then the equilibrium point $\bar{X}$ is stable. If, furthermore, the function $\dot{V}(X)$ is strictly negative for every point (except $\bar{X}$) then the stability is asymptotic.*

Example 5.3. Consider the system

$$\begin{aligned} \dot{x}_1(t) &= x_2(t) \\ \dot{x}_2(t) &= -x_1(t) - x_2(t). \end{aligned}$$

Show that the equilibrium point $(0,0)$ is stable.

To obtain a solution, we define

$$V(x_1, x_2) = x_1^2 + x_2^2.$$

This function is certainly continuous with continuous first partial derivatives. $V(x_1, x_2)$ is clearly minimum at $(0,0)$. The chosen $V(x_1, x_2)$ satisfies the first two requirements of a Liapunov function. We want to check the final requirement.

$$\begin{aligned} \dot{V} &= \frac{\partial V}{\partial x_1}\dot{x}_1 + \frac{\partial V}{\partial x_2}\dot{x}_2 \\ &= 2x_1x_2 + 2x_2(-x_1 - x_2) \\ &= 2x_1x_2 - 2x_1x_2 - 2x_2^2 \\ &= -2x_2^2 < 0 \end{aligned}$$

Therefore, the equilibrium point $(0,0)$ is asymptotically stable since $\dot{V}$ is strictly negative at every non-zero point.

EXERCISE 5.4. Examine the stability of the fixed point at the origin of

$$(i) \qquad \begin{aligned} \dot{x}_1 &= -x_1^3 + x_2^4 \\ \dot{x}_2 &= x_2(2x_1^2 - x_2^2 - x_1x_2^2) \end{aligned}$$

$$(ii) \qquad \begin{aligned} \dot{x}_1 &= x_2 \\ \dot{x}_2 &= -x_1 - x_2^3. \end{aligned}$$

EXERCISE 5.5. Prove that the function

$$V(x_1, x_2) = x_1^2 + x_1^2x_2^2 + x_2^4 \quad (x_1, x_2) \in \mathcal{R}^2$$

is a strong Liapunov function for the system

$$\begin{aligned} \dot{x}_1 &= 1 - 3x_1 + 3x_1^2 + 2x_2^2 - x_1^3 - 2x_1x_2^2 \\ \dot{x}_2 &= x_2 - 2x_1x_2 + x_1^2x_2 - x_2^3. \end{aligned}$$

6. Invariant Sets

The Liapunov function concept and stability theorems can be generalized in several directions to treat special circumstances. One generalization based on the idea of an invariant set is particularly useful in the following cases:

(1) Where a Liapunov function is found and $\dot{V}(X)$ is strictly less than zero for some values of X but not for all values of X. In this case the Liapunov theorem only assures stability. By employing the invariant set concept, however, one can often establish asymptotic stability with the same Liapunov function.
(2) For systems that do not have equilibrium points, but in which the state vector does tend to follow a fixed pattern as time increases.

DEFINITION 6.1. A set G is an invariant set for a dynamic system if whenever a point X on a system trajectory is in G, the trajectory remains in G.

An equilibrium point is the simplest example of an invariant set. Once the system reaches such a point, it never leaves. Also, if a system has several equilibrium points, the collection G of these points is an invariant set.

EXAMPLE 6.2. Show that the circle $x_1^2 + x_2^2 = 1$ is an invariant set of the following system:

$$\begin{aligned} \dot{x}_1 &= x_2 + x_1(1 - x_1^2 - x_2^2) \\ \dot{x}_2 &= -x_1 + x_2(1 - x_1^2 - x_2^2). \end{aligned}$$

The only equilibrium point of the system is $(0, 0)$. The linearized system is

$$\begin{pmatrix} \dot{x}_1 \\ \dot{x}_2 \end{pmatrix} = \begin{pmatrix} 1 & 1 \\ -1 & 1 \end{pmatrix} \begin{pmatrix} x_1 \\ x_2 \end{pmatrix}.$$

The eigenvalue equation is

$$\begin{vmatrix} 1 - \lambda & 1 \\ -1 & 1 - \lambda \end{vmatrix} = 0.$$

with solutions

$$\lambda_1, \lambda_2 = \frac{2 \pm \sqrt{4 - 8}}{2} = 1 \pm i$$

Therefore, the origin is an unstable spiral. The question is "where does the trajectory tend to $t \to \infty$?"

Note that

$$\begin{aligned}x_1\dot{x}_1 + x_2\dot{x}_2 &= x_1x_2 + x_1^2 - x_1^4 - x_1^2x_2^2 - x_1x_2 + x_2^2 - x_1^2x_2^2 - x_2^4 \\ &= x_1^2(1 - x_1^2 - x_2^2) + x_2^2(1 - x_1^2 - x_2^2) \\ &= (x_1^2 + x_2^2)(1 - x_1^2 - x_2^2)\end{aligned}$$

We can write this as

$$(x_1, x_2)\begin{pmatrix}\dot{x}_1 \\ \dot{x}_2\end{pmatrix} = (x_1^2 + x_2^2)(1 - x_1^2 - x_2^2)$$

or

$$< x_1, x_2 > \cdot < \dot{x}_1, \dot{x}_2 >= (x_1^2 + x_2^2)(1 - x_1^2 - x_2^2)$$

where $< x_1, x_2 >$ and $< \dot{x}_1, \dot{x}_2 >$ are respectively the state space vector and velocity vector.

Hence, the velocity vector and the state space vector are orthogonal on the unit circle $1 - x_1^2 - x_2^2 = 0$. The unit circle is an invariant set for the system. To obtain the useful generalized Liapunov results, the concept of invariant sets is combined with another key ideas from the Liapunov stability theorem.

THEOREM 6.3 (Invariant Set Theorem). *Let $V(X)$ be a scalar function with continuous first partial derivatives. Let Ω_s denote the region where $V(X) < s$. Assume that Ω_s is bounded and that $\dot{V}(X) \leq 0$ within Ω_s. Let S be the set of points within Ω_s where $\dot{V}(X) = 0$, and let G be the largest invariant set within S. Then every trajectory in Ω_s tends to G as time increases.*

EXAMPLE 6.4. For the system below, show that the circle $x_1^2 + x_2^2 = 1$ is the invariant set:

$$\begin{aligned}\dot{x}_1 &= x_2 + x_1(1 - x_1^2 - x_2^2), \\ \dot{x}_2 &= -x_1 + x_2(1 - x_1^2 - x_2^2).\end{aligned}$$

Define the function

$$V(x_1, x_2) = (1 - x_1^2 - x_2^2)^2.$$

Then

$$\begin{aligned}\dot{V}(x_1, x_2) &= \frac{\partial V}{\partial x_1}\dot{x}_1 + \frac{\partial V}{\partial x_2}\dot{x}_2 \\ &= 2(-2x_1)(1 - x_1^2 - x_2^2)\dot{x}_1 + 2(-2x_2)(1 - x_1^2 - x_2^2)\dot{x}_2 \\ &= -4(1 - x_1^2 - x_2^2)(x_1\dot{x}_1 + x_2\dot{x}_2) \\ &= -4(x_1^2 + x_2^2)(1 - x_1^2 - x_2^2)^2 \\ &\leq 0.\end{aligned}$$

This result is zero if and only if $x_1^2 + x_2^2 = 1$ on the unit circle. The set S consists of the origin and the unit circle. S is not an invariant set because it contains the origin. The invariant set G is the unit circle.

7. Epidemics Models

7.1. The SIR Model. Let us consider a large population of n individuals and a disease in which infection spreads by contact between individuals. We begin with a simple model whereby individuals who once infected either die or are isolated or recover with immunity. Thus, at any one time the population is comprised of x_1 susceptible individuals, x_2 infected and circulating individuals, and x_3 individuals who either have been removed (by death or isolation) or are immune. We have $x_1 + x_2 + x_3 = n$ for all time.

We assume that the population is subject to some form of homogeneous mixing, and that the rate of contact between susceptibles and infectives is proportional to the product $x_1 x_2$.

The rate of generation of new infectives is therefore $\beta x_1 x_2$, where β is an infection-rate constant. Infectives are assumed to be removed or become immune at the rate proportional to their number with an associated removal rate γ. The governing differential equations are therefore

$$\begin{aligned} \dot{x}_1 &= -\beta x_1 x_2, \\ \dot{x}_2 &= \beta x_1 x_2 - \gamma x_2, \\ \dot{x}_3 &= \gamma x_2. \end{aligned} \tag{7.1}$$

It is easy to verify that this is a constant population model [**1, 2**]. Since x_3 does not appear in the first two equations, we can work with the first two equations

$$\begin{aligned} \dot{x}_1 &= -\beta x_1 x_2, \\ \dot{x}_2 &= \beta x_2 (x_1 - \frac{\gamma}{\beta}) = \beta x_2 (x_1 - \rho), \end{aligned}$$

where $\rho = \dfrac{\gamma}{\beta}$. Obviously, the point $(x_1, x_2) = (c, 0)$ is a fixed point. In fact the x_1-axis is a line of fixed points. Let us examine the nature of one of the fixed points $(c, 0)$. Define

$$y_1 = x_1 - c, \; y_2 = x_2.$$

Then, the system (7.1) becomes

$$\begin{aligned} \dot{y}_1 &= -\beta (y_1 + c) y_2, \\ \dot{y}_2 &= \beta y_2 (y_1 + c - \rho). \end{aligned}$$

When $c = 0$, there is a non-simple fixed point at $(0, 0)$. Again when $c = \rho$, we have another non-simple fixed point at $(\rho, 0)$. Keeping away from these two special fixed points, the linearized equations at $(c, 0)$ are

$$\begin{pmatrix} \dot{y}_1 \\ \dot{y}_2 \end{pmatrix} = \begin{pmatrix} 0 & -\beta c \\ 0 & \beta (c - \rho) \end{pmatrix} \begin{pmatrix} y_1 \\ y_2 \end{pmatrix}.$$

The eigenvalues are $\lambda_1 = 0$, $\lambda_2 = \beta(c - \rho)$. The solution in the neighborhood of $y_1 = 0, y_2 = 0$ is

$$\begin{aligned} y_1 &= C_1 + C_2 e^{\lambda_2 t}, \\ y_2 &= -\frac{1}{\beta c} \dot{y}_1 = -\frac{\lambda_2}{\beta c} C_2 e^{\lambda_2 t}. \end{aligned}$$

Special orbits:

$C_2 = 0$, $y_1 = c\, y_2 = 0$. This is not an orbit. When $C_1 = 0$, we obtain

$$y_1 = -\left(\frac{c-\rho}{c}\right) y_1. \tag{7.2}$$

Equation (7.2) represents a family of straight lines. When $c < \rho$, the straight lines increase as y_1 increases while when $c > \rho$ the straight lines decrease as y_1 increases. The maximum value of x_2 occurs when $x_1 = \rho$. We can express the system (7.1) in the form

$$\frac{\dot{x}_2}{\dot{x}_1} = \frac{\beta x_1 - \gamma}{-\beta x_1}.$$

Upon rearranging, we obtain

$$dx_2 = (-1 + \frac{\rho}{x_1})dx_1, \ \rho = \frac{\gamma}{\beta}.$$

Integrating this gives the solution

$$x_2 = -x_1 + \rho \ln x_1 + Const.$$

At $t = 0$, $x_1(0) = n = x_0$, $x_2(0) = a$ giving

$$x_2 = -x_1 + \rho \ln\left(\frac{x_1}{x_0}\right) + n + a.$$

Several interesting qualitative conclusions can be made from this.

1. The threshold effect: The maximum value of x_2 occurs at the point $x_1 = \rho$. Suppose that a number of infectives $x_2(0)$ is introduced in a population x_0 of susceptibles. If $x_0 > \rho$, the level of infectives will increase until the number of susceptibles is reduced below ρ and will decrease thereafter. If $x_0 < \rho$, the level of infectives will decrease monotonically to zero (no epidemic). Thus, ρ represents a threshold value of susceptibles for the phenomena of an epidemic to occur.
2. The Escape Effect: Since $x_2(0) = -\infty$, it follows that x_2 must vanish at some positive value of x_1. This means that the trajectories terminate on the x_1-axis at a positive value. Therefore, the epidemic terminates for lack of infectives rather than lack of susceptibles, and some individuals escape the disease entirely.
3. Symmetry Effect: For the case $x_1(0) > \rho$ but $x_1(0) - \rho$ is small, the epidemic curves are nearly symmetric with respect to the point $x_1 = \rho$. This means that during the course of the epidemic the number of susceptibles is ultimately reduced to a level below the threshold value ρ as it was initially above this value.

THEOREM 7.1 (The Threshold Theorem). *Let $x_1(0) = \rho + \epsilon$, $\epsilon << \rho$ and suppose that $x_2(0)$ is very small, then ultimately $x_1(0) - x_1(\infty) = 2\epsilon$.*

Proof

$$\frac{dx_2}{dx_1} = \frac{\beta x_1 x_2 - \gamma x_2}{-\beta x_1 x_2} = -1 + \frac{\rho}{x_1}.$$

Integrating, we obtain

$$x_2 = Constant - x_1 + \rho \ln\left(\frac{x_1}{x_0}\right).$$

At $t = 0$, $x_2(0) = Constant - x_1(0)$, thus

$$Constant = x_2(0) + x_1(0).$$

$$x_2 = x_2(0) + x_1(0) - x_1 + \rho \ln\left(\frac{x_1}{x_1(0)}\right)$$

After a very long time

$$x_1(t) \to x_1(\infty), \; x_2(t) \to 0$$

Then

$$0 = x_2(0) + x_1(0) - x_1(\infty) + \rho \ln\left(\frac{x_1(\infty)}{x_1(0)}\right)$$

We can neglect $x_2(0)$ since it is small

$$\begin{aligned}
0 &= x_1(0) - x_1(\infty) + \rho \ln\left(1 - \frac{x_1(0) - x_1(\infty)}{x_1(0)}\right) \\
&= x_1(0) - x_1(\infty) + \rho\left[\frac{x_1(0) - x_1(\infty)}{x_1(0)} + \frac{1}{2}\left(\frac{x_1(0) - x_1(\infty)}{x_1(0)}\right)^2\right] \\
&= (x_1(0) - x_1(\infty))\left[1 - \frac{\rho}{x_1(0)} - \frac{\rho}{2x_1^2(0)}(x_1(0) - x_1(\infty))\right]
\end{aligned}$$

Thus

$$\begin{aligned}
x_1(0) - x_1(\infty) &= 2x_1(0)\left(\frac{x_1(0)}{\rho} - 1\right) \\
&= 2(\rho + \epsilon)\left(\frac{\rho + \epsilon}{\rho} - 1\right) \\
&= 2(\rho + \epsilon)\left(\frac{\epsilon}{\rho}\right) \\
&\approx 2\epsilon
\end{aligned}$$

7.2. Derivation of the basic reproduction number, $\Re_0$. When we are modeling any infectious disease, we want to know the conditions under which it will invade a population. Most epidemic models have a threshold as we demonstrated in the last section where $x_1 = \rho$ was the model threshold. The example in the last section was easy and its threshold was straight forward to determine. In more complex systems, the technique by Van Den Driessche and Watmough (2002) [**7**] may simplify the determination of the model threshold, hereafter called the model reproduction number. In this section we state the technique by Van Den Driessche and Watmough (2002) [**7**] and demonstrate its application with examples. The technique involves the following steps:

(1) Distinguish new infections from other changes in a population. Let $\mathcal{F}_i$ be the rate of appearance of new infections in compartment i, $\mathcal{V}_i^+$ be the rate of transfer of individuals into compartment i and $\mathcal{V}_i^-$ be the rate of

transfer of individuals out of compartment i, then the system (2.2) can be written as in [**7**].

$$\dot{\mathbf{X}} = \mathbf{f}(\mathbf{X}) = \mathcal{F} - \mathcal{V}, \tag{7.3}$$

where

$$\mathcal{V}_i = \mathcal{V}_i^- - \mathcal{V}_i^+, \ \mathcal{F} = (\mathcal{F}_1, ..., \mathcal{F}_n)' \text{ and } \mathcal{V} = (\mathcal{V}_1, ..., \mathcal{V}_n)'.$$

(2) If x_0 is the disease free equilibrium point of (7.3) and the derivatives $D\mathcal{F}(x_0)$ and $D\mathcal{V}(x_0)$ can be partitioned as

$$D\mathcal{F}(x_0) = \begin{pmatrix} F & \mathbf{0} \\ \mathbf{0} & \mathbf{0} \end{pmatrix}, \qquad D\mathcal{V}(x_0) = \begin{pmatrix} V & \mathbf{0} \\ P & Q \end{pmatrix}$$

where F and V are the $m \times m$ matrices defined by

$$F = \left[\frac{\partial \mathcal{F}_i}{\partial x_j}(x_0)\right], \quad \textit{and} \quad V = \left[\frac{\partial \mathcal{V}_i}{\partial x_j}(x_0)\right] \quad \textit{with } 1 \le i, j \le m$$

where m is the number of infectious classes, F is nonnegative, V is a nonsingular M-matrix and all eigenvalues of Q have positive real parts.

(3) Thus, FV^{-1} is the next generation matrix of the model, we can define, the basic reproduction number $\mathfrak{R}_0$ as

$$\mathfrak{R}_0 = \rho(FV^{-1}) \tag{7.4}$$

where $\rho(FV^{-1})$ is the spectral radius of the matrix FV^{-1}.

7.3. Application of van den Driessche-Watmough technique.

EXAMPLE 7.2. Determine the basic reproduction number for the HIV model with treatment of infected individuals:

$$\begin{aligned}
\dot{S} &= \Lambda + b(1-\epsilon)(U+I) - BS - \mu S, \\
\dot{U} &= BS - (\sigma + \mu + \nu_1)U, \\
\dot{I} &= \sigma U + bp\epsilon(U+I) - (\mu + \nu_2)I, \\
\dot{A} &= bq\epsilon(U+I) + \nu_1 U + \nu_2 I - (\mu + \delta)A.
\end{aligned} \tag{7.5}$$

where $N = S + U + I$, $p + q = 1$ and $B = \dfrac{c_0\beta_0 U + c_1\beta_1 I}{N}$. $S-$susceptibles, $U-$ untreated infectives, $I-$treated infectives and $A-$Full blown AIDS cases. The model accounts for the effects of vertical transmission through recruitment of treated infected juveniles of which a proportion p survive to adulthood [**3**].

The disease free equilibrium point is

$$E_0 = \left(\frac{\Lambda}{\mu}, 0, 0\right).$$

Define the disease free states as

$$\mathbf{X_s} = \{U, I \ge 0 \mid U = I = 0\}.$$

We decompose system (7.5) as

$$\dot{X} = \mathcal{F} - \mathcal{V}$$

where $\mathcal{F}$ and $\mathcal{V}$ are define as,

$$\mathcal{F} = \begin{pmatrix} BS \\ 0 \\ 0 \end{pmatrix} \quad \textit{and} \quad \mathcal{V} = \begin{pmatrix} \psi U \\ (\mu + \nu_2)I - \sigma U - bp\epsilon(U+I) \\ (\mu + B)S - \Lambda - b(1-\epsilon)(U+I) \end{pmatrix}, \tag{7.6}$$

where $\psi = \sigma + \mu + \nu_1$. Evaluating $D\mathcal{F}(E_0)$ and $D\mathcal{V}(E_0)$ yields

$$D\mathcal{F}(E_0) = \begin{pmatrix} F & \mathbf{0} \\ \mathbf{0} & \mathbf{0} \end{pmatrix},$$

and

$$D\mathcal{V}(E_0) = \begin{pmatrix} V & \mathbf{0} \\ P & Q \end{pmatrix},$$

where

$$F = \begin{pmatrix} c_0\beta_0 & c_1\beta_1 \\ 0 & 0 \end{pmatrix},$$

$$\begin{aligned} V &= \begin{pmatrix} \psi & 0 \\ -\sigma - bp\epsilon & \mu + \nu_2 - bp\epsilon \end{pmatrix}, \\ &= \begin{pmatrix} \psi & 0 \\ -\sigma - bp\epsilon & (\mu + \nu_2)(1 - R_v) \end{pmatrix}, \quad R_v = \frac{bp\epsilon}{\mu + \nu_2}. \end{aligned}$$

$$P = \begin{pmatrix} c_0\beta_0 - b(1-\epsilon) & c_1\beta_1 - b(1-\epsilon) \end{pmatrix}.$$

$$Q = \mu,$$

The inverse of matrices V and Q are

$$V^{-1} = \begin{pmatrix} \frac{1}{\psi} & 0 \\ \frac{k}{\psi} & \frac{1}{(\mu+\nu_2)(1-R_v)} \end{pmatrix}, \quad k = \frac{\sigma + bp\epsilon}{\mu + \nu_2 - bp\epsilon}.$$

and

$$Q^{-1} = \frac{1}{\mu}.$$

This gives the next generation matrix for the model

$$FV^{-1} = \begin{pmatrix} \frac{c_0\beta_0}{\psi} + \frac{kc_1\beta_1}{\psi} & \frac{c_1\beta_1}{(\mu+\nu_2)(1-R_v)} \\ 0 & 0 \end{pmatrix}$$

with eigenvalues

$$\lambda_1 = 0 \text{ and } \lambda_2 = \frac{c_0\beta_0}{\psi} + \frac{kc_1\beta_1}{\psi}.$$

The dominant eigenvalue (spectral radius) of the next generation operator FV^{-1}, yields the effective reproduction number for the model

$$\mathfrak{R}_0 = \frac{c_0\beta_0}{\psi} + \frac{kc_1\beta_1}{\psi} \tag{7.7}$$

which denotes the "the number of new infections produced by a typical infective individual introduced into a wholly susceptible population in the presence of treatment for infected individuals who may have acquired the disease via horizontal and vertical transmission".

This technique can be used to derive the basic reproduction number for different types of models e.g. multi-group models, staged progression models, multi-strain models and vector-host models. For more examples of this technique study the paper by van den Driessche and Watmough (2002) [**7**].

EXAMPLE 7.3. We consider a population divided into susceptibles (X_1), normal infectives (X_2), normal carriers (X_3), Screened carriers (counselled) (X_4) and AIDS cases (X_5). We assume carriers who have been screened and counselled do not participate in the spread of the disease. The model can be described by a system of ordinary differential equations [**6**].

$$\begin{aligned}\dot{X}_1 &= bN - BX_1 - \mu X_1,\\ \dot{X}_2 &= BX_1 - (\rho_1+\rho_2+\mu)X_2,\\ \dot{X}_3 &= \rho_1 X_2 - (\sigma_1+\mu+\epsilon)X_3,\\ \dot{X}_4 &= \epsilon X_3 - (\sigma_2+\mu)X_4\\ \dot{X}_5 &= \rho_2 X_2 + \sigma_1 X_3 + \sigma_2 X_4 - \mu X_5\end{aligned} \tag{7.8}$$

where $B = \dfrac{\beta X_2 + \gamma X_3}{N}$ and $N = X_1 + X_2 + X_3 + X_4 + X_5$. Adding equations of system (7.8) we obtain

$$\dot{N} = (b-\mu)N.$$

Take $b = \mu$ so that N is constant and define local variables as follows:

$$x_i = \frac{X_i}{N}, \text{ for } i = 1,2,3,4,$$

then, we can rewrite system (7.8) as follows:

$$\begin{aligned}\dot{x}_1 &= b - bx_1 - \bar{B}x_1,\\ \dot{x}_2 &= \bar{B}x_1 - (b+\rho_1+\rho_2)x_2,\\ \dot{x}_3 &= \rho_1 x_2 - (b+\sigma_1+\epsilon)x_3,\\ x_4 &= \epsilon x_3 - (b+\sigma_2)x_4,\\ \dot{x}_5 &= \rho_2 x_2 + \sigma_1 x_3 + \sigma_2 x_4 - bx_5\end{aligned} \tag{7.9}$$

where $\bar{B} = \beta x_2 + \gamma x_3$ and $x_1 + x_2 + x_3 + x_4 + x_5 = 1$. the system (7.9) has two equilibrium points. The disease free equilibrium point (DFE) given by

$$(x_1^*, x_2^*, x_3^*, x_4^*, x_5^*) = (1,0,0,0,0)$$

and the endemic equilibrium point (EEP) given by

$$(x_1^*, x_2^*, x_3^*, x_4^*, x_5^*) = \left(\frac{1}{R}, \frac{b(b+\sigma_1+\epsilon)(R-1)}{D}, \frac{b\rho_1(R-1)}{D}, \frac{b\rho_1\epsilon)(R-1)}{D}\right).$$

where $D = \beta(b+\sigma_1+\epsilon)+\rho_1\gamma$ and $R = \dfrac{\beta(b+\sigma_1+\epsilon)+\rho_1\gamma}{(b+\sigma_1+\epsilon)(b+\rho_1+\rho_2)}$.

Note that the reproduction number R can be expressed in the following way

$$\begin{aligned}R &= \frac{\beta(b+\sigma_1+\epsilon)+\rho_1\gamma}{(b+\sigma_1+\epsilon)(b+\rho_1+\rho_2)}\\ &= \left(\frac{b+\rho_2}{b+\rho_1+\rho_2}\right)\left(\frac{\beta}{b+\rho_2}\right) + \left(\frac{\rho_1}{b+\rho_1+\rho_2}\right)\left(\frac{\gamma}{b+\sigma_1+\epsilon}\right)\\ &= \frac{b+\rho_2}{b+\rho_1+\rho_2}R_0 + \frac{\rho_1}{b+\rho_1+\rho_2}R_c.\end{aligned} \tag{7.10}$$

where

$$R_0 = \frac{\beta}{b+\rho_2} \text{ and } R_c = \frac{\gamma}{b+\sigma_1+\epsilon}.$$

where R_0 denotes the number of secondary infectives due to normal carriers and R_c denotes the number of secondary infectives due to screened carriers. As $\epsilon \to 0$,

$$\begin{aligned} R &= \frac{b+\rho_2}{b+\rho_1+\rho_2} R_0 + \frac{\rho_1}{b+\rho_1+\rho_2} R_c \\ &< \frac{b+\rho_2}{b+\rho_1+\rho_2} R_0 + \frac{\rho_1}{b+\rho_1+\rho_2} R_c^* \end{aligned}$$

where $R_c^* = \dfrac{\gamma}{b+\sigma_1}$ is defined as for the case in the absence of screening. As $\epsilon \to \infty$, $R_c \to 0$ and

$$R \to \frac{b+\rho_2}{b+\rho_1+\rho_2} R_0 < R_0.$$

So that if all carriers are identified and counselled so that they do not influence the dynamics of the disease then the disease can be controlled provided $R_0 < 1$. If $R_0 >> 1$, such that $\dfrac{b+\rho_2}{b+\rho_1+\rho_2} R_0 > 1$, then treatment of normal infectives is imperative to ensure that the disease does not invade the population.

As $\rho_1 \to 0$, $R = R_0$. In this case the carriers do not influence the spread of the disease.

As $\rho_1 \to \infty$, $R = R_c$. In this case as $\epsilon \to \infty$ $R_0 = R_c = 0$. Hence, screening and counselling would ensure that the disease does not invade the population.

7.4. Stability of equilibria. Define local variables

$$y_1 = x_1 - 1,\ y_2 = x_2,\ y_3 = x_3 \text{ and } y_4 = x_4,$$

then, the system (7.9) becomes

$$\begin{aligned} \dot{y}_1 &= -by_1 - \beta y_1 y_2 - \gamma y_1 y_3, \\ \dot{y}_2 &= \beta y_1 y_2 + \gamma y_1 y_3 - (b+\rho_1+\rho_2) y_2, \\ \dot{y}_3 &= \rho_1 y_2 - (b+\sigma_1+\epsilon) y_3, \\ \dot{y}_4 &= \epsilon y_3 - (b+\sigma_2) y_4. \end{aligned} \tag{7.11}$$

The linearized system (7.11) is given by

$$\begin{pmatrix} \dot{y}_1 \\ \dot{y}_2 \\ \dot{y}_3 \\ \dot{y}_4 \end{pmatrix} = \begin{pmatrix} -b & -\beta & -\gamma & 0 \\ 0 & \beta-(b+\rho_1+\rho_2) & \gamma & 0 \\ 0 & \rho_1 & -(b+\sigma_1+\epsilon) & 0 \\ 0 & 0 & \epsilon & -(b+\sigma_2) \end{pmatrix} \begin{pmatrix} y_1 \\ y_2 \\ y_3 \\ y_4 \end{pmatrix}$$

The eigenvalues are

$$\lambda_1 = -b,\ \lambda_2 = -(b+\sigma_1) \text{ and}$$

$$\lambda_{3,4} = \frac{-(\psi_1+\psi_2-\beta) \pm \sqrt{(\psi_1+\psi_2-\beta)^2 - 4\psi_1\psi_2(1-R)}}{2}$$

where $\psi_1 = b+\rho_1+\rho_2$ and $\psi_2 = b+\sigma_1+\epsilon$.

THEOREM 7.4. *The disease free equilibrium is stable if* $R < 1$ *and unstable if* $R > 1$.

THEOREM 7.5. *The disease free equilibrium is globally stable if* $R_0 < 1$ *and* $R_c < 1$.

Proof: Define a Lyapunov function as $V = X_2 + X_3$.
Then

$$\begin{aligned}
\dot{V} &= \dot{X}_1 + \dot{X}_2 \\
&= BX_1 - (\rho_1 + \rho_2 + \mu)X_2 + \rho_1 X_2 - (\sigma_1 + \mu + \epsilon)X_3 \\
&= BX_1 - (\rho_2 + \mu)X_2 - (\sigma_1 + \mu + \epsilon)X_3 \\
&\leq \beta X_2 + \gamma X_3 - (\rho_2 + \mu)X_2 - (\sigma_1 + \mu + \epsilon)X_3 \\
&= (\mu + \rho_2)\left(\frac{\beta}{\mu + \rho_2} - 1\right) X_2 + (\mu + \sigma_1 + \epsilon)\left(\frac{\gamma}{\mu + \sigma_1 + \epsilon} - 1\right) X_3 \\
&= -\left[(\mu + \rho_2)\left(1 - \frac{\beta}{\mu + \rho_2}\right) X_2 + (\mu + \sigma_1 + \epsilon)\left(1 - \frac{\gamma}{\mu + \sigma_1 + \epsilon}\right) X_3\right] \\
&= -\left[(\mu + \rho_2)\left(1 - R_0\right) X_2 + (\mu + \sigma_1 + \epsilon)\left(1 - R_c\right) X_3\right] \\
&\leq 0 \qquad \text{if } R_0 < 1 \text{ and } R_c < 1.
\end{aligned}$$

Thus, establishing theorem 7.5.

References

[1] R.M. Anderson and R.M. May, *Infectious disease of humans: Dynamics and control*, Oxford Univeristy Press, Oxford, UK, 1991.

[2] E. M. Lungu, *Lecture Notes on Mathematical Epidemiology. Course in Mathematical Modelling (MAT 462)*, University of Botswana. 1–113, (2000).

[3] M. Kgosimore and E. M. Lungu, *The effects of vertical transmission on the spread of HIV/AIDS in the presence of treatment*, Mathematical Biosciences and Engineering, **3** (2), (2006). 297–312, .

[4] H. K. Khalil, *Nonlinear systems*, Prentice-Hall, Inc, London, UK. 1996

[5] R. M. M. Mattheij and J. Lolenaar, *Ordinary differential equations in theory and practice*, John Wiley and Sons. New York, USA. 1996.

[6] S. D. Musekwa, *Development of deterministic and stochastic epidemic models with special reference to HIV/AIDS*, PhD Thesis, University of Zimbabwe, Harare. 2005.

[7] P. van den Driessche and J. Watmough, *Reproduction numbers and sub-threshold endemic equilibria for compartmental models of disease transmission*, Mathematical Biosciences, **180** (2002), 29–48.

[8] WHO, *Pandemic (H1N1) 2009 briefing note 4: Preliminary information for understanding the evolving situation*, http://www.who.int/csr/disease/swineflu/notes/h1n1_situation_20090724/en/print.html. accessed 30 July 2009.

[9] WHO/UNAIDS, *AIDS Epidemic Update 2007*, Geneva, 2007.

Department of Mathematics, University of Botswana, P/Bag 0022, Gaborone. Botswana
Current address: Department of Mathematics, University of Botswana, P/Bag 0022, Gaborone. Botswana
E-mail address: lunguem@mopipi.ub.bw

Basic Sciences Department, Botswana College of Agriculture, P/Bag 0027, Gaborone. Botswana
E-mail address: mkgosi@bca.bw

South African Centre of Epidemiological and Analysis, University of Stellenbosch, 19 Jonkershoek Road, Stellnbosch, 7600, South Africa
E-mail address: nyabadzaf@sun.ac.za

DIMACS Series in Discrete Mathematics
and Theoretical Computer Science
Volume **75**, 2010

An Introduction to Optimal Control with an Application in Disease Modeling

Rachael Miller Neilan and Suzanne Lenhart

ABSTRACT. This paper serves as an introduction to the theory of optimal control applied to systems of ordinary differential equations with emphasis on disease models. We outline the steps in formulating an optimal control problem and derive necessary conditions. Several simple examples provide detailed methodology in characterizing the optimal control through use of Pontryagin's Maximum Principle. An SEIR (Susceptible, Exposed, Infected, Recovered) model with control acting as a rate of vaccination is presented and an optimal control problem is formulated to include an isoperimetric constraint on the vaccine supply. Numerical results illustrate how such a constraint alters the optimal vaccination schedule and its effect on the population.

1. Introduction

In an optimal control problem, one adjusts controls in a dynamic system to achieve a goal. The underlying system can have a variety of types of equations such as ordinary differential equations, partial differential equations, discrete equations, stochastic differential equations or integrodifference equations. In this introductory paper, we are considering only systems of ordinary differential equations.

In control of a single ordinary differential equation (ODE), we denote $u(t)$ as the control and $x(t)$ as the state. The state function, $x(t)$, satisfies the ODE modeling the scenario. The control affects the state ODE by

$$x'(t) = g(t, x(t), u(t)),$$

where x' denote the derivative with respect to time t. Both $u(t)$ and $x(t)$ affect the goal, which is called the objective functional. We seek to find an optimal control and corresponding state that achieve the maximum (or minimum) of our objective functional.

For introduction the basic idea of optimal control and the terminology, consider the following example with very simple dynamics. Let $x(t)$ be the number of cancer

---

1991 *Mathematics Subject Classification.* Primary 92D30, 49N05, ; Secondary 34A34.

Key words and phrases. Optimal control, isoperimetric constraint, disease model.

The authors were supported in part by National Science Foundation Grants EF-0832858 (National Institute for Mathematical and Biological Synthesis) and ITR-04274710.

cells in the body at time t and $u(t)$ be the drug concentration in the body at time t. Assume

$$\frac{dx}{dt} = \alpha x(t) - u(t),$$

$$x(0) = x_0$$

where x_0 is known initial data and α is the natural growth rate of the cancer cells. The objective functional is

$$\min_u \left\{ x(T) + \int_0^T u^2(t)\, dt \right\}$$

where the first term represents number of cancer cells at the final time and the second term represents harmful effects of drug on the body. We restrict the values of our control so that $0 \leq u(t) \leq 1$.

The basics of setting up and solving an optimal control problem include

- modeling the situation with a system of ODEs
- choosing format and bounds of controls
- designing an appropriate objective functional
- proving existence of the optimal control
- deriving necessary conditions for the optimal control
- characterizing the optimal control and
- computing the optimal control numerically.

One may also want to prove uniqueness of the optimal control. A crucial step is to investigate how the optimal control depends on various parameters in the model. One should first understand how the parameters affect the model without control and then consider the control case. See [**2, 17**] for techniques for parameter sensitivity and analysis and [**18**] for such techniques used in combination with an optimal control problem for cholera. See also [**19**] for an illustration showing the dependence of the optimal control on parameters in a leukemia model.

To design an appropriate objective functional, one must balance opposing factors in the functional and decide whether or not to include terms at the final time. Opposing factors in the goal may include maximizing benefit while minimizing the cost of implementing the control. Choosing the format of an objective functional is crucial because your optimal control results strongly depend on that format. If the objective functional has more than two factors to consider, then one may want to give weights (balancing coefficients) to those factors depending on their relative importance. See [**3, 14, 19**] to illustrate this point about balancing coefficients.

In this introductory paper, we emphasize how to characterize the optimal control when an optimal control is known to exist. See the book by Fleming and Rishel [**5**] for assumptions to guarantee the existence of an optimal control. For an introduction to optimal control theory, see [**12, 16**].

In the next section, we derive necessary conditions that the optimal control and the corresponding state must satisfy. In the following section we give three simple examples and in the last section we present an epidemiological example in more detail.

2. Necessary conditions

Consider the optimal control problem where the objective functional is

$$\max_u \int_0^T f(t, x(t), u(t))\, dt \tag{2.1}$$

subject to

$$x'(t) = g(t, x(t), u(t)) \tag{2.2}$$

$$\text{where } x(0) = x_0 \text{ and } x(T) \text{ is free.} \tag{2.3}$$

We assume that the controls are piecewise continuous functions with values in a set U_1. However, one can also use Lebesgue measurable functions.

The optimal control, denoted by $u^*(t)$, achieves the maximum. One can substitute $u^*(t)$ into the state ODE (2.2) and obtain the corresponding optimal state $x^*(t)$. We say $u^*(t)$, $x^*(t)$ is an optimal pair. Presented next is a brief derivation of the necessary conditions. That is, if $u^*(t)$, $x^*(t)$ is an optimal pair, then these conditions will hold. These necessary conditions for optimal control theory for ODEs was developed by Pontryagin and his collaborators around 1950. They developed the key idea of introducing the adjoint function to attach the differential equation to the objective functional. This idea is similar to Lagrange multipliers that attach the constraints when finding the maximum of a function in multi-dimensional calculus subject to some equation constraints.

Suppose u^*, x^* is an optimal pair for the problem defined by (2.1)-(2.3). Let $h(t)$ be a variation function, $a \in \mathbb{R}$, and $u^*(t) + ah(t)$ be another control. Then $y(t, a)$ is the state corresponding to $u^* + ah$ and

$$\frac{dy(t,a)}{dt} = g\left(t, y(t,a), u^*(t) + ah(t)\right).$$

At $t = 0$, $y(0, a) = x_0$ since all trajectories start at the same position. Furthermore, $y(t, 0) = x^*(t)$ when $a = 0$ and the control is u^*.

We can write our objective functional as a function of a as we consider variations on the control u^*. Consider the function

$$J(a) = \int_0^T f\left(t, y(t,a), u^*(t) + ah(t)\right) dt.$$

The maximum of J with respect to a occurs at $a = 0$, which gives

$$\left.\frac{dJ}{da}\right|_{a=0} = 0.$$

Furthermore, a differentiable function, $\lambda(t)$, called the adjoint is introduced such that

$$\int_0^T \frac{d}{dt}\left(\lambda(t) y(t,a)\right) dt = \lambda(T) y(T,a) - \lambda(0) y(0,a)$$

$$\Rightarrow \int_0^T \frac{d}{dt}\left(\lambda(t) y(t,a)\right) dt + \lambda(0) y(0,a) - \lambda(T) y(T,a) = 0.$$

Adding the value zero written in the form above to our $J(a)$ gives

$$
\begin{aligned}
J(a) &= \int_0^T \left[f(t, y(t,a), u^*(t) + ah(t)) + \frac{d}{dt}\left(\lambda(t) y(t,a)\right) \right] dt \\
&\quad + \lambda(0) y(0,a) - \lambda(T) y(T,a) \\
&= \int_0^T \left[f(t, y(t,a), u^*(t) + ah(t)) + \lambda'(t) y(t,a) \right. \\
&\qquad \left. + \lambda(t) g(t, y, u^*(t) + ah(t)) \right] dt + \lambda(0) x_0 - \lambda(T) y(T,a).
\end{aligned}
$$

Here we used product rule and the fact that $g = dy/dt$. Differentiating J with respect to a yields

$$
\begin{aligned}
\frac{dJ}{da} &= \int_0^T \left[f_x \frac{\partial y}{\partial a} + f_u \frac{\partial (u^* + ah)}{\partial a} + \lambda'(t) \frac{\partial y}{\partial a} \right. \\
&\qquad \left. + \lambda(t) \left(g_x \frac{\partial y}{\partial a} + g_u \frac{\partial (u^* + ah)}{\partial a} \right) \right] dt - \lambda(T) \frac{\partial}{\partial a} y(T,a)
\end{aligned}
$$

where the arguments of f, g terms are $(t, y(t,a), u^*(t) + ah(t))$. Evaluating this differential at $a = 0$ gives

$$
\begin{aligned}
0 &= \left. \frac{dJ}{da} \right|_{a=0} \\
&= \int_0^T \left[(f_x + \lambda g_x + \lambda') \left. \frac{\partial y}{\partial a} \right|_{a=0} + (f_u + \lambda g_u) h \right] dt - \lambda(T) \frac{\partial y}{\partial a}(T, 0)
\end{aligned}
$$

where the arguments of f, g terms are $(t, x^*(t), u^*(t))$.

In order for the above to hold true, we choose $\lambda(t)$ such that

$$
\begin{aligned}
&\lambda'(t) = -\left[f_x(t, x^*, u^*) + \lambda(t) g_x(t, x^*, u^*) \right], \\
&\lambda(T) = 0, \ \text{and} \\
&0 = \int_0^T (f_u + \lambda g_u)\, h(t)\, dt \quad \text{for } h(t) \text{ arbitrary.}
\end{aligned}
$$

The last line implies

$$
f_u(t, x^*, u^*) + \lambda(t) g_u(t, x^*, u^*) = 0 \quad \text{for all } 0 \le t \le T.
$$

One can state the first order necessary conditions in the simplest form by Pontryagin's Maximum Principle [**20**]. In practice before applying this principle, one should show that an optimal control exists using a compactness argument. Such an argument depends on the specificset of controls used, frequently piecewise-continuous or bounded Lebesgue measurable functions. After showing the objective functional is bounded for all controls, then one can construct a maximizing (or minimizing) sequence of controls and corresponding state sequences and show convergence in the appropriate space. See [**5, 4**] for details of existence results.

THEOREM 2.1. **Pontryagin's Maximum Principle** *If $u^*(t)$ and $x^*(t)$ are optimal for problem (2.1)-(2.3), then there exists adjoint variable $\lambda(t)$ such that*

$$
H(t, x^*(t), u, \lambda(t)) \le H(t, x^*(t), u^*(t), \lambda(t)),
$$

at each time, for all u with values in U_1 where the Hamiltonian H is defined by

$$
H(t, x(t), u(t), \lambda(t)) = f(t, x(t), u(t)) + \lambda(t) g(t, x(t), u(t))
$$

and

$$\lambda'(t) = -\frac{\partial H(t, x(t), u(t), \lambda(t))}{\partial x}$$
$$\lambda(T) = 0.$$

The final time condition on the adjoint variable is called the transversality condition. This principle converted the problem of finding a control which maximizes the objective functional subject to the state ODE and initial condition to the problem of optimizing the Hamiltonian pointwise. As stated above, the Hamiltonian is defined by

$$\begin{aligned} H(t, x, u, \lambda) &= f(t, x, u) + \lambda g(t, x, u) \\ &= \text{(integrand of the objective functional)} + \text{(adjoint)} \times \text{(RHS of ODE)}. \end{aligned}$$

One can generate the necessary conditions by maximizing H with respect to u at u^*. They are

$$\frac{\partial H}{\partial u} = 0 \Rightarrow f_u + \lambda g_u = 0 \text{ (optimality equation),}$$
$$\lambda' = -\frac{\partial H}{\partial x} \Rightarrow \lambda' = -\left(f_x + \lambda g_x\right) \text{ (adjoint equation), and}$$
$$\lambda(T) = 0 \text{ (transversality condition).}$$

We note that this theorem is stated in a simple case where there are no constraints (like upper and lower bounds) on the controls.

We can also consider second order conditions. For maximization, we have

$$\frac{\partial^2 H}{\partial u^2} \leq 0 \quad \text{at } u^*$$

and for minimization,

$$\frac{\partial^2 H}{\partial u^2} \geq 0 \quad \text{at } u^*$$

We started with two unknowns, u^* and x^*, and we introduced an adjoint λ (similar to a Lagrange multiplier). Now we have three unknowns, u^*, x^* and λ. Frequently, when the control enters into the problem in a nonlinear way, we can set $H_u|_{u=u^*} = 0$ and solve for u^* in terms of x^* and λ. Then we have two unknowns x^* and λ with two ODEs and two boundary conditions (an initial condition for the state and a final time condition for the adjoint).

In many biological or physical problems, the controls will have bounds imposed due to the specific application. Pontryagin's Maximum Principle still holds when the controls are constrained within the bounds

$$a \leq u(t) \leq b.$$

In this case of bounded controls, solving for the optimal control can be more difficult when H is linear with respect to u. For example, $\frac{\partial H}{\partial u}$ would not contain u. Thus the maximum of H might occur always at the extremes of the control set, i.e.

$$u(t) = a \text{ or } b$$

at all times. This case with optimal controls taking values only at the upper or lower bounds is called a bang-bang scenario. Another possibility is that

$$\frac{\partial H}{\partial u} = 0$$

might occur over some interval of time within our whole time interval. In this situation, called the singular case, one can not easily solve for an optimal control from the optimality condition, thus requiring other techniques. We will not treat the case when the control problem is linear in u in this introductory article. We refer the reader to [**16, 21**] for this case.

3. Examples

We present three simple examples to illustrate the techniques of optimal control. It is important to note that an optimal control depends on initial conditions, parameters values and length of time. We do not investigate the results of changes in these in this paper, but one should consider dependence of results on "data" and parameters in a detailed research example.

3.1. Example 1.

Consider the simple problem

$$\min_u \int_0^1 u(t)^2 \, dt$$

subject to

$$\begin{aligned} x'(t) &= x(t) + u(t), \\ x(0) &= 1. \end{aligned}$$

What optimal control is expected? The goal is artificial because it does not depend on the state x, but it only emphasizes having a low value of u^2. One would expect the optimal control to be identically zero and now we show this with our new tool. The Hamiltonian is

$$\begin{aligned} H &= (\text{integrand}) + (\text{adjoint}) \times (\text{RHS of ODE}) \\ &= u^2 + \lambda(x + u). \end{aligned}$$

The first and second order necessary conditions with respect to the control are

$$\begin{aligned} \left.\frac{\partial H}{\partial u}\right|_{u=u^*} &= 2u^* + \lambda = 0 \\ &\Rightarrow u^* = -\frac{\lambda}{2}, \\ \frac{\partial^2 H}{\partial u^2} &= 2 > 0. \end{aligned}$$

The adjoint equation and transversality condition are

$$\lambda' = -\frac{\partial H}{\partial x} = -\lambda, \qquad \lambda(1) = 0.$$

Solving the adjoint differential equation yields

$$\lambda = \lambda_0 e^{-t}$$

where λ_0 is a constant. The final time condition $\lambda(1) = 0$ implies $\lambda_0 = 0$ and then $\lambda \equiv 0$. Therefore, $u^* \equiv 0$ and $x^* = e^t$ for all $t \in [0, 1]$.

3.2. Example 2. Consider the problem

$$\min_u \int_0^2 x(t) + \frac{1}{2}u(t)^2\, dt$$

subject to

$$x'(t) = x(t) + u(t),$$
$$x(0) = \frac{1}{2}e^2 - 1.$$

What optimal control is expected? Here we seek to pull x down while keeping u^2 small. We expect a negative optimal control. The Hamiltonian is

$$H = x + \frac{1}{2}u^2 + \lambda(x + u).$$

The adjoint equation and transversality condition are

$$\lambda'(t) = -\frac{\partial H}{\partial x} = -1 - \lambda, \qquad \lambda(2) = 0$$

implying

$$\lambda(t) = e^{2-t} - 1.$$

The optimality condition leads to

$$0 = \left.\frac{\partial H}{\partial u}\right|_{u=u^*} = u^* + \lambda$$
$$\Rightarrow \quad u^*(t) = -\lambda = 1 - e^{2-t}.$$

The second order condition is

$$\frac{\partial^2 H}{\partial u^2} = 2 > 0.$$

The associated state is

$$x^*(t) = \frac{1}{2}e^{2-t} - 1.$$

3.3. Example 3. In the next section, we give an epidemic model in some detail. Since we will have more than one ODE, we will have several states, one corresponding to each ODE. Each state then has its corresponding adjoint. It is also possible to have multiple controls affecting the dynamics. Suppose we have an n-dimensional vector of states and an m-dimensional vector of controls. Consider the problem for a system of ODEs where

$$\max_{\vec{u}} \int_{t_0}^{t_1} f(t, \vec{x}(t), \vec{u}(t))\, dt + \phi(\vec{x}(t_1))$$
$$\text{subject to} \quad \vec{x}\,'(t) = \vec{g}(t, \vec{x}(t), \vec{u}(t)),$$
$$\vec{x}(t_0) = \vec{x}_0,\ \vec{x}(t_1) \text{ is free.}$$

The Hamiltonian becomes

$$H(t, \vec{x}, \vec{u}, \vec{\lambda}) = f(t, \vec{x}, \vec{u}) + \vec{\lambda}(t) \cdot \vec{g}(t, \vec{x}, \vec{u}).$$

Note that the dot product gives a sum of the λ_i terms multiplied by the RHS of the ODE of i-th state. The corresponding necessary conditions are

$$x_i'(t) = g_i(t, \vec{x}, \vec{u}), \ x_i(t_0) = x_{i0} \text{ for } i = 1, ..., n,$$

$$\lambda_j'(t) = -\frac{\partial H}{\partial x_j}, \ \lambda_j(t_1) = \phi_{x_j}(\vec{x}(t_1)) \text{ for } j = 1, ..., n, \text{ and}$$

$$0 = \frac{\partial H}{\partial u_k} \text{ at } u_k^* \text{ for } k = 1, ..., m.$$

Consider the example problem

$$\min_u \int_0^1 x_2(t) + u^2(t)dt$$

subject to

$$x_1' = x_2, \qquad x_1(0) = 0, \qquad x_1(1) = 1,$$
$$x_2' = u, \qquad x_2(0) = 0, \qquad x_2(1) \text{ is free.}$$

We introduce two adjoint variables, one for each state variable, and form the Hamiltonian,

$$H = x_2 + u^2 + \lambda_1 x_2 + \lambda_2 u.$$

The adjoint equations are

$$\lambda_1'(t) = -\frac{\partial H}{\partial x_1} = 0,$$
$$\lambda_2'(t) = -\frac{\partial H}{\partial x_2} = -\lambda_1 - 1, \qquad \text{with } \lambda_2(1) = 0.$$

Note that if a state has two boundary conditions, then its adjoint has no boundary condition. In this example, λ_1 does not have a boundary condition, since x_1 has two boundary conditions.

Solving the adjoint ODEs yields

$$\lambda_1(t) \equiv C,$$
$$\lambda_2(t) = -(C+1)(t-1)$$

for some constant C. Using the optimality condition, we have

$$0 = \left.\frac{\partial H}{\partial u}\right|_{u=u^*} = 2u^* + \lambda_2,$$
$$\Rightarrow \quad u^* = -\frac{\lambda_2}{2} = \frac{C+1}{2}(t-1).$$

The state equations become

$$x_2' = u \Rightarrow x_2(t) = \frac{C+1}{2}\left(\frac{t^2}{2} - t\right) \qquad \text{since } x_2(0) = 0,$$
$$x_1' = x_2 \Rightarrow x_1(t) = \frac{C+1}{2}\left(\frac{t^3}{6} - \frac{t^2}{2}\right) \qquad \text{since } x_1(0) = 0.$$

Noting that $x_1(1) = 1$, it follows $C = -7$. Thus, the optimal solution set is

$$u^*(t) = 3 - 3t, \quad x_1^*(t) = \frac{3}{2}t^2 - \frac{1}{2}t^3, \quad x_2^*(t) = 3t - \frac{3}{2}t^2.$$

4. SEIR Model with Isoperimetric Constraint

4.1. Background. Controlling the spread of an infectious disease can be achieved through various vaccination strategies. Using optimal control techniques, it is possible to find the vaccination schedule that minimizes the number of infectious individuals and the overall cost of the vaccination during a fixed time. We consider the case when vaccination supplies are limited and find the optimal vaccination schedule such that only a given number of people are vaccinated. For background on such models, see [**7, 8**]. For other work on optimal control of disease models, see [**1, 9, 15, 11, 4**].

We focus on a microparasitic infectious disease. This includes any viruses, bacteria, or fungi. Such diseases can be characterized by their small size, ability to reproduce directly within individual host, and relatively short duration of infection. See the book by Keeling and Rohani [**13**] for a variety of such models coming from microparasites; disease models discussed there include tick-borne diseases, measles, and malaria. Vaccinated individuals, along with those who have been infected and have recovered, produce an immune response to the disease. Immunity is not hereditary and therefore everyone is born susceptible.

4.2. Model. We present a SEIR model to illustrate the use of optimal control. We did not choose this to represent a particular disease, but just to illustrate the control techniques. For the SEIR model presented here, see related work [**10, 16**]. In this model, the host population is divided into susceptible, exposed, infected, and immune (recovered or vaccinated) classes. The exposed class contains those who have the disease but remain latent for some time before becoming infectious. We let $S(t)$, $E(t)$, $I(t)$, and $R(t)$ denote the number of individuals in the susceptible, exposed, infectious, and immune classes at time t. The total population at time t is represented by $N(t) = S(t) + E(t) + I(t) + R(t)$. The differential equations governing these classes are

$$S'(t) = bN(t) - dS(t) - cS(t)I(t) - u(t)S(t) \tag{4.1}$$

$$E'(t) = cS(t)I(t) - (e+d)E(t) \tag{4.2}$$

$$I'(t) = eE(t) - (g+a+d)I(t) \tag{4.3}$$

$$R'(t) = gI(t) - dR(t) + u(t)S(t) \tag{4.4}$$

$$N'(t) = (b-d)N(t) - aI(t). \tag{4.5}$$

The control is denoted by $u(t)$, the percentage of susceptible individuals being vaccinated per unit of time. It is assumed the vaccine is always effective so that all vaccinated susceptibles become immune. We bound the control with $0 \le u(t) \le .9$ to eliminate the case where the entire susceptible population is vaccinated. Let b be the natural exponential birth rate of the population and d be the natural exponential death rate. Incidence or frequency of the disease is described by the term $cS(t)I(t)$. The parameter e is the rate at which the exposed individuals become infectious and g is the rate at which infectious individuals recover. The parameter a denotes the death rate due to the disease in an infected individual.

If one would apply optimal control to a model for a particular disease, one should check for the model without control that the basic reproductive number R_0

is greater than one for the parameter ranges to consider. Thus the disease is not expected to die out without intervention strategies.

We extend this model to consider the situation in which a limited supply of vaccine is available. If X denotes the total number of susceptible people we can vaccinate over T years, then we have an integral constraint,

$$\int_0^T S(t)u(t)dt = X.$$

Such constraints are called isoperimetric [**12**] and can be handled by creating another state variable, $W(t)$, such that

$$W'(t) = S(t)u(t) \tag{4.6}$$
$$W(0) = 0 \tag{4.7}$$
$$W(T) = X. \tag{4.8}$$

Our goal is to minimize the number of infectious individuals and the overall cost of the vaccination over T years. The problem is stated as

$$\min_u \int_0^T AI(t) + u^2(t)dt \tag{4.9}$$

where the set of controls is

$$U = \{u : [0, T] \to [0, .9] \quad | \ u \text{ is Lebesgue measurable } \}$$

subject to (4.1)-(4.3), (4.5)-(4.8) and the conditions

$$S(0) = S_0, \qquad E(0) = E_0, \qquad I(0) = I_0, \qquad N(0) = N_0, \tag{4.10}$$

$$S(T), E(T), I(T), N(T) \text{ are free.} \tag{4.11}$$

Notice that the variable R appeared only in the R' equation (4.4) and $R(t) = N(t) - S(t) - E(t) - I(t)$. Therefore, we ignored R when creating the optimality system. The value A in the objective functional is a balancing parameter, which determines the relative importance of the two factors.

Using Pontryagin's Maximum Principle [**20**] to find the optimal vaccination schedule, we first define the Hamiltonian as

$$\begin{aligned} H = AI + u^2 + \lambda_S(bN - dS - cSI - uS) + \lambda_E(cSI - (e + d)E) \\ + \lambda_I(eE - (g + a + d)I) + \lambda_N((b - d)N - aI) + \lambda_W(Su). \end{aligned} \tag{4.12}$$

The values λ_S, λ_E, λ_I, λ_N, and λ_W are the associated adjoints for the states S, E, I, N, and W respectively. By differentiating the Hamiltonian with respect to each state variable, we find the differential equation for the associated adjoint. Also, because S, E, I, and N do not have fixed values at the final time, the values of the associated adjoints at the final time are zero. Since W has initial and terminal conditions, λ_W has no transversality condition. Therefore, the adjoint system is

(4.13) $\lambda'_S = \lambda_S(d + cI + u) - \lambda_E cI - \lambda_W u, \qquad \lambda_S(T) = 0$

(4.14) $\lambda'_E = \lambda_E(e + d) - \lambda_I e, \qquad \lambda_E(T) = 0$

(4.15) $\lambda'_I = -A + \lambda_S cS - \lambda_E cS + \lambda_I(g + a + d) + \lambda_N a, \qquad \lambda_I(T) = 0$

(4.16) $\lambda'_N = -\lambda_S b + \lambda_N(d - b), \qquad \lambda_N(T) = 0$

(4.17) $\lambda'_W = 0.$

By the optimality condition, we have

$$\frac{\partial H}{\partial u}|_{u^*} = 0$$

on the interior of the control set, where u^* denotes the optimal control. Solving for u^* on the interior of the control set gives

$$u^*(t) = \frac{S(t)(\lambda_S(t) - \lambda_W(t))}{2}. \tag{4.18}$$

Taking the bounds into account, we conclude

$$u^*(t) = \min[0.9, \max[0, \frac{S(t)(\lambda_S(t) - \lambda_W(t))}{2}]]. \tag{4.19}$$

The state and adjoint differential equations together with the above control characterization are solved numerically to illustrate our control results. Because state equations have initial conditions and adjoint equations have conditions at the final time, an iterative program wass created to numerically simulate solutions. Given an initial guess for the control, to compute the optimal state values, the program solves (4.1)-(4.3),(4.5),(4.6) with initial conditions (4.7) and (4.10) forward in time using a Runge Kutta method of the fourth order. Resulting state values are placed in adjoint equations (4.13)-(4.16). These adjoint equations with given final conditions are then solved backwards in time. Again, a fourth order Runge Kutta method is employed. Both state and adjoint values are used to update the control using the characterization (4.19) and the entire process repeats itself. This iterative process terminates when current state, adjoint, and control values are sufficiently close to successive values. For convergence results for such iterative methods, see [**6**].

Because of (4.17), $\lambda_W(t) = k$ for all $t \in [0, T]$ where k is an unknown constant. The value of $\lambda_W(t) = k$ directly affects the value of $W(t)$. The Matlab program finds the appropriate value of k whose optimal solutions satisfy both endpoint conditions, $W(0) = 0$ and $W(T) = X$. We start with $k = 0$ and compute the optimal state, control, and adjoint values as explained above. Because the state equations are solved forward in time, the condition $W(0) = 0$ is always satisfied and we need only worry about $W(T)$. For all sets of tested parameters, we have found that larger k values correspond to small values of $W(T)$.

Depending on the value of $W(T)$ associated with $k = 0$, we increase or decrease k. Again, optimal state, adjoint, and control values are computed, the value of $W(T)$ is compared to the inputted value of X, and k is increased/decreased accordingly. When $W(T) = X$ is reasonably satisfied, the current k value and its associated control, states and adjoints are chosen as optimal.

Once the correct k value and optimal state, adjoint, and control values have been found, we substitute them into the R' equation (4.4). Using the updated

TABLE 1. Parameter Values

Value	**Description**
$S_0 = 1000$	initial susceptible population
$E_0 = 100$	initial exposed population
$I_0 = 50$	initial infected population
$R_0 = 15$	initial recovered population
$b = 0.525$	birth rate
$d = 0.5$	death rate
$c = 0.001$	incidence coefficient
$e = 0.5$	exposed to infectious rate
$g = 0.1$	recovery rate
$a = 0.2$	disease induced death rate
$A = 0.1$	weight parameter
$T = 20$	number of years

equation and the inputted initial condition R_0, we solve for R using a fourth order Runge Kutta.

4.3. Numerical Example. To understand the impact of the added constraint, we first look at the optimal vaccination schedule given the objective functional in 4.9 and no constraint placed on the number of susceptible people being vaccinated. With the absence of the isoperimetric constraint, we remove the state variable $W(t)$ from the optimal control problem and create a Matlab program to solve the new optimality system.

Running the new program with the values in Table 1 produces the optimal vaccination schedule and corresponding population dynamics displayed as solid curves in Figure 1. The dashed curve in the infectious class represents dynamics in absence of vaccination. With this optimal vaccination schedule, 4508 susceptible individuals are vaccinated, which was calculated from $\int_0^T S(t)u(t)dt$.

Now, suppose we have the same parameters as above, but are limited to only 2500 vaccinations. We run the original program with $X = 2500$. The program terminates at $k = .0019$, corresponding to $W(T) = 2500$. The optimal vaccination schedule and corresponding population dynamics are displayed as solid curves in Figure 2. The dashed line again represents the infectious class in absence of vaccination. With this optimal schedule, 2500 susceptibles are vaccinated over the 20 years. This is approximately 2000 fewer vaccinations than that in the optimal schedule of Figure 1.

Compare the two optimal vaccination schedules. The schedule in Figure 1 requires maximum vaccination initially, then a gradual decrease over the next twenty years. The optimal schedule in Figure 2 also starts with maximum initial vaccination. However, the vaccination rate decreases quickly until its termination in the eighth year. Because of this, the recovered population in Figure 2 declines quickly after the eighth year. Both figures show successful control of the infected class during the 20-year time period.

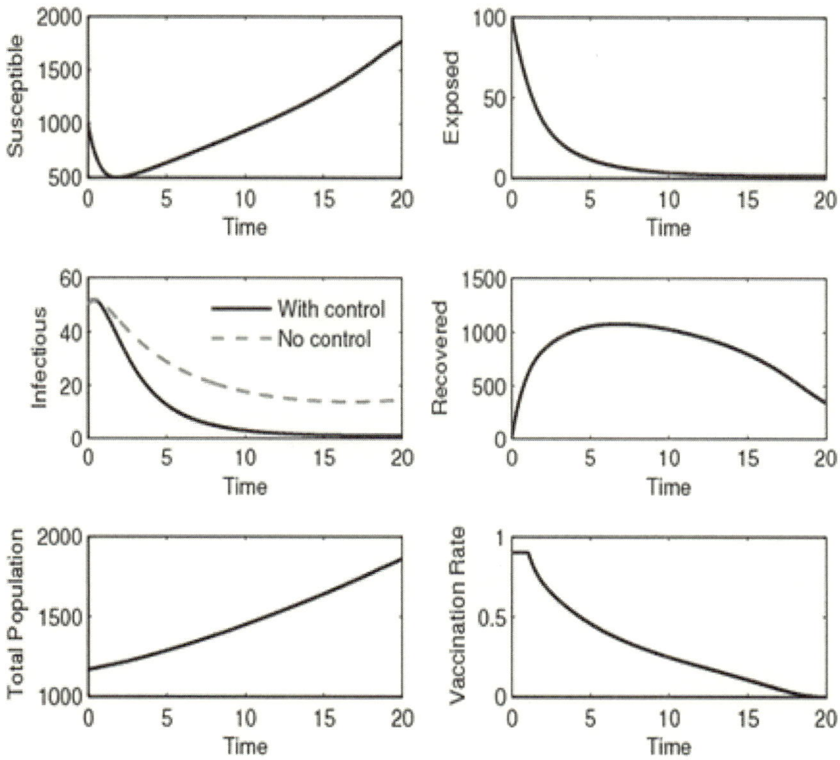

FIGURE 1. Optimal vaccination schedule without constraint

For further comparison, we look at the value of the objective functional,

$$\int_0^T AI(t) + u^2(t)dt$$

for the optimal values given in both Figure 1 and Figure 2. A left point Reimann Sum is incorporated into the programs to approximate both values. For optimal values given in Figure 1, the objective functional is 24.2463. For optimal values in Figure 2, the objective functional is 25.4745. We expect the objective functional of Figure 1 to be lower because Figure 1 represents the optimal schedule without a constraint. The schedule in Figure 2 represents the most optimal schedule which satisfies the integral constraint.

5. Conclusions

We have outlined the steps in setting up an optimal control problem for a system of ordinary differential equations. Pontryagin's Maximum Principle summarizes the

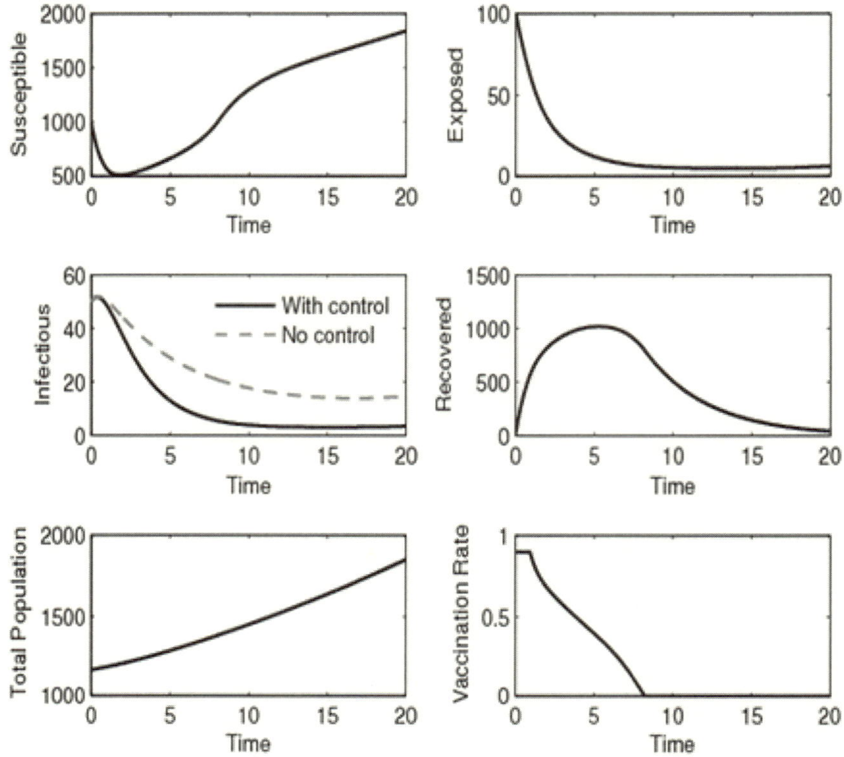

FIGURE 2. Optimal vaccination schedule with constraint

necessary conditions for such problems. We provided several examples using this principle to characterize an optimal control. These simple examples were chosen to illustrate basic optimal control methodology.

In greater detail, we presented an SEIR epidemic model where the control enters as a rate of vaccination. In the associated optimal control problem, the goal is to characterize the vaccination schedule which minimizes the number of infected individuals and the cost of vaccination over some finite time period. In addition, we placed a constraint on the vaccine supply. We showed that isoperimetric constraints on the control can be handled by creating an additional state variable. Numerical results illustrate the optimal vaccination schedule with and without the constraint. Both strategies indicate successful short-term control of the disease. The methods outline in this paper allow one to compute optimal control schemes, assess the relative cost, and determine resulting population dynamics. This is an invaluable tool for policy makers needing immediate insight in designing cost-effective strategies for disease control.

References

[1] Behncke, H., *Optimal control of deterministic epidemics*, Optim. Control Appl. Meth., **21** (2000), p. 269-285.

[2] Blower, S. M., and H. Dowlatabadi, Sensitivity and uncertainity analysis of complex models of disease transmission: an HIV model, as an example, Int. Stat. Rev. 2(1994), p. 229-243.

[3] Bodine, E. , L. J. Gross, and S. Lenhart, Optimal control applied to a model of species augmentation, Mathematical Biosciences and Engineering 5(4) 2008, p. 669-680.

[4] Fister, K. R., Lenhart, S. and Mc Nally, J. S., Optimizing Chemotherapy in an HIV Model, *Electron. J. Diff. Eqns.*, **32**, 1-12 (1998).

[5] Fleming, W. H. and R. W. Rishel, *Deterministic and Stochastic Optimal Control*, Springer Verlag, New York, 1975.

[6] Hackbusch, W. K. *A Numerical Method for Solving Parabolic Equations with Opposite Orientations*, Computing, **20**(1978), p. 229-240 .

[7] Hethcote, H. W. *An immunization model for a heterogeneous population,* Theor. Pop. Biol. **14** (1978), p. 338-349.

[8] Hethcote, H. W., and Waltman, P. *Optimal vaccination schedules in a deterministic epidemic model,* Math. Biosci. **18** (1973), p. 365-381.

[9] Joshi, H. R. *Optimal Control of an HIV Immunology Model*, Optim. Control Appl. Meth., bf 23(2002), p. 199-213.

[10] Joshi, H. R., S. Lenhart, M. Li, and L. Wang, Optimal Control Methods Applied to Disease Models, AMS proceeding volume on Emerging Diseases, Contemporary Mathematics 410 (2006), p. 187-207.

[11] Jung, E., S. Lenhart, and Z. Feng, *Optimal control of treatments in a two-strain tuberculosis model*, Discrete Contin. Dyn. Syst. Ser. B 2 (2002), no. 4, p. 473-482.

[12] Kamien, M. I. and N. L. Schwartz, Dynamic Optimization: The Calculus of Variations and Optimal Control in Economics and Management, 2nd ed, New York, Elsevier Science, 1991.

[13] Keeling, M. J., and P. Rohani, Modeling Infectious Diseases in Humans and Animals, Princeton University Press, Princeton, 2008.

[14] Kern, D. L., S. Lenhart, R. Miller and J. Yong, Optimal Control applied to native-invasive population dynamics, J. of Biological Dynamics 1 (4), 2007, p. 379-393.

[15] Kirschner, D., S. Lenhart, and S. Serbin, *Optimal Control of the Chemotherapy of HIV*, J. Math. Biol, **35**(1997), p. 775-792.

[16] Lenhart S. and J. Workman, Optimal Control Applied to Biological Models, Boca Raton, Chapman Hall/CRC, 2007.

[17] Marino, S., I. B. Hogue, C. J. Ray, and D. E. Kirschner, A methodology for performing global uncertainity and sensitivity analysis in systems biology, J. Theor. Bio. 254 (2008), p. 178-196.

[18] Miller Neilan, R. L., E. Schaefer, H. Gaff, K. R. Fister, and S. Lenhart, Modeling optimal intervention strategies for cholera, preprint.

[19] Nanda, S., S. Lenhart, and H. Moore, Optimal Control of a Chronic Myelogenous Leukemia Model, Math. Biosciences 210(1) 2007, p. 143-156.

[20] Pontryagin, L. S., V. G. Boltyanskii, R. V. Gamkrelize, and E. F. Mishchenko, The Mathematical Theory of Optimal Processes, New York, Wiley, 1962.

[21] Sethi, S. P. and G. L. Thompson, *Optimal Control Theory: Applications to Management Science and Economics*, Kluwer, Boston, 2nd edition, 2000.

Department of Mathematics, University of Tennessee, Knoxville, Tennessee 37996

Current address: Department of Oceanography & Coastal Sciences, Louisiana State University, Baton Rouge, Louisiana 70803

E-mail address: `rmill48@lsu.edu`

Department of Mathematics, University of Tennessee, Knoxville, Tennessee 37996

E-mail address: `lenhart@math.utk.edu`

DIMACS Series in Discrete Mathematics
and Theoretical Computer Science
Volume **75**, 2010

Introduction to discrete-time epidemic models

Abdul-Aziz Yakubu

ABSTRACT. We use simple discrete-time SIS and SEIS epidemic models to introduce a framework for studying disease transmission dynamics in populations that exhibit compensatory (contest competition) and overcompensatory (scramble competition) dynamics with and without the strong Allee effect. We compute the basic reproductive number, $\Re_0$, and use it to predict the (uniform) persistence or extinction of the infective population, where the population dynamics are compensatory and the strong Allee mechanism is either present or absent. We use the SIS model to explore the relationship between the demographic equation and the epidemic process, where the total population dynamics are overcompensatory. In particular, we show that the demographic dynamics drive both the susceptible and infective dynamics.

1. Introduction

In 2001, Castillo-Chavez and Yakubu, provided a framework for studying disease dynamics in the presence of complex dynamics [10 - 13]. In their model framework, the total population at generation t, denoted by $T(t)$, is governed by the one-dimensional equation

$$T(t+1) = f_\gamma(T(t)) = f(T(t)) + \gamma T(t), \tag{1}$$

where $\gamma \in (0,1)$ is the constant "probability" of surviving per generation, and $f : \mathbb{R}_+ \to \mathbb{R}_+$ models the birth or recruitment process [5, 10-13, 20, 21, 26, 32, 34-36]. The set of iterates of

$$f_\gamma : \mathbb{R}_+ \to \mathbb{R}_+$$

is equivalent to the set of density sequences generated by Model (1). We use f_γ to describe the dynamics of Model (1).

When $f(T) = Tg(T)$ and the density-dependent function $g(T)$ is the per-capita growth rate, then $f_\gamma(T) = T\left(g(T) + \gamma\right)$. Traditionally, density-dependent vital rates are classified as depensatory, compensatory or overcompensatory. If

$$\frac{dg(T)}{dT} > 0$$

for some $T > 0$, then the per-capita growth rate g is said to exhibit *depensation* or *Allee effect* [14]. The Allee effect, a biological phenomenon named after W. C. Allee, describes a positive relation between population density and the per capita growth rate of species. In the presence of the Allee effect, there is a decrease in population growth rate at low population sizes. That is, species that exhibit the Allee effect do not thrive at low population densities. However, the effect usually saturates or disappears as populations get larger. Presence of the Allee effect in populations may be due to any number of causes. In some species, reproduction or finding a mate is increasingly difficult as the population density decreases [13, 14, 34, 37].

The per-capita growth rate, g, is said to be *compensatory* if

$$\frac{dg(T)}{dT} \leq 0,$$

$$\frac{df(T)}{dT} \geq 0$$

and

$$\lim_{T \to \infty} f(T) = K > 0.$$

When g is compensatory the decline in the per-capita growth rate with density is exactly compensated for by the increase in density so that the net growth rate is asymptotically constant [13, 14, 26].

The per-capita growth rate, g, is said to be *overcompensatory* if

$$\lim_{T \to \infty} f(T) = 0.$$

When g is overcompensatory the increase in T is not enough to compensate for the decrease in $g(T)$ at high densities [13, 14, 26].

Scramble and contest competition are two extreme forms of intraspecific competition for resources [8, 13]. Systems that exhibit scramble competition try to support all individuals including those who are non-reproductive. In scramble competition, the resources are equally divided among individuals, so that, beyond a threshold density, none can get enough of a share of the resource to survive and reproduce. Models that are subject to overcompensatory dynamics, such as the Ricker model, provide examples of systems where new recruits experience scramble competition [8, 13]. In contest competition, some individuals get a big enough share of the resource to survive and reproduce at the expense of the rest. Models that are subject to compensatory dynamics, such as the Beverton-Holt model (a special case of Smith-Slatkin model), provide examples of systems where new recruits experience contest competition [8, 13].

As in [34], we use a simple discrete-time SIS epidemic model and precise mathematical definitions to extend the framework of Castillo-Chavez and Yakubu to include population dynamics under *compensatory* (non-oscillatory) and *overcompensatory* (oscillatory and chaotic) dynamics with and without the *strong Allee effect.*

As in [1-6, 10-13, 15], we assume that a disease invades and subdivides the target population into two classes: susceptibles (non-infectives) and infectives. Prior to the time of disease invasion, the population dynamics are assumed to be compensatory or overcompensatory (where the strong Allee effect is either present or absent) or growing at a geometric rate. The transition from susceptible to infective is a function of the contact rate α between susceptibles and the proportion of infectives (prevalence) in the population. To simplify our analysis, we assume that the disease is non-fatal and individuals (infected and susceptible) have equal probability of surviving one generation. Mild viral infections, such as most infections from rhinoviruses (causative agents of the common cold) are examples of such non-fatal infections. Since rhinovirus infection occurs primarily in humans and other higher primates, it does not quite fit our model framework. However, it is illustrative of the type of diseases being modeled. Our primary focus is on the impact of infected individuals, the strong Allee effect, compensatory and overcompensatory dynamics on the persistence or control of infectious diseases.

We compute $\Re_0$ and used it to predict disease persistence or extinction when the population dynamics are compensatory and the strong Allee effect is either present or absent and when the total population is growing at a geometric rate [4-6, 15, 19, 22, 32, 33]. As in [10-13], when the demographic dynamics are overcompensatory, we numerically explore the relationship between the demographic equation and the epidemic process. Franke and Yakubu have shown that, in periodic environments it is possible for the infective population to be on a chaotic attractor while the demographic dynamics are oscillatory but non-chaotic [21].

To demonstrate that our framework can also be used to study other infectious diseases, we also introduce a Susceptible-Exposed-Infectious-Susceptible (SEIS) epidemic model. As in [5], we compute $\Re_0$ for the SEIS model and use it to predict disease persistence and extinction.

The paper is organized as follows. In Section 2, we introduce the demographic equation for the study. The equation, a discrete-time model, describes the dynamics of the (total) population before disease invasion. We introduce in Section 2, precise mathematical definitions of *compensatory dynamics*, *overcompensatory dynamics*, and the *strong Allee effect*. The discrete-time SIS epidemic model is constructed in Section 3. When the recruitment function is either a positive constant or the Beverton-Holt model [7-13, 16-18, 20-32, 34-37], then the population dynamics are compensatory, the total population is uniformly persistent and lives on a globally attracting positive fixed point (no strong Allee effect). When the recruitment function is a modified Beverton-Holt model, then the population has the strong Allee effect. However, when the recruitment function is the Ricker model [27-29], then the population dynamics are overcompensatory, and the demographic equation is capable of supporting complex dynamics such as period-doubling bifurcations route to chaos. In Section 4, the basic reproductive number $\Re_0$ is introduced and used to predict the (uniform) persistence or extinction of the infective population, where the population dynamics are compensatory with or without the strong Allee effect. Also in Section 4, we analyze the SIS epidemic model under geometric demographic dynamics. In Section 5, we illustrate that it is possible for the demographic dynamics to drive both the *S-dynamics* and *I-dynamics* as it undergoes period-doubling bifurcations. The SEIS model is introduced in Section 6, and the implications of our results are discussed in Section 7.

2. Demographic equation

When the recruitment rate is constant per generation, then $f(T(t)) = k(1-\gamma)$ and Model (1) becomes the linear difference equation

$$T(t+1) = k(1-\gamma) + \gamma T(t). \tag{2}$$

Hence,

$$T(t) = (T(0) - k)\,\gamma^t + k$$

and

$$\lim_{t\to\infty} T(t) = T_\infty = k.$$

That is, the total population is asymptotically constant and demographic effects eventually vanish.

When the recruitment function is proportional to the total population and μ is the constant per-capita birth rate, then $f(T(t)) = \mu T(t)$ and Model (1) becomes the linear difference equation

$$T(t+1) = (\mu + \gamma)\, T(t). \tag{3}$$

Hence,

$$T(t) = (\mu + \gamma)^t\, T(0).$$

In this case, it is useful to introduce the demographic basic reproductive number,

$$\Re_d = \frac{\mu}{1-\gamma}.$$

When $\Re_d > 1$, the population invades at a geometric rate and when $\Re_d < 1$ the population goes extinct at a geometric rate.

Next, we introduce two types of density dependent demographic dynamics commonly found in the literature, *compensatory* and *overcompensatory* dynamics with and without the *strong Allee effect* (see definitions below).

Definition 1 [26, 34]. *The demographic dynamics in Model (1) are compensatory in an open interval J whenever all positive population sizes in J approach the unique positive equilibrium at $T_\infty \in J$ monotonically under f_γ iterations.*

For example, when the recruitment function is the classic Beverton-Holt model,

$$f(T) = \frac{(1-\gamma)\mu k T}{(1-\gamma)k + (\mu - 1 + \gamma)T}, \tag{4}$$

then the demographic dynamics in Model (1) are compensatory in $J = (0, \infty)$, where $\mu > 1$ and $T_\infty = k > 0$ (see Figure 1) [24, 26, 31, 34].

Definition 2 [26, 34]. *The demographic dynamics in Model (1) are overcompensatory in an open interval J containing the positive equilibrium T_∞ whenever $f_\gamma'(T_\infty) < 0$.*

When the recruitment function is the classic Ricker model,

$$f(T) = Te^{r-T}, \tag{5}$$

then the demographic dynamics in Model (1) are overcompensatory in $J = (0, \infty)$, whenever

$$r > \frac{1}{1-\gamma} + \ln(1-\gamma)$$

and $T_\infty = r - \ln(1-\gamma)$ (see Figure 1) [26-29, 31, 34].

We will use the following definition to demonstrate the persistence of infective populations in an SIS epidemic model. In the definitions, $f_\gamma^t(T) = \underbrace{f_\gamma \circ f_\gamma \circ \cdots \circ f_\gamma(T)}_{t \text{ compositions}}$ is the composition map evaluated at the point T.

Definition 3 [20, 34]. *The total population is persistent for all initial population sizes in J if*

$$\lim_{t\to\infty} \inf f_\gamma^t(T) > 0$$

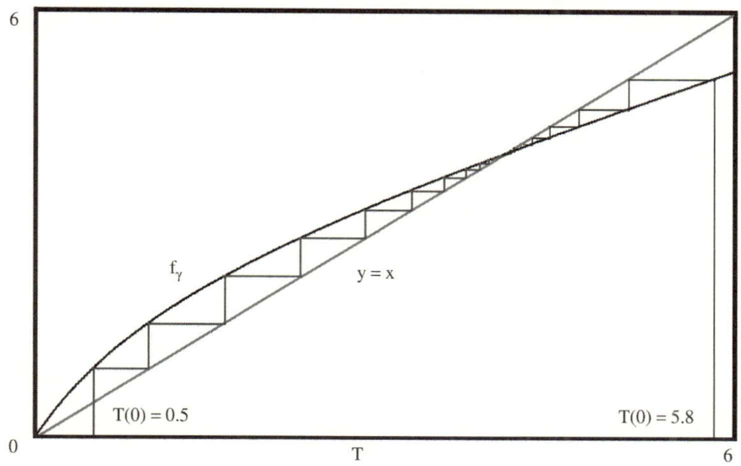

FIGURE 1. The initial conditions $T(0) = 0.5$ (red) and $T(0) = 5.8$ (blue) converge to the postive equilibrium point $T_\infty = 4$ monotonically (compensatory dynamics) in Model (1), where $f(T) = \frac{(1-\gamma)\mu kT}{(1-\gamma)k+(\mu-1+\gamma)T}$, $\gamma = 0.5, \mu = 2$ and $k = 4$.

for each $T \in J$, where $f_\gamma^t = \underbrace{f_\gamma \circ f_\gamma \circ \cdots \circ f_\gamma}_{t \text{ compositions}}$. The total population is uniformly persistent for all initial population sizes in J if there exists a positive constant η such that

$$\liminf_{t\to\infty} f_\gamma^t(T) \geq \eta$$

for each $T \in J$.

These definitions imply that, when the dynamics are compensatory in J then the total population is uniformly persistent (and hence, persistent) in J. For example, when $f(T) = \frac{(1-\gamma)\mu kT}{(1-\gamma)k+(\mu-1+\gamma)T}$ then $T_\infty = k$, the dynamics are compensatory in $(0, \infty)$ and the total population is uniformly persistent (and hence, persistent) in $(0, \infty)$.

Definition 4 [34]. *The total population has the strong Allee effect if there exists a positive number t_∞ such that $\lim_{t\to\infty} f_\gamma^t(T) = 0$ for all $T \in [0, t_\infty)$, and the total population is uniformly persistent on a subset of (t_∞, ∞).*

These definitions imply that, when $\{0\}$ is a locally asymptotically stable fixed point of f_γ and the dynamics are compensatory in an interval $J \subset (t_\infty, \infty)$, then

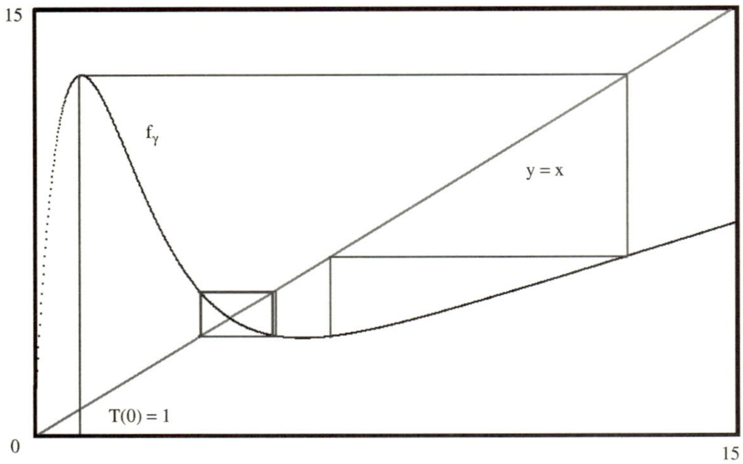

FIGURE 2. The initial condition $T(0) = 1$ converges to the 2-cycle attractor (overcompensatory dynamics) at $\{3.584 \to 5.088\}$ in Model (1), where $f(T) = Te^{r-T}$, $\gamma = 0.5$ and $r = 3.5$.

the strong Allee effect is present in the population. For example, when

$$f(T) = \frac{\eta T^2}{1 + \lambda T^2}$$

and $\eta > 2(1-\gamma)\sqrt{\lambda} > 0$, then the strong Allee effect is present in the total population. That is, all positive initial population sizes smaller than $t_\infty = \frac{\eta - \sqrt{\eta^2 - 4\lambda(1-\gamma)^2}}{2\lambda(1-\gamma)}$ are attracted to zero monotonically, while all positive initial population sizes bigger than t_∞ converge *monotonically* (compensatory dynamics) to the attracting positive fixed point, $T_\infty = \frac{\eta + \sqrt{\eta^2 - 4\lambda(1-\gamma)^2}}{2\lambda(1-\gamma)}$ (see Figure 3).

When

$$f(T) = T^\eta \exp(r - T)$$

and $\eta > 1$, then it is possible to have the Allee effect in the presence of overcompensatory population dynamics in Model (1) (see Figure 4) [34].

3. Discrete-time SIS epidemic model

In this section, we construct a simple two epidemiological class discrete-time *susceptible-infective-susceptible* (SIS) epidemic process on the demographic equation, Model (1). Let $S(t)$ denote the population of susceptibles; $I(t)$ denotes the population of the infected, assumed infectious; $T(t) \equiv S(t) + I(t)$ denotes the total population size at generation t; T_∞ denotes the demographic positive steady state

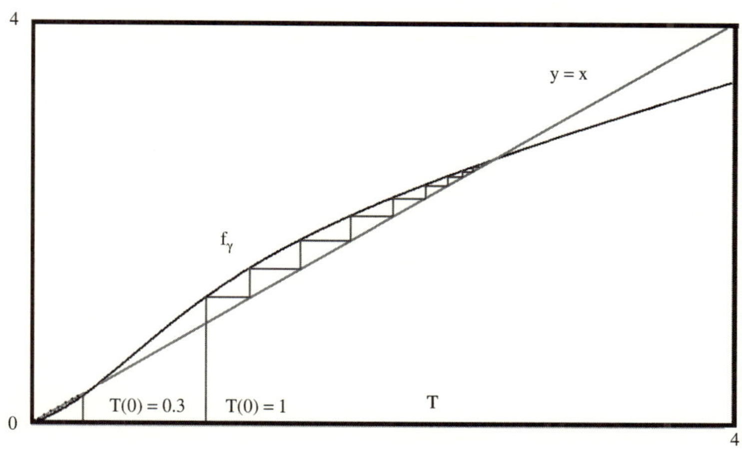

FIGURE 3. The initial condition $T(0) = 0.3$ (blue) converges to zero and $T(0) = 1$ (red) converges monotonically (compensatory dynamics and the strong Allee effect) to the postive equilibrium point $T_\infty = 2.618$ in Model (1), where $f(T) = \frac{\eta T^2}{1+\lambda T^2}$, $\gamma = 0.5, \lambda = 1$ and $\eta = 1.5$.

or attracting population and $\overline{T}_0$ the initial point on a globally attracting cycle, when they exist. We assume that susceptible (respectively, infected) individuals survive with constant probability γ_1 (respectively, γ_2) per generation, and infected individuals recover with constant probability $(1-\sigma)$.

Let $\phi : [0, \infty) \to [0, 1]$ be a monotone concave probability function with $\phi(0) = 1, \phi'(T) < 0$ and $\phi''(T) \geq 0$ for all $T \in [0, \infty)$. At generation t, we assume the susceptible individuals become infected with nonlinear probability $\left(1 - \phi\left(\frac{\alpha I(t)}{T(t)}\right)\right)$ per generation, where the transmission constant α is positive. That is, α models the impact of prevalence on ϕ. When infections are modeled as Poisson processes, then $\phi\left(\frac{\alpha I(t)}{T(t)}\right) = e^{-\frac{\alpha I(t)}{T(t)}}$ [5, 10-13].

Our assumptions and notation lead to the following SIS epidemic model:

$$\left.\begin{aligned} S(t+1) &= f(T(t)) + \gamma_1 \phi\left(\frac{\alpha I(t)}{T(t)}\right) S(t) + \gamma_2(1-\sigma)I(t) \\ I(t+1) &= \gamma_1 \left(1 - \phi\left(\frac{\alpha I(t)}{T(t)}\right)\right) S(t) + \gamma_2 \sigma I(t) \end{aligned}\right\} \quad (6)$$

where $0 < \gamma_i, \sigma < 1$ and $T(t) > 0$ for each $i \in \{1, 2\}$. We summarize our model parameters and functions in Table 1.

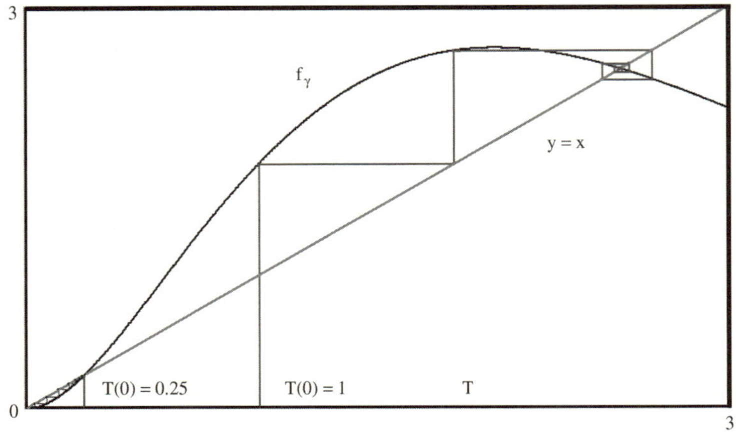

FIGURE 4. The initial condition $T(0) = 0.25$ (blue) converges to zero and $T(0) = 1$ (red) oscillates (overcompensatory dynamics and the strong Allee effect) about the postive equilibrium point $T_\infty = 2.544$ and converges to it in Model (1),where $f(T) = T^2 e^{r-T}$, $\gamma = 0.01$ and $r = 1.6$.

Table 1: Model Parameters and Functions

Parameter	**Description**
γ_1	Survival "probability" of susceptible individuals per generation;
γ_2	Survival "probability" of infective individuals per generation;
α	Transmission constant;
$(1-\sigma)$	Recovery "probability" of infective individuals per generation;
ϕ	Frequency-dependent escape "probability" function;
f	Birth or recruitment function;
$\Re_d$	Demographic basic reproductive number.

Below, we summarize some of the underlying assumptions in Model (6).

(a)	The disease increases mortality but does not affect fecundity;
(b)	There is no acquired immunity;
(c)	There is no latent period (or it is very short);
(d)	Transmission is frequency dependent rather than density dependent.

Theoretical and empirical investigations have been done on comparing these assumptions. In continuous-time epidemic models, it is known that these assumptions are not universally applicable [4, 21].

Model (6) is a deterministic SIS epidemic model and has no "probability" of transmission. The assumption of deterministic dynamics is valid in a large population, where stochasticity is unimportant. This assumption places a constraint on the applicability of the model. Stochastic transmission (including a Poisson process) in a small population (close to extinction), for example, would not be described by the SIS model.

In [10-13], Castillo-Chavez and Yakubu, studied discrete-time SIS models under the assumption that susceptible and infected individuals have equal probability of surviving one generation ($\gamma_1 = \gamma_2 = \gamma$). In a recent paper, Franke and Yakubu studied a non-autonomous discrete-time SIS model with $\gamma_1 > \gamma_2$ [21].

The total population in generation $t+1$, $S(t+1)+I(t+1)$, the sum of the two equations of Model (6), is the following equation:

$$T(t+1) = f(T(t)) + \gamma_1 S(t) + \gamma_2 I(t). \tag{7}$$

That is,

$$f(T(t)) + (\min\{\gamma_1, \gamma_2\})\, T(t) \leq T(t+1) \leq f(T(t)) + (\max\{\gamma_1, \gamma_2\})\, T(t). \tag{8}$$

When an infected individual is less likely than a susceptible individual to survive one generation, then Inequality (8) becomes

$$f(T(t)) + \gamma_2 T(t) \leq T(t+1) \leq f(T(t)) + \gamma_1 T(t). \tag{9}$$

In Inequality (9), the $T-$ *dynamics* generated by Model (6) are bounded by the $T-$*dynamics* generated by the demographic equation, Model (1), where γ is either γ_1 or γ_2. To simplify our analysis, we assume throughout that the disease is non-fatal and all susceptible and infected individuals have equal probability of surviving one generation. That is, $\gamma = \gamma_1 = \gamma_2$ and Model (6) assumes that a non-fatal disease has invaded the total population and partitioned the population into susceptibles and infectives, where the total population in generation $t+1$, $T(t+1) = S(t+1) + I(t+1)$. That is, the sum of the two equations of Model (6) is the demographic equation, Model (1).

Although Model (6) has no disease-induced mortality, the population does experience death via density dependence. In the demographic equation, this form of regulation has been shown to have complex population dynamics such as period-doubling bifurcations and chaos [10-13, 20, 21, 27-29].

4. Disease extinction versus disease persistence

Here, we introduce the epidemic threshold parameter, the basic reproductive number, $\Re_0$, for Model (6). We use $\Re_0$ to study Model (6) with or without the Allee effect, where the total population is under compensatory dynamics.

4.1. Compensatory dynamics. When the recruitment function is either $f(T(t)) = k(1-\gamma)$ (constant) or $f(T(t)) = \frac{(1-\gamma)\mu k T(t)}{(1-\gamma)k+(\mu-1+\gamma)T(t)}$ (the classic Beverton-Holt model), then Allee effect is not present and the dynamics are compensatory. That is, the long-term demographic effects disappear in Model (1) and $\lim_{t\to\infty} T(t) = T_\infty > 0$. In this case, letting $S(t) = T_\infty - I(t) \geq 0$ in the $I-$*equation* of Model (6) gives rise to the following one-dimensional equivalent autonomous "limiting system" [8, 20, 38].

$$I(t+1) = \gamma\left(1 - \phi\left(\alpha\frac{I(t)}{T_\infty}\right)\right)(T_\infty - I(t)) + \gamma\sigma I(t), \tag{10}$$

where $I(t) \leq T_\infty$ for all $t \in \{0,1,2,...\}$. Others have proved mathematical theorems on the qualitative dynamics equivalence of autonomous and nonautonomous systems, such as Model (6) and Equation (10) [8, 20, 38].

The basic reproductive number is

$$\Re_0 = \frac{-\alpha\gamma\phi'(0)}{1-\gamma\sigma}.$$

In $\Re_0$, $\frac{1}{1-\gamma\sigma} = 1 + \gamma\sigma + (\gamma\sigma)^2 + \cdots$ is the product of the average death adjusted infectious period in generations; γ is the proportion that can be invaded by the disease (survival first then infection); and $-\alpha\phi^{'}(0)$ is the maximum rate of infection of susceptible individuals per infective. Thus, $\Re_0$ gives the average number of secondary infections due to small initial infective individuals over their life-time.

In Equation (10), if $\Re_0 > 1$ and the strong Allee effect is absent in the total population, then the strong Allee effect is not present in the infective population and the infective population persists uniformly on a unique endemic equilibrium. However, if the strong Allee effect is present in the total population and $\Re_0 > 1$, then the strong Allee effect is present in the infective population. That is, the infective population persists uniformly on a unique endemic equilibrium when the infective population is large while it goes extinct when the population size is small. If $\Re_0 < 1$, then the infective population decreases to zero; regardless of initial population sizes. We summarize these results in Theorem 1 and Corollary 1.

Theorem 1. *Let the demographic dynamics in Model (6) be compensatory in* $(0,\infty)$ *(that is,* $\lim_{t\to\infty} T(t) = T_\infty > 0$ *whenever* $T(0) > 0$*) and* $\gamma = \gamma_1 = \gamma_2$.

(a) If $\Re_0 < 1$, *then* $\lim_{t\to\infty} I(t) = 0$ *in Model (6),*
whenever $I(0) \leq T(0)$. *That is, the disease goes extinct.*
(b) If $\Re_0 > 1$, *then Model (6) has a unique endemic equilibrium*
I^* *such that* $\lim_{t\to\infty} I(t) = I^* > 0$ *whenever* $T(0) \geq I(0) > 0$.
That is, the infective population persists uniformly on a fixed point attractor.

Proof. Let

$$F(I) = \gamma\left(1 - \phi\left(\alpha\frac{I}{T_\infty}\right)\right)(T_\infty - I) + \gamma\sigma I.$$

Then,

$$F(I(t)) = I(t+1).$$

That is, the set of iterates of the map F is equivalent to the set of density sequences generated by Equation (10).

Differentiating F with respect to I gives

$$\begin{aligned} F^{'}(I) &= -\gamma\left(1-\phi\left(\alpha\tfrac{I}{T_\infty}\right)\right) - \tfrac{\alpha\gamma}{T_\infty}\phi'\left(\alpha\tfrac{I}{T_\infty}\right)(T_\infty - I) + \gamma\sigma. \\ F^{''}(I) &= \tfrac{2\alpha\gamma}{T_\infty}\phi'\left(\alpha\tfrac{I}{T_\infty}\right) - \tfrac{\alpha^2\gamma}{T_\infty^2}\phi''\left(\alpha\tfrac{I}{T_\infty}\right)(T_\infty - I). \end{aligned}$$

To prove the result, we will show that $\Re_0 < 1$ implies $0 < F^{'}(0) < 1$, $\Re_0 > 1$ implies $F^{'}(0) > 1$, and $F^{''}(I) < 0$ for $I \in (0, T_\infty]$.

When $0 < \Re_0 < 1$, then

$$0 < F^{'}(0) = -\alpha\gamma\phi^{'}(0) + \gamma\sigma < 1.$$

Therefore, the fixed point $\{0\}$ is locally asymptotically stable under $F-$*iterations*. Notice that $\phi' < 0$ and $\phi'' \geq 0$ imply that $F^{''} < 0$ for $I \in (0, T_\infty]$. Moreover, the monotonicity condition on ϕ' and the fact that $F^{'}(0) < 1$ imply $F^{'}(I) < 1$ or $F(I) < I$ for $I \in (0, T_\infty]$. Consequently, $\{I(t)\}_{t \geq 0}$, is a strictly decreasing sequence bounded below by zero that converges to the only fixed point of F in $[0, T_\infty]$, $\{0\}$. This proves that $\Re_0 < 1$ implies $\lim_{t\to\infty} I(t) = 0$.

When $\Re_0 > 1$, then

$$F^{'}(0) = -\alpha\gamma\phi'(0) + \gamma\sigma > 1,$$

and $\{0\}$ is a locally unstable fixed point of F. Let I^* denote the smallest positive fixed point of F in $[0, T_\infty]$. Notice that

$$F(T_\infty) = \gamma\sigma T_\infty < T_\infty.$$

As a result, the Intermediate Value Theorem guarantees the existence of the positive fixed point I^* in $(0, T_\infty)$ satisfying $F(I^*) = I^*$, and $F(I) > I$ for $I \in (0, I^*)$. Therefore, $F^{'}(I^*) \leq 1$. $F^{''}(I) < 0$ implies that $F^{'}(I) < F^{'}(I^*) \leq 1$ for $I \in (I^*, T_\infty)$. This implies that

$$\int_{I^*}^{I} F^{'}(x)dx < \int_{I^*}^{I} dx.$$

Hence, $F(I) > I$ for $I \in (0, I^*)$ and $F(I) < I$ for $I \in (I^*, T_\infty]$.

To prove that the positive fixed point I^* is globally attracting in $(0, T_\infty]$, we first prove the non-existence of non-trivial two-cycles of F. That is, we show that $1 + F^{'}(I) > 0$. Notice that

$$\begin{aligned} 1 + F^{'}(I) &= 1 - \gamma\left(1 - \phi\left(\alpha\frac{I}{T_\infty}\right)\right) - \frac{\alpha\gamma}{T_\infty}\phi'\left(\alpha\frac{I}{T_\infty}\right)(T_\infty - I) + \gamma\sigma \\ &\geq 1 - \gamma + \gamma\sigma > 0. \end{aligned}$$

That is, $1 + F^{'}(I) \neq 0$ for $I \in (0, T_\infty]$. Suppose F has a non-trivial 2-cycle $\{I_1, I_2\}$, where I_1, $I_2 \in (0, T_\infty]$. Then $F(I_1) = I_2$ and $F(I_2) = I_1$, where $I_1 \neq I_2$. By the Mean Value Theorem, there exists a point J between I_1 and I_2 satisfying $F^{'}(J) = \frac{F(I_1) - F(I_2)}{I_1 - I_2} = -1$, a contradiction to $1 + F^{'}(J) > 0$. Hence, F has no non-trivial 2-cycles in $[0, T_\infty]$. Applying the results of Cull [16], McCluskey and Muldowney [30], the non-existence of non-trivial two-cycles of F implies the global stability of the positive fixed point I^* in $(0, T_\infty]$. That is, if $\Re_0 > 1$ then $\lim_{t\to\infty} I(t) \geq I^*$ whenever $T_\infty \geq I(0) > 0$. This completes the proof of the theorem.

$\Re_0 = \frac{-\alpha\gamma\phi'(0)}{1-\gamma\sigma}$ is an increasing function of the transmission constant α. Consequently, high disease transmission among susceptible individuals can lead to disease invasion while low transmissions lead to disease extinction. An obvious way to decrease $\Re_0$ is to decrease the disease transmission. That is, transmission rate in susceptibles as well as the survival and recovery rates are critical parameters for the persistence or control of the disease in Model (6) whenever the total population is asymptotically constant. The relative sensitivities of $\Re_0$ to the recovery and survival rates satisfy

$$\frac{\frac{\partial \Re_0}{\partial \gamma}}{\frac{\partial \Re_0}{\partial \sigma}} = \frac{1}{\gamma^2} > 1.$$

Thus, in Model (6), $\Re_0$ is more sensitive to survival than to recovery.

Corollary 1. *Let the total population have the strong Allee effect, where the demographic dynamics under* f_γ *iterations are compensatory in* (t_∞, ∞), $\{0\}$ *is globally attracting in* $[0, t_\infty)$ *and* $\gamma = \gamma_1 = \gamma_2$.

(a) *If* $T(0) < t_\infty$, *then* $\lim_{t\to\infty} T(t) = I(t) = S(t) = 0$ *in Model (6).*
That is, small initial population sizes lead to extinction of the total population.
(b) *If* $T(0) > t_\infty$, *then* $\lim_{t\to\infty} T(t) = T_\infty > 0$ *in Model (6).*
That is, large initial population sizes lead to uniform persistence of the total population on a fixed point attractor.
(c) *If* $\Re_0 > 1$ *and* $T(0) > t_\infty$, *then Model (6) has a unique endemic equilibrium* I^* *such that* $\lim_{t\to\infty} I(t) = I^* > 0$ *whenever* $T(0) \geq I(0) > 0$.
That is, the infective population persists uniformly on a fixed point attractor.

Proof: Since $\{0\}$ is globally attracting in $[0, t_\infty)$ under f_γ iterations, $T(0) < t_\infty$ implies that $\lim_{t\to\infty} T(t) = 0$. $T(t) = S(t) + I(t)$ and $T(t) = 0$ imply $I(t) = S(t) = 0$. By compensatory dynamics in (t_∞, ∞), we have $\lim_{t\to\infty} T(t) = T_\infty > 0$. Now, proceed exactly as in the proof of Theorem (1) to establish the result.

The presence of the Allee effect in the total population guarantees the Allee effect in the infective population whenever $\Re_0 > 1$ (Corollary 1). Hence, disease control measures should allow for the Allee effect in the infective population whenever there is evidence of the Allee effect in the total population. Now, we use the modified Beverton-Holt model and Corollary 1 to illustrate the Allee effect in a specific SIS discrete-time model.

Example 1. *In Model (6), let*

$$f(T) = \frac{\eta T^2}{1 + \lambda T^2} \text{ and } \phi\left(\frac{\alpha I}{T_\infty}\right) = e^{-\frac{\alpha I}{T_\infty}},$$

where

$$\eta = 2,\ \lambda = 1,\ \alpha = 10,\ \gamma = 0.1 \text{ and } \sigma = 0.5.$$

With our choice of the Modified Beverton-Holt function f, the map f_γ has compensatory dynamics in the open interval $(0.627, \infty)$, where the origin is locally attracting. That is, Example 1 has the strong Allee effect and the population dynamics are compensatory in (t_∞, ∞), where $t_\infty = 0.627$, $T_\infty = 1.595$ and $\Re_0 = 10.526$. By Corollary 1, $\Re_0 > 1$ implies that $\lim_{t\to\infty} I(t) = 0.014$, and the infective population persists whenever the initial total population size is bigger than 0.627. However, the infective population goes extinct whenever the initial total population size is smaller than 0.627. That is, a strong Allee effect in the demographic equation implies the strong Allee effect in the $I - equation$ whenever $\Re_0 > 1$.

4.2. Geometric growth. When $f(T(t)) = \mu T(t)$, then new recruits arrive at the constant per-capita birth rate μ and the total population in Model (1) is under geometric growth. Next, we use proportions to study Model (6) under geometric growth. That is, we introduce the new variables

$$s(t) = \frac{S(t)}{T(t)},$$

and

$$i(t) = \frac{I(t)}{T(t)}.$$

In the new variables, Model (6) with $f(T(t)) = \mu T(t)$ and $\gamma = \gamma_1 = \gamma_2$ becomes

$$\left.\begin{array}{lcl} s(t+1) & = & \frac{\mu}{(\gamma+\mu)} + \frac{\gamma}{(\gamma+\mu)}\phi\left(\alpha i(t)\right)s(t) + \frac{\gamma}{(\gamma+\mu)}(1-\sigma)i(t), \\ i(t+1) & = & \frac{\gamma}{(\gamma+\mu)}\left(1-\phi\left(\alpha i(t)\right)\right)s(t) + \frac{\gamma\sigma}{(\gamma+\mu)}i(t). \end{array}\right\} \tag{11}$$

Since

$$s(t) + i(t) = 1$$

for all t, all solutions of Model (11) are on the invariant line

$$\{(s,i) \in [0,\infty) \times [0,\infty) \mid s + i = 1\}.$$

Using the substitution $s = 1 - i$, the i-equation in Model (11) reduces to the "one-dimensional" difference equation

$$i(t+1) = \frac{\gamma}{(\gamma+\mu)}\left(1-\phi\left(\alpha i(t)\right)\right)\left(1-i(t)\right) + \frac{\gamma\sigma}{(\gamma+\mu)}i(t) \tag{12}$$

where $i(t) \leq 1$ for all $t \in \{0,1,2,...\}$. Using "linearization" technique in Equation (12), at the disease free equilibrium point $i_\infty = 0$, we obtain that

$$i(t+1) \approx \frac{\gamma}{(\gamma+\mu)}\left(-\alpha\phi'(0) + \sigma\right)i(t).$$

Hence, the basic reproductive number for Model (11) is

$$\Re_0 = \frac{-\alpha\gamma\phi'(0)}{(1-\gamma)\left(\Re_d - 1\right) + (1-\gamma\sigma)}.$$

When $\Re_d = 1$, then the demographic effects disappear and $\Re_0$ reduces to

$$\Re_0 = \frac{-\alpha\gamma\phi'(0)}{1-\gamma\sigma}.$$

As in the case of bounded asymptotic growth (Theorem 1), we show that if $\Re_0 > 1$, then the proportion of infectives in the total population persists uniformly on a positive endemic equilibrium while if $\Re_0 < 1$ the proportion of infectives in the total population decreases to zero; regardless of initial population sizes. We summarize these results in the following theorem.

Theorem 2. *Let*

$$f(T(t)) = \mu T(t)$$

in Model (1), where $\gamma = \gamma_1 = \gamma_2$.

(a) If $\Re_d > 1$ *and* $\Re_0 < 1$, *then* $\lim_{t\to\infty}(s(t), i(t)) = (1, 0)$ *in Model (11).*
That is, the proportion of infectives in the total population goes to zero while the total population is increasing at a geometric rate.
(b) If $\Re_d > 1$ *and* $\Re_0 > 1$, *then Model (11) has a unique endemic equilibrium* i^* *such that* $\lim_{t\to\infty} i(t) = i^* > 0$ *whenever* $T(0) \geq i(0) > 0$.
That is, the proportion of infectives in the total population persists uniformly on a fixed point attractor while the total population is increasing at a geometric rate.
(c) If $\Re_d < 1$ *and* $\Re_0 < 1$, *then* $\lim_{t\to\infty}(s(t), i(t)) = (1, 0)$ *in Model (11).*
That is, the proportion of infectives in the total population goes to zero while the total population is decreasing at a geometric rate.
(d) If $\Re_d < 1$ *and* $\Re_0 > 1$, *then Model (11) has a unique endemic equilibrium* i^* such that $\lim_{t\to\infty} i(t) \geq i^* > 0$ *whenever* $T(0) \geq i(0) > 0$.
That is, the proportion of infectives in the total population persists uniformly on a fixed point attractor while the total population is decreasing at a geometric rate.

Proof. Since $f(T(t)) = \mu N(t)$, we have $T(t+1) = (\gamma + \mu)T(t)$ and $\Re_d = \frac{\mu}{1-\gamma}$. Consequently, T increases geometrically when $\Re_d > 1$ while it decreases geometrically when $\Re_d < 1$. To establish the result, we prove that if in addition $\Re_0 < 1$, then all solutions $(s(t), i(t))$ of Model (11) converge to the disease-free equilibrium point $(1, 0)$ as $t \to \infty$. However, if $\Re_0 > 1$ we proceed exactly as in the proof of Theorem 1 to prove that as $t \to \infty$ all positive solutions $(s(t), i(t))$ of Model (11) converge to a unique endemic equilibrium, $(s^*, i^*) \in (0, \infty) \times (0, \infty)$.

For the proof of this result, define

$$F : [0, 1] \to [0, 1]$$

by

$$F(i) = \frac{\gamma}{(\gamma + \mu)}(1 - \phi(\alpha i))(1 - i) + \frac{\gamma\sigma}{(\gamma + \mu)}i.$$

Now, proceed exactly as in the proof of Theorem 1 to establish the result.

5. Overcompensatory dynamics in SIS models

Model (1), the discrete-time demographic equation, is capable of supporting periodic or chaotic dynamics. In [10-13], Castillo-Chavez and Yakubu showed complex dynamics in Model (1) where new recruits are subject to *overcompensatory* dynamics and are governed by the Smith-Slatkin model. If new recruits are governed by the classic Ricker model (Equation (5)), then Model (1) becomes

$$T(t+1) = T(t)e^{r-N(t)} + \gamma T(t), \tag{13}$$

where the inherent intrinsic growth rate $r > 0$. In this section, we use the Ricker model to illustrate complex dynamics in Model (1) and the SIS model, Model (8). In particular, we numerically illustrate that the demographics dynamics drive the disease dynamics whenever $\Re_0 > 1$.

When

$$0 < r < \frac{2}{1-\gamma} + \ln(1 - \gamma),$$

the total population in Model (13) is asymptotically constant and assumes the positive steady state,

$$T_\infty = r - \ln(1 - \gamma).$$

If in addition $\Re_0 > 1$, then the infective population persists uniformly on a globally attracting positive fixed point while if $\Re_0 < 1$ the infective population goes extinct (Theorem 1). However, as r increases past $\frac{2}{1-\gamma} + \ln(1-\gamma) > 0$, the dynamics are overcompensatory and the positive fixed point undergoes period-doubling bifurcations route to chaos (see FIG. 5).

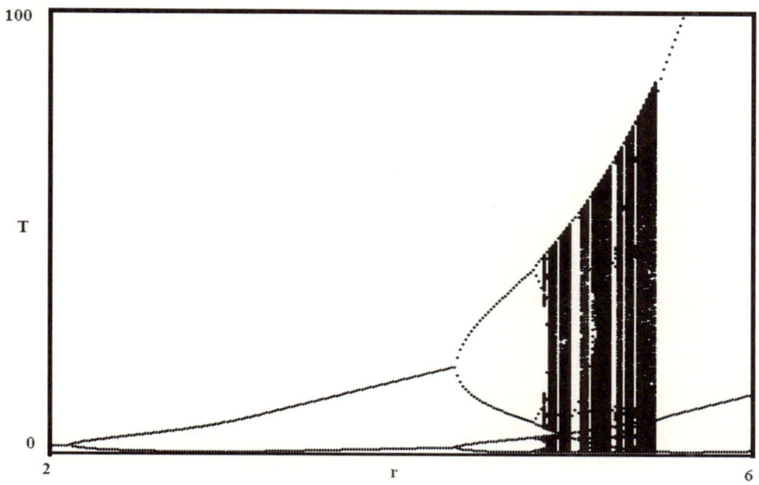

FIGURE 5. In Model (1), the total population undergoes period-doubling bifurcation route to chaos as r is varied between 2 and 6, where $f(T) = Te^{r-T}$ and $\gamma = 0.1$. On the horizontal axis, $2 \leq r \leq 6$ and on the vertical axis, $0 \leq T \leq 100$.

Elaydi and Yakubu proved that non-trivial periodic orbits of autonomous models such as Models (1) and (6) are never globally attracting [18]. That is, when the dynamics are overcompensatory and the total population is on either a cyclic (non-chaotic) or a chaotic attractor, then the ultimate disease outcome depends on initial population sizes; with and without the strong Allee effect.

In Example 2, we demonstrate that when the infective population is non-zero and the demographic T-dynamics are overcompensatory, then the T-dynamics "drive" both the S-dynamics and I-dynamics (see FIG. 5-7).

Example 2. *In Model (2), let*

$$f(T) = Te^{r-T} \text{ and } \phi\left(\alpha\frac{I}{T_\infty}\right) = e^{-\alpha\frac{I}{T_\infty}},$$

where

$$2 \leq r \leq 6,\ \alpha = 10,\ \gamma = \gamma_1 = \gamma_2 = 0.1 \text{ and } \sigma = 0.5.$$

In Example 2, the recruitment function is the Ricker model and infection is modeled as a Poisson process [1-2, 10-13]. With our choice of the Ricker function f, the map f_γ has overcompensatory dynamics in the open interval $(0,\infty)$, where the Allee effect is missing. When $r = 2.0$, then $T_\infty = 2.105$ and $\Re_0 = 10.526 > 1$. As predicted by Theorem 1, Model (8) has the endemic equilibrium $(2.087, 0.018)$ and the disease persists on a fixed point attractor. As r is varied between 2 and 6, FIG. 5-7 show that both the S-dynamics and I-dynamics follow the T-dynamics as it undergoes period-doubling bifurcations route to chaos. However, $T = S+I$ implies that the amplitudes of oscillations in the S-dynamics and I-dynamics are different from that of the T-dynamics whenever the disease is endemic. In Example 2, the survival rate $\gamma = 0.1$ is much smaller than the recovery rate $(1-\sigma) = 0.5$, and the transmission constant is $\alpha = 10$. Our choice of parameters and the frequency-dependent escape Poisson function led to a large variation in S magnitude, $[0, 100]$ (Figure 6), and a small one in I magnitude, $[0, 0.05]$ (Figure 7).

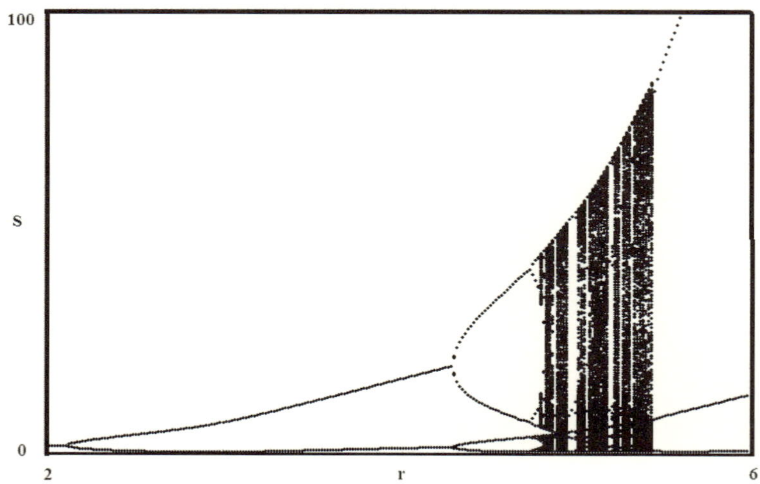

FIGURE 6. In Example 2, the susceptible population dynamics follows the total population dynamics and undergoes period-doubling bifurcation route to chaos as r is varied between 2 and 6. On the horizontal axis, $2 \le r \le 6$ and on the vertical axis, $0 \le S \le 100$.

6. Discrete-time SEIS epidemic model

In this section, we introduce a three epidemiological class *susceptible-exposed-infectious-susceptible* ($SEIS$) model. The three classes are: *susceptibles* (individuals that do not have the disease or have recovered from it), *exposed* (individuals who have the disease but do not transmit it), and *infectious* (individuals who have

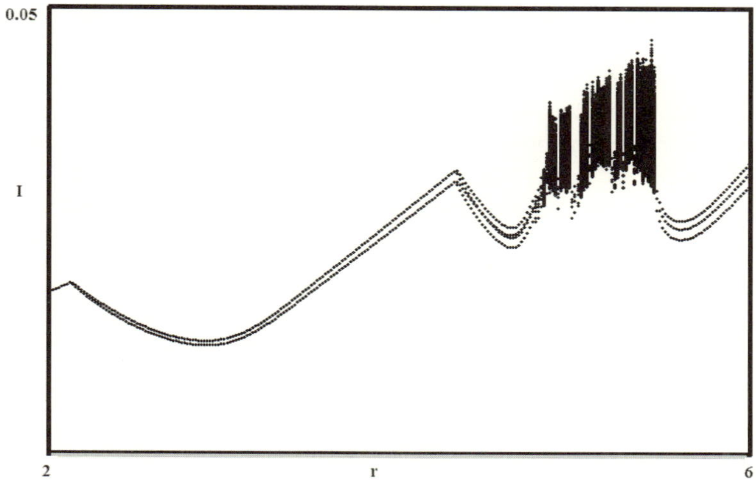

FIGURE 7. In Example 2, the infective population dynamics follows the total population dynamics and undergoes period-doubling bifurcation route to chaos as r is varied between 2 and 6. On the horizontal axis, $2 \leq r \leq 6$ and on the vertical axis, $0 \leq I \leq 0.05$.

the disease and transmit it). The dynamics of the total population size in generation t, denoted by $T(t) \equiv S(t) + E(t) + I(t)$, is governed by Model (1), where $E(t)$ denotes the population of exposed; as in Model (6), $S(t)$ denotes the population of susceptibles and $I(t)$ denotes the population of infected, assumed infectious; and, $T_\infty \equiv \lim_{t\to\infty} T(t)$ denotes the demographic steady state for the total population whenever it exists. Individuals are assumed to survive with constant probability γ (die with probability $1-\gamma$) each generation, and then change class (or not); that is, the demographic dynamics happen before the disease dynamics. The probability that an exposed individual stay exposed is σ, and δ is the probability that an infected individual does not recover. As in Model (6), it is assumed that susceptible individuals become exposed with probability $1 - \phi$ per generation (remain susceptible with non-constant probability function ϕ), where $\phi \equiv \phi(\alpha \frac{I(t)}{T(t)})$ is a frequency dependent monotone concave map with $\phi(0) = 1; \phi' < 0$ (that is, the probability that a susceptible does not become exposed decreases), $\phi'' \geq 0$ for, and $\alpha > 0$. To simplify the analysis, we assume that the disease is not lethal and does not give partial or permanent immunity (that is, an infectious individual becomes susceptible to the disease again after treatment). Also, we assume that a susceptible individual has to be in the exposed class before becoming infectious. Similarly, an exposed individual must become infectious before recovering and becoming susceptible. These assumptions and notation lead to the following discrete-time single

SEIS disease transmission model.

$$\left.\begin{array}{rcl} S(t+1) & = & f(T(t)) + \gamma\phi(\alpha\frac{I(t)}{T(t)})S(t) + \gamma(1-\delta)I(t), \\ E(t+1) & = & \gamma(1-\phi(\alpha\frac{I(t)}{T(t)}))S(t) + \gamma\sigma E(t), \\ I(t+1) & = & \gamma(1-\sigma)E(t) + \gamma\delta I(t). \end{array}\right\} \quad (14)$$

Model (14) was studied by Arreola *et al.* at the Mathematical and Theoretical Biology Institute of Cornell University summer undergraduate research program under our supervision [5]. As in the SIS model, it is possible to use Model (14) to investigate disease transmission dynamics in species that exhibit compensatory and overcompensatory population dynamics with and without the strong Allee effect.

6.1. Geometric growth in SEIS model. We assume that new recruits arrive at the positive per-capita rate μ per generation, that is, the recruitment function is $f(T(t)) = \mu T(t)$. Consequently, $T(t) = (\mu+\gamma)^t T(0)$ (that is population is under geometric growth) and recall that the demographic basic reproductive number is defined by

$$\Re_d = \frac{\mu}{1-\gamma}.$$

Let $x(t) = \frac{S(t)}{T(t)}$, $y(t) = \frac{E(t)}{T(t)}$ and $z(t) = \frac{I(t)}{T(t)}$. In the new variables, Model (14) reduces to the following system of three nonlinear difference equations.

$$\left.\begin{array}{rcl} x(t+1) & = & (1-\frac{\gamma}{\mu+\gamma}) + \frac{\gamma}{\mu+\gamma}\phi(\alpha z(t))x(t) + \frac{\gamma(1-\delta)}{\mu+\gamma}z(t), \\ y(t+1) & = & \frac{\gamma}{\mu+\gamma}(1-\phi(\alpha z(t)))x(t) + \frac{\gamma\sigma}{\mu+\gamma}y(t), \\ z(t+1) & = & \frac{\gamma(1-\sigma)}{\mu+\gamma}y(t) + \frac{\gamma\delta}{\mu+\gamma}z(t). \end{array}\right\} \quad (15)$$

Since $x(t) = 1 - y(t) - z(t)$, Model (14) reduces to the following system of two nonlinear equations.

$$\left.\begin{array}{rcl} y(t+1) & = & \frac{\gamma}{\mu+\gamma}(1-\phi(\alpha z(t)))(1-y(t)-z(t)) + \frac{\gamma\sigma}{\mu+\gamma}y(t), \\ z(t+1) & = & \frac{\gamma(1-\sigma)}{\mu+\gamma}y(t) + \frac{\gamma\delta}{\mu+\gamma}z(t). \end{array}\right\} \quad (16)$$

6.1.1. $\Re_0$ *for SEIS model.* For Model (15), we apply the next generation matrix approach in [3] to calculate the basic reproduction $\Re_0$. The unique disease-free equilibrium, DFE, is given by $\overline{x} = 1$, where $\overline{y} = \overline{z} = 0$. Let

$$\eta = \frac{\gamma}{\mu+\gamma}.$$

Ordering the states as (y, z, x) and calculating the Jacobian matrix J evaluated at the DFE, we obtain

$$J(0,0,1) = \begin{pmatrix} F+T & O \\ A & C \end{pmatrix},$$

where the submatrices are

$$F = \eta \begin{pmatrix} 0 & -\alpha\phi'(0) \\ 0 & 0 \end{pmatrix},$$

$$T = \eta \begin{pmatrix} \sigma & 0 \\ (1-\sigma) & \delta \end{pmatrix},$$

$$A = \begin{pmatrix} 0 & \eta((1-\delta)+\alpha\phi'(0)) \end{pmatrix},$$

$$C = \eta \text{ and } O = \begin{pmatrix} 0 \\ 0 \end{pmatrix}.$$

It is straightforward to see that the matrices F and T are nonnegative, $F+T$ is irreducible, the spectral radius of C and that of T are less than one. By Theorem 2.1 in [3], the basic reproductive number of Model (15), $\Re_0$, is the spectral radius of the product matrix $F(I-T)^{-1}$. Hence,

$$\Re_0 = \frac{-\eta^2 \alpha \phi'(0)(1-\sigma)}{(1-\eta\delta)(1-\eta\sigma)}.$$

Furthermore, the DFE of Model (15) is locally asymptotically stable if $\Re_0 < 1$ and unstable if $\Re_0 > 1$. That is, Theorem 2.1 of [3] gives the *local* stability of the DFE. However, one can show that it is *globally* stable whenever $\Re_0 < 1$ (that is, whenever it is locally asymptotically stable). The proof of this result uses the *Lyapunov function* theorem of La Salle [17]. To define a Lyapunov function, we consider the very general first order discrete-time model

$$x(t+1) = F(x(t)) \tag{17}$$

where the function $F : U \subset \Re^2 \to \Re^2$ is continuous. Let x_∞ be a fixed point of F.

A real valued function

$$V : U \subset \Re^2 \to \Re$$

is said to be a *Lyapunov function for System (17) on U* if V is continuous and $V(F(x)) \leq V(x)$ whenever both x and $F(x) \in U$. The Lyapunov function V is said to be *positive definite* at x_∞ if $V(x) > 0$ for all x in an open ball around x_∞, and V is said to be *negative definite* at x_∞ if $-V$ is positive definite at x_∞. We now state the Lyapunov function theorem of La Salle [17].

Theorem 3. *Suppose that V is a positive definite Lyapunov function defined on an open ball around a fixed point x_∞ of a continuous map $F : U \subset \Re^2 \to \Re^2$. Then, x_∞ is stable. If in addition, $V(F(x)) < V(x)$ whenever both $x \neq x_\infty$ and $F(x) \in U$, then x_∞ is asymptotically stable on U. Moreover, if $U = \Re^2$ and $V(x) \to \infty$ as $\mid x \mid \to \infty$, then x_∞ is globally asymptotically stable.*

The proof of Theorem 3 is in [17] and is omitted. The reduced $S-E-I-S$ epidemic model, Model (16), has a unique endemic equilibrium whenever $\Re_0 > 1$. We summarize these results in the following theorem.

Theorem 4. *If* $\Re_0 < 1$, *then* $\lim_{t\to\infty} y(t) = z(t) = 0$ and the disease-free equilibrium is globally stable *in Model (16). That is, the disease goes extinct. However, if $\Re_0 > 1$ then the disease-free equilibrium is unstable and Model (16) has a unique endemic equilibrium.*

Proof: Define the reproduction function of Model (16), $F : [0,1] \times [0,1] \to [0,1] \times [0,1]$, by

$$F(y,z) = \left(\frac{\gamma}{\mu+\gamma}(1-\phi(\alpha z))(1-y-z) + \frac{\gamma\sigma}{\mu+\gamma}y, \frac{\gamma(1-\sigma)}{\mu+\gamma}y + \frac{\gamma\delta}{\mu+\gamma}z\right).$$

Now, define $V : [0,1] \times [0,1] \to [0,1]$ by

$$V(y,z) = y - \frac{\eta\alpha\phi'(0)z}{1-\eta\delta}$$

where $\eta = \frac{\gamma}{\mu+\gamma}$. We will show that V is a Lyapunov function for F. V is continuous, $V(0,0) = 0$ and $V(y,z) > 0$ for all $(y,z) \neq (0,0)$ in $[0,1] \times [0,1]$.

Notice that $V(0,0) = 0$. Since $\eta\alpha\phi'(0) < 0$ and $1 - \eta\delta > 0$, $V(y,z) = y - \frac{\eta\alpha\phi'(0)z}{1-\eta\delta} > 0$ for all $(y,z) \neq (0,0)$ in $[0,1] \times [0,1]$. Furthermore,

$$\Re_0 = \frac{-\eta^2\alpha\phi'(0)(1-\sigma)}{(1-\eta\delta)(1-\eta\sigma)} < 1$$

is equivalent to the inequality

$$(\frac{\eta\sigma(1-\eta\delta) - \eta^2\alpha\phi'(0)(1-\sigma)}{1-\eta\delta}) < 1.$$

Next, we show that $V(F(y,z)) < V(y,z)$ for all points $(y,z) \in (0,1] \times (0,1]$. It is useful to note that since $\phi(0) = 1$, $\phi'(\alpha z) < 0$ and $\phi''(\alpha z) \leq 0$ we have

$$0 \leq 1 - \phi(\alpha z) \leq -\alpha\phi'(0)z.$$

$$\begin{aligned} V(F(y,z)) &= \eta((1-\phi(\alpha z))(1-y-z)+\sigma y) - \eta\tfrac{\eta\alpha\phi'(0)}{1-\eta\delta}((1-\sigma)y+\delta z) \\ &\leq \eta(1-\phi(\alpha z)) + \eta(\sigma - \tfrac{\eta\alpha\phi'(0)(1-\sigma)}{1-\eta\delta})y - \eta\tfrac{\eta\delta\alpha\phi'(0)z}{1-\eta\delta} \\ &\leq \eta(\sigma - \tfrac{\eta\alpha\phi'(0)(1-\sigma)}{1-\eta\delta})y - \eta\alpha\phi'(0)(1+\tfrac{\eta\delta}{1-\eta\delta})z \\ &\leq (\tfrac{\eta\sigma(1-\eta\delta)-\eta^2\alpha\phi'(0)(1-\sigma)}{1-\eta\delta})y - \tfrac{\eta\alpha\phi'(0)}{1-\eta\delta}z < V(y,z). \end{aligned}$$

By the Lyapunov function theorem of La Salle, the disease free equilibrium point is globally stable [15].

The endemic equilibrium (y_∞, z_∞) is a solution of the following pair of equations:

$$y_\infty = \eta((1-\phi(\alpha z))(1-y_\infty-z_\infty)+\sigma y_\infty) \tag{18}$$

$$z_\infty = \eta(1-\sigma)y_\infty + \eta\delta z_\infty \tag{19}$$

Let $\tau = \frac{\eta(1-\sigma)}{1-\eta\delta}$. Then Equation (19) reduces to

$$z_\infty = \tau y_\infty. \tag{20}$$

Substituting for z_∞ in Equation (18) we obtain

$$(1-\eta\sigma)y_\infty = \eta(1-\phi(\tau\alpha y_\infty))(1-(1+\tau)y_\infty). \tag{21}$$

Now, let

$$M(y_\infty) = (1-\eta\delta)y_\infty,$$

and

$$H(y_\infty) = \eta(1-\phi(\tau\alpha y_\infty))(1-(1+\tau)y_\infty).$$

Then the endemic equilibrium exists whenever the two functions, $H(y_\infty)$ and $M(y_\infty)$ intersect at $y_\infty \in (0,1)$.

The graph of $M(y_\infty)$ is a line through the origin with slope $(1-\eta\delta)$. The graph of $H(y_\infty)$ also passes through the origin, $H(y) \geq 0$ and $\lim_{y\to\infty} H(y) = -\infty$. As a result, we have at least one endemic equilibrium whenever $M^{'}(0) < H^{'}(0)$. That is, whenever

$$(1-\eta\sigma) < -\eta\tau\alpha\phi'(0).$$

Therefore, an endemic equilibrium exists when

$$\Re_0 = \frac{-\eta\tau\alpha\phi'(0)}{(1-\eta\sigma)} > 1.$$

For uniqueness, observe that whenever y_∞ exists it is in the open interval $(0,1)$, and $M(y_\infty) > 0$. Thus, we must have $H(y_\infty) > 0$. This gives rise to

$$0 < 1 - (1+\tau)y_\infty \text{ or } y_\infty < \frac{1}{1+\tau} < 1.$$

$H^{''}(y_\infty) < 0$ implies that $H(y_\infty)$ is concave down and $H^{'}(y_\infty)$ is decreasing. This gives the uniqueness of y_∞.

As in Model (6), an obvious way to decrease $\Re_0$ is to decrease the disease transmission in Model (16). The sensitivity of $\Re_0$ to changes in the exposed probability σ is

$$\frac{\partial \Re_0}{\partial \sigma} = \frac{\alpha(1-\eta)\eta^2\phi'(0)}{(1-\eta\delta)(1-\eta\sigma)^2} < 0.$$

Thus, $\Re_0$ decreases (respectively, increases) with increasing (respectively, decreasing) values of σ. However, the sensitivity of $\Re_0$ to changes in the "not recovered" probability δ is

$$\frac{\partial \Re_0}{\partial \delta} = -\frac{\alpha(1-\sigma)\eta^3\phi'(0)}{(1-\eta\sigma)(1-\eta\delta)^2} > 0$$

and the sensitivity of $\Re_0$ to changes in the survival probability γ is

$$\frac{\partial \Re_0}{\partial \gamma} = -\frac{\alpha(1-\sigma)\eta(1-\eta)^2\left(2-\eta\sigma-\eta\delta\right)\phi'(0)}{(1-\eta\sigma)^2(1-\eta\delta)^2\mu} > 0.$$

Therefore, the relative sensitivities of $\Re_0$ to the exposed and survival rates satisfy

$$\frac{\frac{\partial \Re_0}{\partial \gamma}}{\frac{\partial \Re_0}{\partial \delta}} = \frac{(1-\eta)^2\left(2-\eta\sigma-\eta\delta\right)}{(1-\eta\sigma)\mu\eta^2}.$$

Thus, $\Re_0$ is more sensitive to survival than to disease exposure if

$$\gamma < \sqrt{\mu} \text{ and } \sigma < \frac{(1-\eta)^2\left(2-\eta\delta\right)-\mu\eta^2}{\eta\left((1-\eta)^2-\mu\eta^2\right)},$$

which is true for malaria in children of most of the malaria endemic geographic regions of Africa.

Now, we use a specific example to illustrate the impact of increasing values of the transmission constant α on disease persistence or extinction in Model (16).

Example 3. *In Model (16), let*

$$\phi\left(\alpha z\right) = e^{-\alpha z}$$

where

$$\alpha \in [200, 300],\ \gamma = \delta = 0.1,\ \mu = 1 \text{ and } \sigma = 0.5.$$

In Example 3, $\gamma = 0.1 < \sqrt{\mu} = 1$ and $\sigma = 0.5 < \frac{(1-\eta)^2(2-\eta\delta)-\mu\eta^2}{\eta((1-\eta)^2-\mu\eta^2)} = 22.01$. Thus, with our choice of constants, $\Re_0$ is more sensitive to survival than to disease exposure. Furthermore, $\alpha < 228.9$ implies $\Re_0 < 1$ and $\alpha > 228.9$ implies $\Re_0 > 1$. As predicted by Theorem 4, Figure 8 shows that $\{(0,0)\}$ is asymptotically stable when $\alpha < 228.9$. That is, the disease goes extinct when $\Re_0 < 1$. In addition, Figure 8 shows that $(0,0)$ is unstable and the system has a stable unique endemic equilibrium when $\alpha > 228.9$. That is, the disease persists on a stable positive equilibrium when $\Re_0 > 1$.

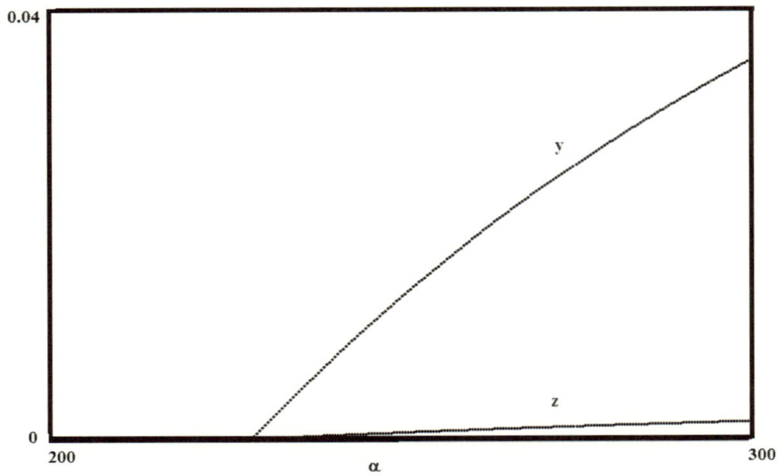

FIGURE 8. In Example 3, $\alpha < 228.9$ implies $\Re_0 < 1$ and $\alpha > 228.9$ implies $\Re_0 > 1$. On the horizontal axis, $200 \leq \alpha \leq 300$ and on the vertical axis, $0 \leq y, z \leq 0.04$.

7. Conclusion

Some animal populations experience strong fluctuations due to a variety of factors that include but are not limited to scramble intraspecific competition. In this article, we use a simple discrete-time SIS epidemic model to introduce a framework for investigating disease transmission dynamics in species that exhibit compensatory (contest competition) and overcompensatory (scramble competition) population dynamics with and without the strong Allee effect, where individuals (infected and susceptibles) have equal probability of surviving one generation. We compute the basic reproductive number $\Re_0$, and use it to predict the (uniform) persistence or extinction of the infective population, where the population dynamics are compensatory with or without the strong Allee effect. The transmission rate of susceptibles as well as the survival and recovery rates are critical model parameters for the persistence or control of the disease. The presence of the strong Allee effect in the total population implies its presence in the infective population whenever $\Re_0 > 1$.

In our simple SIS model, the *T-dynamics*, *S-dynamics* and *I-dynamics* are qualitatively the same when $\Re_0 > 1$. That is, the differences between the *S-dynamics* and *I-dynamics* are limited to their variation in "amplitude".

In addition, we use an SEIS model to demonstrate that the discrete-time epidemic model framework of Castillo-Chavez and Yakubu can be used to study a wide class of infectious diseases.

Acknowledgment

The author thanks the referees for useful comments and suggestions. This study is partially supported by funds from the NOAA-NEFSC in Woods Hole, MA and the National Science Foundation-Cornell University Contract #6103.

8. References

(1) L. Allen and A. M. Burgin, Comparison of deterministic and stochastic SIS and SIR models in discrete-time, *Math. Biosci.* 163, 1 (2000).

(2) L. Allen, Some discrete-time SI, SIR and SIS models, *Math. Biosci.* 124, 83 (1994).

(3) L. Allen and P. van den Driessche, The basic reproduction number is some discrete-time epidemic models, *J. Diff. Eqns. & Appl.*, 14(10-11), 1127-1147 (2008).

(4) R. M. Anderson and R. M. May, Infectious diseases of humans: Dynamics and control, *Oxford University, Oxford* (1992).

(5) Arreola, R., Crossa, A., Velasco, M. C. Discrete-time S-E-I-S models with dispersal between two patches, *Biometric Department, MTBI Cornell University Technical Report,* (2000).

(6) N. T. J. Bailey, The simple stochastic epidemic: a complete solution in terms of known functions, Biometrika 50, 235 (1963)

(7) M. Begon, J. L. Harper and C. R. Townsend, Ecology: individuals, populations and communities, *Blackwell Science Ltd* (1996).

(8) J. Best, C. Castillo-Chavez and A.-A. Yakubu, Hierarchical competition in discrete time models with dispersal, *Fields Institute Communications,* 36, 59-86 (2003).

(9) R. J. H. Beverton and S. J. Holt, On the dynamics of exploited fish populations, H. M. Stationery Off., London, *Fish. Invest.,* 2, 19 (1957).

(10) C. Castillo-Chavez and A. Yakubu, Dispersal, disease and life-history evolution, *Math. Biosc.,* 173, 35-53 (2001).

(11) C. Castillo-Chavez and A. Yakubu, Epidemics on attractors, *Contemporary Math.,* 284, 23-42 (2001).

(12) C. Castillo-Chavez and A. Yakubu, Discrete-time S-I-S models with complex dynamics, *Nonlin. Anal. TMA,* 47(7), 4753-4762 (2001).

(13) C. Castillo-Chavez and A. A.Yakubu, Intraspecific competition, dispersal and disease dynamics in discrete-time patchy environments in: Carlos Castillo-Chavez with Sally Blower, Pauline van den Driessche, Denise Kirschner and Abdul-Aziz Yakubu (Ed.), *Mathematical Approaches For Emerging and Reemerging Infectious Diseases: An Introduction to Models, Methods and Theory,* Springer-Verlag, New York (2002).

(14) H. Caswell, Matrix population models: construction, analysis and interpretation, *Sinauer Associates Inc* (2001).

(15) K. L. Cooke and J. A. Yorke, Some equations modelling growth processes of gonorrhea epidemics, *Math. Biosc.,* 16, 75 (1973).

(16) P. Cull, Local and global stability for population models, *Biol. Cybern.*, 54, 141 (1986).

(17) S. N. Elaydi, Discrete Chaos. *Chapman & Hall/CRC,* Boca Raton, FL, 2000.

(18) S. N. Elaydi and A.-A. Yakubu, Global Stability of Cycles: Lotka-Volterra Competition Model With Stocking, *J. Diff. Equations Appl. 8(6), 537-549 (2002).*
(19) P. W. Ewald, Evolution of infectious disease, *Oxford University*, Oxford, NY (1994).
(20) J. E. Franke and A.-A. Yakubu, Discrete-Time SIS Epidemic Model In a Seasonal Environment, *SIAM J. Appl. Math.,* Vol 66, No. 5, 1563-1587 (2006).
(21) J. E. Franke and A.-A. Yakubu, Disease-Induced Mortality In Density-Dependent Discrete-Time SIS Epidemic Models, *J. Math. Biol.,* 57, 755-790 (2008).
(22) K. P. Hadeler and P. van den Driessche, Backward bifurcation in epidemic control, *Math. Biosc.*146, 15 (1997).
(23) M. P. Hassell, The dynamics of competition and predation, *Studies in Biol.* 72, The Camelot Press Ltd. (1976).
(24) M. P. Hassell, J. H. Lawton and R. M. May, Patterns of dynamical behavior in single species populations, *J. Anim. Ecol.* 45, 471-486 (1976).
(25) V. L. Kocic and G. Ladas, Global behavior of nonlinear difference equations of higher order with applications, *Mathematics and its Applications,* 256, Kluwer Academic Publishers Group, Dordrecht, 1993.
(26) M. S. Kulenovic and A.-A. Yakubu, Compensatory versus overcompensatory dynamics in density-dependent Leslie models, *J. Diff. Eqns. & Appl.*, 10(13-15), 1251-1265 (2004).
(27) R. M. May and G. F. Oster, Bifurcations and dynamic complexity in simple ecological models, *Amer. Naturalist* 110, 573-579 (1976).
(28) R. M. May, Simple mathematical models with very complicated dynamics, *Nature* 261, 459-469 (1977).
(29) R. M. May, Stability and complexity in model ecosystems, *Princeton University Press* (1974).
(30) C. C. McClusky and J. C. Muldowney, Bendixson-Dulac criteria for difference equations, *J. Dyn. Diff. Eqns.,* 10, 567 (1998).
(31) A. J. Nicholson, Compensatory reactions of populations to stresses, and their evolutionary significance, *Aust. J. Zool.* **2**, 1-65 (1954).
(32) K. R. Rios-Soto, C. Castillo-Chavez, M. G. Neubert, E. S. Titi and A. Yakubu, Epidemic spread in populations at demographic equilibrium,), Contemporary Mathematics, *AMS volume 410,* Mathematical Studies on Human Disease Dynamic: Emerging Paradigms and Challenges, 297-309 (2006).
(33) P. van den Driessche and J. Watmough, A simple SIS epidemic model with a backward bifurcation, *J. Math. Biol.*, 40, 525 (2000).
(34) A.-A. Yakubu, Allee effects in a discrete-time SIS epidemic model with infected newborns, *Journal of Difference Equations and Appl.*, Vol. 13, No. 4, 341-356 (2007).
(35) A.-A. Yakubu, Discrete-time Metapopulation Dynamics and Unidirectional Dispersal, *J. Diff. Eqns. & Appl.*, 9(7), 633-653 *(2003)*.
(36) A.-A. Yakubu and M. Fogarty, Spatially discrete metapopulation models with directional dispersal, *Math. Biosc.,* 204, 68-101 (2006).

(37) P. Yodzis, Introduction to Theoretical Ecology, *Harper & Row*, Publishers, New York (1989).
(38) X.-Q. Zhao, Asymptotic behavior for asymptotically periodic semiflows with applications, *Comm. Appl. Nonl. Anal.* 3, 43-66 (1996).

Howard University, Washington, DC 20059
E-mail address: ayakubu@howard.edu

DIMACS Series in Discrete Mathematics
and Theoretical Computer Science
Volume **75**, 2010

Introduction to Optimal Control for Discrete Time Models with an Application to Disease Modeling

Wandi Ding and Suzanne Lenhart

ABSTRACT. This paper serves as an introduction to the theory of optimal control applied to systems of discrete time models with an emphasis on disease models. We outline the steps in solving such optimal control problems and discuss the necessary conditions. A simple disease example provides detailed methodology in charactering the optimal control through the use of Pontryagin's Maximum Principle. Numerical results are given to illustrate several cases.

1. Introduction

For many populations, births and growth occur in regular times each year (or each cycle). Discrete time models or difference equations are well suited to describe the life histories of organisms with discrete reproduction and/or growth. For example, the Beverton-Holt stock-recruitment [**7**] model for a population N_t at time t is

$$N_{t+1} = rN_t \left(1 + N_t \frac{r-1}{K}\right)^{-1}.$$

Another application involves a population which is divided into separate discrete age classes. At each time step, a certain proportion of each class may survive and enter the next age class. Individuals in the first age class originate through reproduction from other classes

$$\begin{aligned} N_1(t+1) &= f_1 N_1(t) + f_2 N_2(t) + f_3 N_3(t) \\ N_2(t+l) &= p_1 N_1(t) \\ N_3(t+1) &= p_2 N_2(t). \end{aligned}$$

For more background on discrete models, see the paper by Yakubu [**13**] in this volume and see the book by Caswell [**3**] and the edited volume by Abello and Cormode [**1**].

1991 *Mathematics Subject Classification.* Primary 39A10, 49N05 .
Key words and phrases. Optimal control, discrete time models, disease model.
The authors were supported in part by National Science Foundation Grants EF-0832858 (National Institute for Mathematical and Biological Synthesis) and ITR-04274710.

For examples involving disease models in discrete time, see [**2, 4, 6**]. We remark that in discrete time models, the order of events within a time step is crucial, so one should keep that in mind when building a discrete model. See [**5**] for an epidemic which is discrete in time and space and in which the order of events is important.

In an optimal control problem, one adjusts controls in a dynamic system to achieve a goal. The underlying system can have a variety of types of equations such as ordinary differential equations, partial differential equations, difference equations, stochastic differential equations or integrodifference equations. In this paper, we are considering only systems of equations which are discrete in time.

In control of a single difference equation, with discrete time steps, we denote $u = (u_0, u_1, \ldots, u_{T-1})$ as the control and $x = (x_0, x_1, \ldots, x_T)$ the state. Given x_0, the state function satisfies the difference equation modeling the scenario. The control affects the state difference equation,

$$x_{k+1} = g(x_k, u_k, k)$$

for $k = 0, 1, 2, \ldots, T-1$ and with x_0 as given. Both the control and the state usually affect the goal, which is called the objective functional. We seek to find an optimal control and corresponding state that achieve the maximum (or minimum) of our objective functional.

Let's start with a simple example of optimal control of a discrete time model to illustrate the ideas.

$$\begin{aligned} &\min_u \sum_{k=0}^{2} \frac{1}{2}\left[x_k^2 + Bu_k^2\right] \\ \text{subject to}\quad &x_{k+1} = x_k + u_k \qquad \text{for } k = 0, 1, 2, \\ &x_0 = 5. \end{aligned}$$

The state has 4 components, x_0, x_1, x_2, x_3 while the control has one fewer component, u_0, u_1, u_2. Here the goal is to minimize the square of the state terms and the square of the control terms. The coefficient B is a weight factor, that gives the relative importance of the two terms in the goal.

Now we formulate a control problem in more generality. Given a control $u = (u_0, u_1, \ldots, u_{T-1})$ and initial state x_0, the state equation is given by the difference equation

$$x_{k+1} = g(x_k, u_k, k)$$

for $k = 0, 1, 2, \ldots, T-1$. Note that the state has one more component than the control

$$x = (x_0, x_1, \ldots, x_T).$$

We have the following objective functional, which represents our goal:

$$J(u) = \phi(x_T) + \sum_{k=0}^{T-1} f(x_k, u_k, k).$$

The term, $\phi(x_T)$, represents a type of 'salvage' term; for example, one may want the population to be large at the final time T. The objective functional can be maximized or minimized over controls u. In the minimization case, the goal is to find an optimal control u^* such that

$$J(u^*) = \min_u J(u),$$

where the minimization is over a class of vectors with bounded components (with bounds specified to fit the situation.)

Necessary conditions, that an optimal control and corresponding state must satisfy, can be derived similarly to the case of ordinary differential equations, using a generalization of Pontryagin's Maximum Principle [**9**]. To see more detail about the derivation of the necessary conditions, see the book by Lenhart and Workman [**8**]. The key idea is introducing the adjoint function to attach the difference equation to the objective functional, resulting in the formation of a function called the Hamiltonian. This principle converts the problem of finding the control to optimize the objective functional subject to the state difference equation with initial condition to finding the control to optimize Hamiltonian pointwise (with respect to the control).

Now we have the Hamiltonian at each time step k, where our adjoint function is $\lambda = (\lambda_0, \lambda_1, \ldots, \lambda_T)$:

$$H_k = f(x_k, u_k, k) + \lambda_{k+1} g(x_k, u_k, k), \quad \text{for } k = 0, 1, \ldots, T-1.$$

Notice the indexing on the adjoint; it is one step ahead of the other terms. The necessary condition states that the Hamiltonian is maximized at each step with respect to the control u_k at the optimal control u_k^*. The adjoint equations and corresponding final time conditions (transversality conditions) are also given. If we do not have any constraints on our control, the necessary conditions are

$$\begin{aligned} \lambda_k &= \frac{\partial H_k}{\partial x_k} \\ \lambda_T &= \phi'(x_T^*) \\ \frac{\partial H_k}{\partial u_k} &= 0 \text{ at } u^*. \end{aligned}$$

Notice that the adjoint function has final time conditions while the state function has initial time conditions. Suppose that the controls are bounded, which is quite usual in biological examples. Suppose $a \leq u_k \leq b$ for each k, then these bounds need to be imposed after you solve the optimality equation

$$\frac{\partial H_k}{\partial u_k} = 0 \text{ at } u^*$$

for each component of the control at each time step.

2. Simple Illustrative Example

Next we consider a simple example [**8**] to illustrate the solution technique. Our objective functional is

$$\begin{aligned} &\min_u \sum_{k=0}^{2} \frac{1}{2}\left[x_k^2 + u_k^2\right] \\ \text{subject to} \quad & x_{k+1} = x_k + u_k \qquad \text{for } k = 0, 1, 2, \\ & x_0 = 5. \end{aligned}$$

At each time step, the control u_k is the input, that will result in the growth or decline of the state. What optimal control is expected? We are seeking to minimize the state and the size of control. We expect the optimal control to be negative or zero.

Starting with the Hamiltonian,

$$H_k = \frac{1}{2}\left[x_k^2 + u_k^2\right] + \lambda_{k+1}(x_k + u_k),$$

our necessary conditions are:

$$\begin{aligned}
\lambda_k &= \frac{\partial H_k}{\partial x_k} = x_k + \lambda_{k+1} \quad \text{for } k = 0, 1, 2,\\
\lambda_3 &= 0,\\
0 &= \frac{\partial H_k}{\partial u_k} = u_k + \lambda_{k+1} \quad \text{at } u_k^*.
\end{aligned}$$

Thus the optimal control satisfies

$$u_k = -\lambda_{k+1},$$

which gives

$$x_{k+1} = x_k - \lambda_{k+1} \quad \text{for } k = 0, 1, 2.$$

Our transversality condition is

$$\lambda_3 = 0,$$

since we do not have a salvage term, meaning there is no dependence on the state at the final time in the objective functional.

Combining above conditions yields

$$x_3 = x_2$$

and four equations in $x_1, x_2, \lambda_1, \lambda_2$,

$$x_1 = 5 - \lambda_1, \qquad x_2 = x_1 - \lambda_2$$

$$\lambda_1 = x_1 + \lambda_2, \qquad \lambda_2 = x_2.$$

After solving these algebraic equations, the optimal state values are

$$x_1^* = 2, x_2^* = 1, x_3^* = 1$$

and the optimal control values are

$$u_0^* = -3, u_1^* = -1, u_2^* = 0.$$

We see in this simple case, only the controls are making changes in the states.

3. System Case

Next we state the necessary conditions in the case of a system of difference equations:

$$x_{j,k+1} = g_j(x_{1,k}, \ldots, x_{n,k}, u_{1,k}, \ldots, u_{m,k}, k),$$

with

$$x_j = (x_{j,0}, x_{j,1}, \ldots, x_{j,T}).$$

for $k = 0, 1, 2, \ldots, T-1, j = 1, 2, \ldots, n$. Note that k is the index for the time steps and j is the index for the states. There are m controls, n states, and T time steps. Define the objective functional as

$$J(u) = \phi(x_{1,T}, \ldots, x_{n,T}) + \sum_{k=0}^{T-1} f(x_{1,k}, \ldots, x_{n,k}, u_{1,k}, \ldots, u_{m,k}, k)$$

Now we have one adjoint variable for each state variable and form the Hamiltonian,

$$\begin{aligned} H_k &= f(x_{1,k}, \ldots, x_{n,k}, u_{1,k}, \ldots, u_{m,k}, k) \\ &+ \sum_{j=1}^{n} \lambda_{j,k+1} g_j(x_{1,k}, \ldots, x_{n,k}, u_{1,k}, \ldots, u_{m,k}, k), \end{aligned}$$

we can obtain the necessary conditions,

$$\lambda_{j,k} = \frac{\partial H_k}{\partial x_{j,k}}$$

$$\lambda_{j,T} = \frac{\partial \phi}{\partial x_{j,T}}(x_{1,T}, \ldots, x_{n,T})$$

$$\frac{\partial H_k}{\partial u_{i,k}} = 0 \text{ at } (u^*_{1,k}, \ldots, u^*_{m,k}).$$

for $k = 0, 1, 2, \ldots, T-1, j = 1, 2, \ldots, n$ and $i = 0, 1, 2, \ldots, m$.

We illustrate the system case in the following disease example.

4. Disease Example

We illustrate the techniques of optimal control using a simple epidemic example. This volume contains many examples of epidemic models and the emphasis in this article is on control techniques.

Consider an SIR system, in which the state variables are S, susceptibles, I, infecteds and R, immune individuals. Our stae equations are:

$$\begin{aligned} S_{k+1} &= S_k(1-u_k) - \beta\Big(S_k(1-u_k)\Big)I_k, \\ I_{k+1} &= I_k + \beta S_k(1-u_k)I_k - d_2 I_k, \\ R_{k+1} &= R_k + u_k S_k, \end{aligned} \tag{4.1}$$

where $k = 1, 2, \ldots, T-1$, β is the transmission rate and d_2 is the additional death rate due to infection. The control variable is u with $0 \leq u_k \leq 1-d$, with $d > 0$. The control can be interpreted as the proportion to be vaccinated, so we can see that $u_k S_k$ individuals move from the susceptible class to the immune class at time step k. Notice the order of the events in this model. Here the vaccination happens first, meaning that a proportion of susceptibles $u_k S_k$ is moved from the susceptible class to the immune class. Then the interaction of the non-immune susceptibles with the infecteds, which is why the infectivity term has the format,

$$\beta S_k(1-u_k)I_k.$$

The remaining susceptibles, after the movement of the vaccinated susceptibles to the immune class,

$$S_k(1-u_k),$$

are interacting with the infecteds, I_k. Note that infected individuals have the disease and are able to transmit it.

Note that positivity of the components of a discrete model can be an issue in a discrete model. We are using a small number of time steps here since we are considering control actions reacting to an outbreak of a disease in short time. Thus the sizes of our parameters and the number of time steps insures the positivity of the S, I, R classes here.

The goal is to minimize our objective functional,

$$\sum_{k=1}^{T-1}(I_k + Bu_k^2 + B_1 u_k) + I_T,$$

where T is the final time. The constants B and B_1 are the cost coefficients. We are minimizing the number of infected individuals during the time steps $k = 1$ to $T-1$ and at the final time and also minimizing the cost of administering the control. We are assuming the cost of administering the control is quadratic for simplicity. See [**8**] for other formats of controls in objective functionals.

4.1. The adjoints. The Hamiltonian at time step k is

$$\begin{aligned} H_k = I_k + Bu_k^2 + B_1u_k &+ \lambda_{1,k+1}\Big(S_k(1-u_k) - \beta\Big(S_k(1-u_k)\Big)I_k\Big) \\ &+ \lambda_{2,k+1}\Big(I_k + \beta S_k(1-u_k)I_k - d_2 I_k\Big) \\ &+ \lambda_{3,k+1}\Big(R_k + u_k S_k\Big). \end{aligned} \tag{4.2}$$

The equations for the adjoint variables for $k = 1, 2, \ldots, T-1$ are

$$\begin{aligned} \lambda_{1,k} = \frac{\partial H_k}{\partial S_k} &= \lambda_{1,k+1}\Big(1 - u_k - \beta(1-u_k)I_k\Big) \\ &+ \lambda_{2,k+1}\Big(\beta(1-u_k)I_k\Big) + \lambda_{3,k+1}u_k, \end{aligned} \tag{4.3}$$

$$\begin{aligned} \lambda_{2,k} = \frac{\partial H_k}{\partial I_k} &= 1 + \lambda_{1,k+1}\Big(-\beta S_k(1-u_k)\Big) \\ &+ \lambda_{2,k+1}\Big(1 + \beta S_k(1-u_k) - d_2\Big) + \end{aligned} \tag{4.4}$$

$$\lambda_{3,k} = \frac{\partial H_k}{\partial R_k} = \lambda_{3,k+1}. \tag{4.5}$$

Our transersality conditions give at time T, we have $\lambda_{1,T} = \lambda_{3,T} = 0$, since S_T and R_T are not in the objective functional. But notice that $\lambda_{2,T} = 1$ since

$$\phi(I_T) = I_T \text{ and } \frac{\partial \phi}{\partial I} = 1.$$

For $k = 1, 2, \ldots, T-1$, the control characterization is derived from

$$\frac{\partial H_k}{\partial u_k} = 2Bu_k + B_1 + \lambda_{1,k+1}\Big(-S_k + \beta S_k I_k\Big) + \lambda_{2,k+1}\Big(-\beta S_k I_k\Big) + \lambda_{3,k+1}S_k = 0, \tag{4.6}$$

subject to the lower and upper bounds for u. For $k = 1, 2, \ldots, T-1$, the characterization becomes

$$u_k^* = \min\Big(1-d, \max\Big(0, [\lambda_{1,k+1r}(S_k - \beta S_k I_k) + \lambda_{2,k+1}(\beta S_k I_k) - \lambda_{3,k+1}S_k - B_1]/2B\Big)\Big).$$

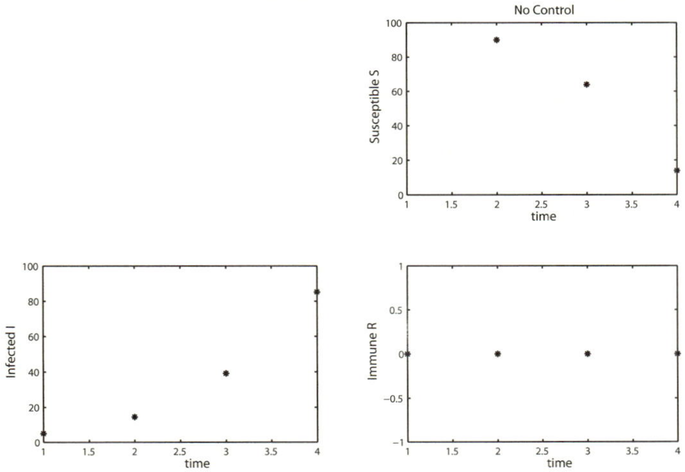

FIGURE 1. S, I, R without control

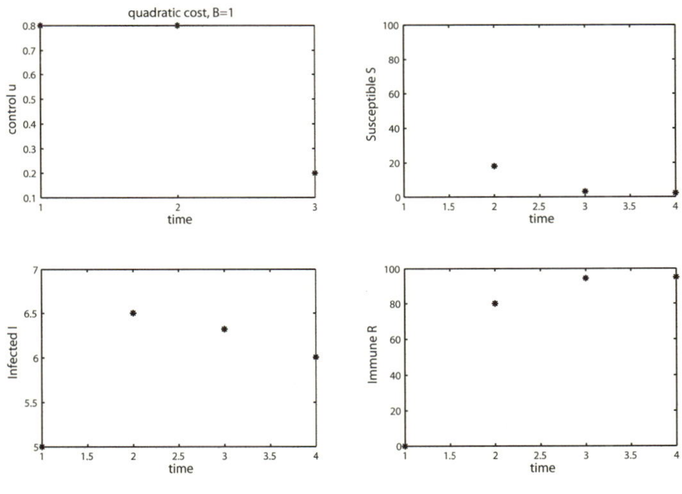

FIGURE 2. Case 1: S, I, R with $B = 1$

4.2. Numerical Examples. The optimality system consists of the state system, adjoint system, initial and final time conditions, and the control characterization. We solve the optimality system by an iterative method with forward solving of the state system followed by backward solving of the adjoint system. We start with an initial guess for the control at the first iteration and then before the next iteration, we update the control by using the characterization. We continued until convergence of successive iterates is achieved.

We illustrate two cases of changing of the parameters in the objective functional. Case 1. Quadratic Cost ($B_1 = 0$)

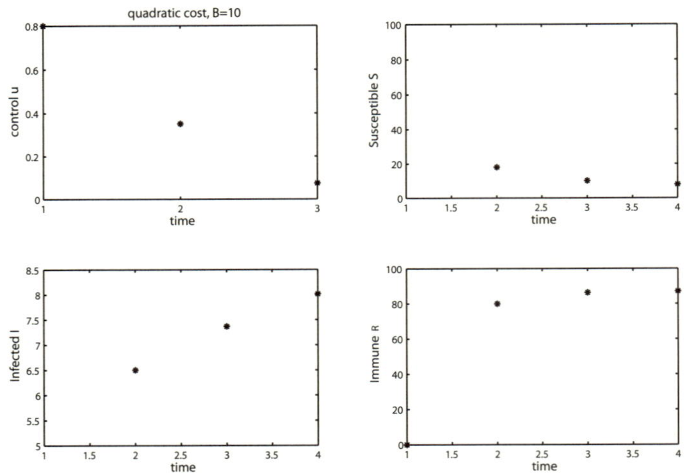

FIGURE 3. Case 1: S, I, R with $B = 10$

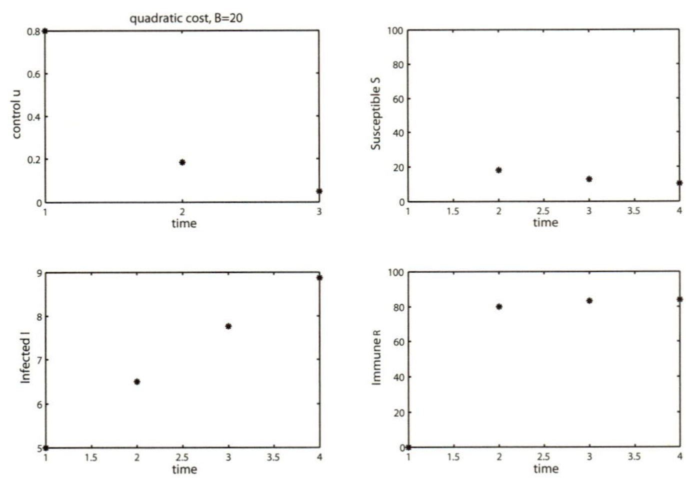

FIGURE 4. Case 1: S, I, R with $B = 20$

We choose $S(1) = 100, I(1) = 5, \beta = 0.02, d_2 = 0.1, d = 0.2$ and $T = 4$. First we give the numerical results without any control in Figure 1. Then we vary cost coefficient $B = 1, 10, 20, 50$ in J to see how it affects the control and the susceptible, infected and immune populations in Figures 2-5. We can see the number of infecteds are reduced significantly. As B gets bigger, it is more costly to apply the control, so the control effort is decreasing.

Case 2. Approximate Linear Cost

We still use the same parameters for $S(1), I(1), \beta, d_2, d$ and T. For Figure 6, we take $B = 0.01$ and $B_1 = 1$ in J to approximate the linear cost. The control for the first two time steps reaches the upper bound, then reduces to the lower bound

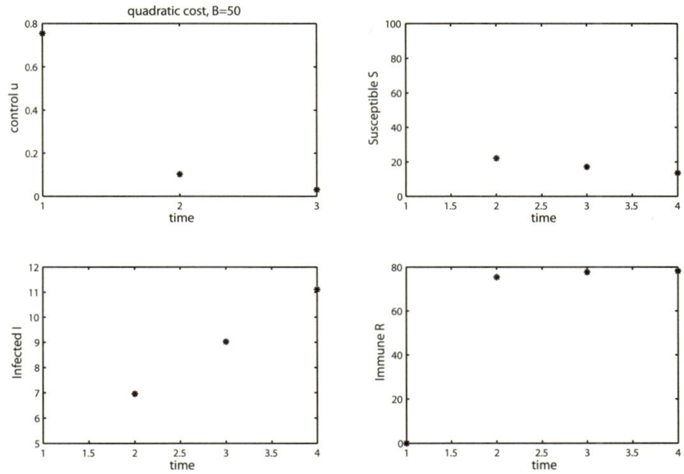

FIGURE 5. Case 1: S, I, R with $B = 50$

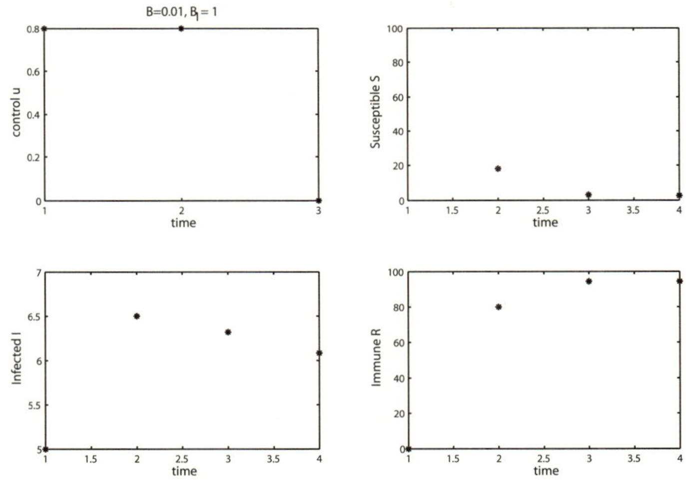

FIGURE 6. Case 2: S, I, R with $B = 0.01, B_1 = 1$

for the third time step. In Figure 7, we take $B_1 = 10, B = 0.01$ and see the control for the first time step reaches the upper bound, then reduces to the lower bound for the second and third time steps. So the control is a "bang-bang" control, which means the optimal control values are only at the upper and lower bounds. Note the differences in the optimal controls and the states between the two cases, illustrating that parameters in the objective functional make an impact.

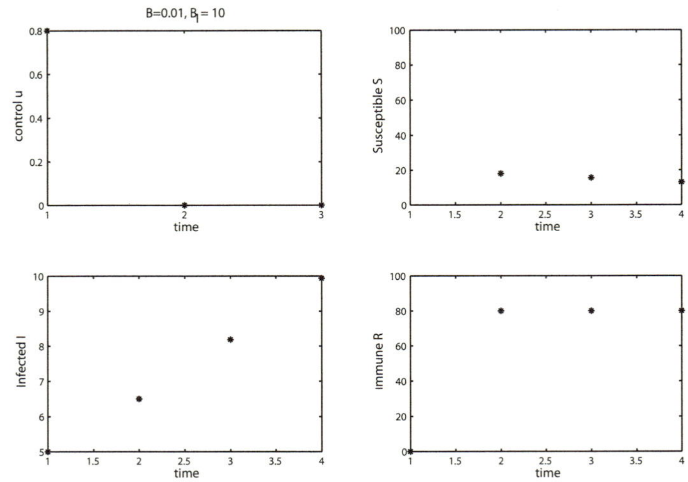

FIGURE 7. Case 2: S, I, R with $B = 0.01, B_1 = 10$

5. Conclusion

Here we have presented the techniques of optimal control on some simple examples of discrete models. Given a model with a control, the format of an optimal control depends on the format of the objective functional and the corresponding parameters. We illustrate in section 4 how changing parameters in an objective functional can affect the optimal controls.

For further examples of optimal control with discrete time, see [**10, 11, 12**].

References

[1] J. Abello and G. Cormode, editors, Discrete Methods in Epidiemology, DIMACS Series in Discrete Mathematics and Theoretical Computer Science, American Mathematical Society, Providence RI, 2006,

[2] L. J. S. Allen and D. A. Flores and R. K. Ratnayake and J. R. Herbold, Discrete-time deterministic and stochastic models for the spread of rabies, Applied Mathematics and Computation, 132 (2002), 132, 271–292.

[3] H. Caswell, Matrix Population Models: Construction, Analysis and Interpretation, Sinauer Press, Sunderland, MA 2001.

[4] C. Castillo-Chavez and A. Yakubu, Discrete time S-I-S models with complex dynamics, Nonlinear Analysis TMA, 47 (2001), 4753-4762.

[5] W. Ding, L. J. Gross, K. Langston, S. Lenhart and L. S. Real, Rabies in Raccoons: Optimal Control for a Discrete Time Model on a Spatial Grid, J. of Biological Dynamics 1(4), 2007, 379-393.

[6] J. E. Franke and A-A. Yakubu, Disease-induced mortality in density-dependent discrete-time SIS epidemic models, J. Math. Biol. 57 (2008), 755-780.

[7] M. Kot, Elements of Mathematical Ecology, Cambridge, MA 2001.

[8] S. Lenhart and J. Workman, Optimal Control Applied to Biological Models, Boca Raton, Chapmal Hall/CRC, 2007.

[9] L.S. Pontryagin, V.G. Boltyanskii, R.V. Gamkrelize, and E.F. Mishchenko, The Mathematical Theory of Optimal Processes, New York, Wiley, 1962.

[10] Sethi, S. P., and Thompson, G. L., *Optimal Control Theory: Applications to Management Science and Economics*, Kluwer, Boston, 2nd edition, 2000.

[11] A. Whittle, S. Lenhart and L. T. Gross, Optimal Control for Management of an Invasive Plant Species, Mathematical Biosciences and Engineering 4(1), 2007, 101-112.

[12] A. Whittle, S. Lenhart and J. White, Optimal Control of Gypsy Moth populations, the Bulletin of Mathematical Biology 70 (2008), 398-411.

[13] A-A. Yakubu, Introduction to discrete-time models, this volume to appear.

Department of Mathematical Sciences, Middle Tennessee State University, Murfreesboro, Tennessee 37132

E-mail address: wding@math.mtsu.edu

Department of Mathematics, University of Tennessee, Knoxville, Tennessee 37996

E-mail address: lenhart@math.utk.edu

DIMACS Series in Discrete Mathematics
and Theoretical Computer Science
Volume **75**, 2010

Incorporating stochasticity in simple models of disease spread

Jonathan Dushoff

As we have seen in earlier chapters, simple models of infectious diseases in homogeneous populations have produced many important insights. The most basic of these is the basic reproductive number R_0, and its corollaries: the population (or 'herd') immunity threshold; and the qualitative shape of the relationship between R_0, disease parameters and endemic levels of disease. Another key idea is the cyclic tendency of epidemic outbreaks, and the natural tendency of these oscillations to be damped.

Although such models have produced important insights, it is important to bear in mind that they are simple (albeit useful) approximations to a much more complex reality. Thus, it is also useful to consider what the key simplifications of these models are, and ways in which their predictions might change when various complications are added. Several such complications may be loosely grouped under the classification of "heterogeneities": populations in the simple models we have learned about are fundamentally homogeneous.

Examples of heterogeneities not accounted for in simple models include "parametric heterogeneity", "geographic heterogeneity" and "demographic heterogeneity." Parametric heterogeneity refers to individual differences in transmission parameters for a particular disease; for example, differences among individuals in contact rate, susceptibility to infection, or tendency to transmit disease. Starting with the work of Hethcote and Yorke [**11**], parametric heterogeneity has been shown to pervasively affect the relationship between risk factors and disease – on the whole, tending to make disease levels less sensitive to increases and decreases in risk [**8**].

Geographic heterogeneity refers to the geometry of interaction networks between people; people do not mix homogeneously, but instead mixing is structured by spatial location, social networks, and other factors. The effects of geographic heterogeneity on disease spread is an active research area, which is further divided (loosely) into spatial models (see, e.g., [**15**]) and network models (e.g.,[**4**]). This chapter will focus on demographic heterogeneity. A good source for further reading on this subject is [**1**].

This work was supported by the National Science and Engineering Research Council of Canada.

1. Modeling demographic heterogeneity

Demographic heterogeneity refers to the heterogeneity introduced simply by treating individuals as individuals. To see what this means, we first ask what happens in a classic, ODE model of disease, if we introduce a single infectious individual to a susceptible population. If $R_0 > 1$, after a short period of time, we deterministically find something like 1.1 infectious individuals, whereas if $Ro < 1$, after a short period of time we have 0.9 infectious individuals.

In reality, of course, a single infectious individual does not increase smoothly to 1.1 infectious individuals. Instead, the system will take a discrete jump, either to 2 infectious individuals or to 0. We cannot reasonably expect to specify a model of disease transmission in enough detail that we can predict exactly when the next event of each type will occur. Instead, simple models that include discrete events are fundamentally stochastic; even in theory we don't know when the next event will occur, nor even what it will be.

Thus, if we treat individuals as individuals, we necessarily introduce "demographic" stochasticity, defined as stochasticity caused by the existence of individual people and discrete events. Stochasticity may also operate at a larger scale; we refer to events outside our model that affect more than one person at a time as "environmental" stochasticity. In a model of disease spread in human populations, sources of environmental stochasticity would include weather and economic change, for example.

This is illustrated in Figure 1. The deterministic trajectory starts from a single introduction and increases smoothly to around 2.5 infectious individuals. In contrast, the stochastic trajectories move in discrete, unpredictable jumps. Some of them randomly increase to as high as 8 or 9 infectious individuals, while in one case, the disease goes extinct before the end of the week.

2. Describing a demographic model

Interestingly, there is a natural way of translating a simple ODE model directly into an analogous discrete-individual model. This being so, it is useful to investigate how the behavior and predictions SIR models are changed by the inclusion of this realistic effect.

To create a discrete-events model, we describe our system in terms of the *probability rates* of events happening. If the rate of event E is $r_E(t)$, the probability of the event occurring in the time interval $(t, t + dt)$ is $r_E(t)dt$. If the system is *Markovian*, $r_E(t)$ depends only on the state of the system at time t. If the system is *non-Markovian* $r_E(t)$ can depend (for example) on how long the system has been in a particular state.

The Markovian assumption allows us to specify the state of our system with a much smaller amount of information, but it can have unwanted consequences. In particular, assuming that residence in a particular state is independent of history is equivalent to assuming that the residence time in that state is exponentially distributed. This assumption is often strikingly unrealistic – for example, in a human population with exponentially distributed lifetimes and a mean lifetime of 70 years, 5% of people will live to be over 200 years old! Thus, we must question the extent to which our results depend on this extremely convenient, but unrealistic, assumption.

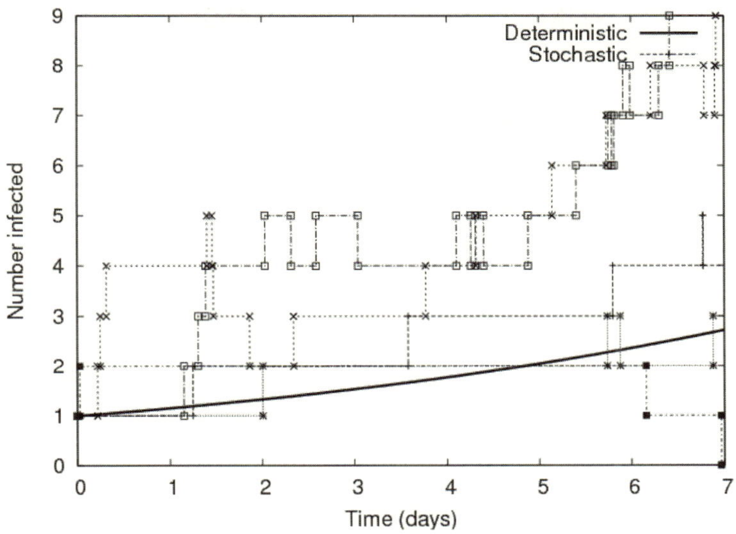

FIGURE 1. The deterministic trajectory from a simple SIR model (2.1) is compared with several trajectories from an analogous stochastic model (Table 1). Parameters are $R_0 = 2$, $\rho = 0.01$. The disease generation time is 7 days.

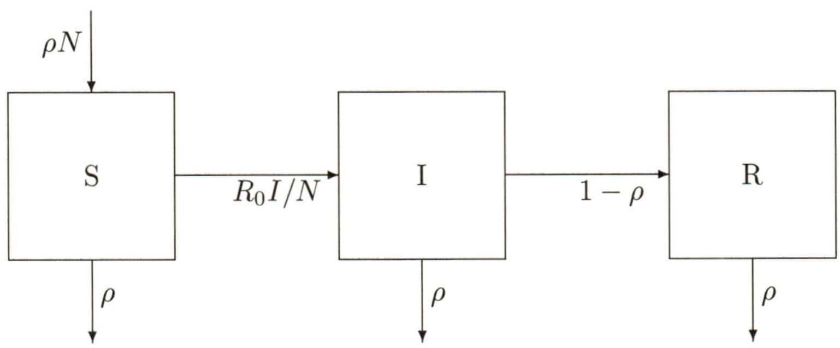

FIGURE 2. A diagrammatic model of the spread of an infectious disease. Individuals may be **S**usceptible, **I**nfectious, or **R**esistant. Susceptible individuals move to the infectious category at a rate proportional to the number of infectious individuals present. Births, deaths and recovery from disease into the Resistant class occur at constant rates.

Figure 2 shows a diagram of an infectious disease model. By counting time in units of infectious disease generations, and populations as fractions of the total population, we can reduce this simple, but by no means trivial, model to only two parameters, the basic reproductive number R_0; and ρ, which represents the ratio between the two fundamental time scales of the model: the average infectious period, and the average duration of immunity following infection.

$$\begin{aligned} \dot{x} &= \rho(1 - x) - R_0 xy \\ \dot{y} &= R_0 xy - y \end{aligned} \tag{2.1}$$

Event	**transition**	**rate**	**Effect** (S, I)
Infection	$S \to I$	R_0SI/N	$(-1, 1)$
Recovery	$I \to R$	$(1-\rho)I$	$(0, -1)$
Rebirth	$R \to S$	$\rho(N-S-I)$	$(1, 0)$
Rebirth	$I \to S$	ρI	$(1, -1)$

TABLE 1. We specify a demographic model by describing the events that can occur; the way that the rates of these events depend on the state of the system; and the effect of these events on the variables that describe the state of our system.

Here, x; y refer to the proportion of the population infectious; susceptible. Since we assume a constant population, we are free to drop the equation for the proportion in the removed class. The dots refer to derivatives with respect to time.

Table 1 shows how we re-cast the model in Figure 2 as a demographic model, reflecting a population composed of discrete individuals. Each arrow represents an event that can occur stochastically, affecting a discrete individual, with a probabilistic rate that corresponds to the deterministic rate in (2.1). We will discuss below how this stochastic model of the disease system in Figure 2 can be either simulated, or analyzed. Note that the model given by Table 1 cannot be parameterized as simply as the one in (2.1); if individuals are discrete, the population size N will fundamentally affect the behavior of the model.

The demographic model is an exact analogue of the deterministic one, both conceptually, and in the technical sense that as the population size $N \to \infty$ in the demographic model, its behavior converges to that of the deterministic model. Although we can convert a demographic model to a deterministic model simply by allowing the population size to go to infinity, translating a deterministic model to a demographic one requires us to make choices about how to group the terms in our model into events. For example, the two transmission terms in our simple model – the contribution of $-R_0xy$ to $\dot{x}$, and the contribution of R_0xy to $\dot{y}$ – clearly refer to the same event: an individual moves from the susceptible class to the infectious class. Less clear is the interpretation of birth and death terms. We could choose to interpret the model (2.1) as having independent birth and death events – and thus, stochastic fluctuations in population size – or we can choose (as we do in Table 1) to link these birth and death events, and keep the population constant.

Having described a model that takes demographic stochasticity into account, we can now begin to ask questions about the expected effects of demographic stochasticity on disease dynamics. In particular, we can now ask questions about the *probability* of establishment or persistence of diseases with $R_0 > 1$. We can also ask how we expect demographic stochasticity to affect temporal dynamics of diseases, and how much variability we expect to see due to demographic stochasticity.

3. The behavior of a stochastic model

We have experience in interpreting the behavior of deterministic models. Given parameters, and a starting point, we examine the predicted trajectory of the model. We also have techniques for combining information from different starting points into phase planes, and information using different parameter sets into bifurcation diagrams.

Simulating a realization

- Given a state of the system:
  - List possible events, and associated rates.
  - Randomly select the time and nature of the next event:
    - Calculate the total rate r_T
    - the next event will happen after an exponential waiting time with mean $1/r_T$.
    - The probability of event E is r_E/r_T.
  - Change the system state appropriately.
- Repeat forever.
- Or until disease is extinct.
- Or until you are tired

TABLE 2. Steps in simulating a demographic model.

For stochastic models, we must re-evaluate what we mean by the "behavior" of a system. Given parameters, and a starting point, we do not know what the trajectory of the model will be. We can attempt to simulate a random sample of what the model might do. Such an example of a single trajectory is called a *realization.* We can attempt to characterize the universe of all possible such realizations; this is called the *ensemble*; we can imagine the ensemble as an infinity of realizations running simultaneously. Less ambitious than attempting to characterize the whole ensemble, we could ask about the probability distribution that describes what state we expect the population to be in at any given time; this is called the *ensemble distribution.*

We have a variety of techniques available to interpret a stochastic dynamical system. 1) Most straightforwardly, we can simulate one or many realizations. 2) We can simulate the entire ensemble distribution; this technique is restricted to systems with relatively small population size, since such simulations require that we keep track of one state variable for each possible state of the system. 3) We can solve the ensemble distribution dynamics exactly; this is possible only in special cases, but these solutions can be enlightening. 4) We can construct analytic *approximations* to the ensemble distribution.

3.1. Simulating individual realizations. Continuous-time models with discrete events can be simulated in a straightforward manner, outlined below Table 2. This method has been known for at least half a century, and is attributed to Kendall by [**6**]. It was explicated in detail by Gillespie [**10**], and is often referred to as the Gillespie method. Briefly, given that rates are known, we can infer the distribution of the waiting time to the next event, as well as the probability that the next event is of any particular type. By iterating, we can simulate a stochastic realization.

3.2. Simulating the ensemble distribution. We model the ensemble distribution by creating one conceptual 'box' for each possible state of the system, and asking what is the probability that the system is in each box. Conceptually, this approach is surprisingly simple; the catch is that there may be a lot of boxes – in fact, one for each possible state of the system. In an SIS model with fixed

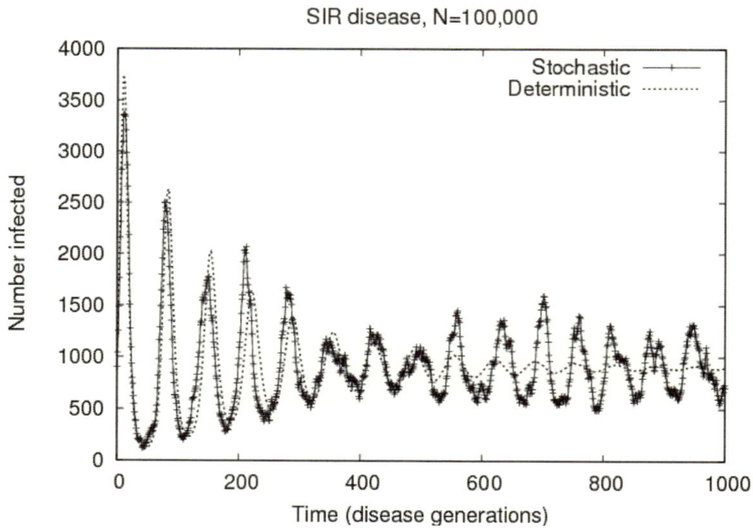

FIGURE 3. The deterministic trajectory from a simple SIR model (2.1) is compared with a typical stochastic trajectory from an analogous stochastic model (Table 1). Parameters are $R_0 = 10$, $\rho = 0.001$, $N = 1,000,000$. The system was started relatively close to the endemic equilibrium (with 120,000 susceptibles) to avoid too violent a first epidemic.

population size, we might have effectively only one state parameter in the deterministic model. In this case, the number probabilities to model in the ensemble distribution is of order N, the population size. In an SIR model, we need at least two deterministic state variables, so the number of discrete state probabilities will be of order N^2 – or N^3 if we allow population size to vary, or take disease latency into account ....

Since the human global population is on the order of 10^{10} individuals, with major cities having $> 10^5$ individuals, this approach quickly becomes prohibitive. Nonetheless, we may gain valuable information from our investigations of simpler cases.

Although often difficult in practice, simulating an ensemble distribution is conceptually straightforward. Given our event rates, we can determine the rate of *direct* transit between any to states S and S'. This rate will of course be zero in many cases. It is then straightforward to write equations for how the probabilities of being in a given state $p(S)$ change through time:

$$\dot{p}_S = \sum_{S'} p_{S'} r_{S' \to S} - p_S \sum_{S'} r_{S \to S'} \tag{3.1}$$

4. Analytic approaches

In addition to simulating equations of the form (3.1), we may also seek analytic understanding. Rather remarkably, in some cases equations of this form can be solved exactly for interesting biological systems. Although these examples are necessarily very limited, such exact solutions can be very illuminating.

We might also seek approximate analytic solutions to increase our understanding. These two approaches are related, since an exact solution to a simplified problem may in some cases serve as an approximate solution to the original problem. In addition to such simplifications, analytic approximation techniques that can be applied include moment approximations and diffusion approximations.

Two of the most useful tools for understanding deterministic disease models are based on linearizations. We linearize around the disease-free equilibrium to investigate what factors control whether the disease can invade and persist. We linearize around the endemic equilibrium to investigate the system's tendency to cycle, and the characteristic period and damping time of cycles. Both of these methods have analogues in demographic models (see below): the linear birth-death model is based on linearizing about the disease-free equilibrium, and diffusion approximations are based on linearizing about the endemic equilibrium.

4.1. The fate of an introduced disease. Consider for a moment the long-term fate of a realizations of our demographic system (Table 1). The total population always remains fixed, but on reflection we will see that *eventually* the disease will always go extinct: however large N, and however low the (average) probability of recovery before the next infection, in infinite time, we will always eventually throw H tails in a row, so to speak.

From a biological point of view, this fact may not seem very interesting, since the expected time to extinction of disease in our model will often dwarf the expected lifetime of the universe. Mathematically speaking, however, it poses serious obstacles. Investigating equilibria is a vitally useful mathematical technique, but the only real equilibrium of this system is the disease-free equilibrium. Below, we will see how this concept is addressed with the concept of the quasi-equilibrium.

Beyond the observation that the disease must go extinct eventually, it is useful to categorize qualitatively different *ways* in which it might go extinct. Based on the behavior of our system, we can identify either three (if we are mathematicians) or four (if biologists) such routes to extinction:

Fizzle: the disease fails to cause an epidemic. We will make this concept precise below

Burnout: the disease causes an epidemic, which reduces the number of susceptibles below the threshold required, and goes extinct before the level of susceptibles recovers (after the first epidemic)

Fadeout: the disease causes several epidemics, and approaches "quasi-equilibrium" (see below) before going extinct.

Persistence: the disease fades out, but after a biologically unreasonable period of time. There is no convenient *mathematical* distinction between fadeout and persistence, but biologically it may make sense to make an arbitrary distinction.

4.2. Equilibrium and quasi-equilibrium. We define equilibrium in our demographic system as an ensemble distribution that does not change with time. As noted above, the only equilibrium of the system is then the disease-free equilibrium. As long as any populations not extinct, proportion extinct will increase. In particular, there is no equilibrium corresponding to the endemic equilibrium of the deterministic system. This is deeply inconvenient, since we would like to study such an equilibrium, to characterize how the system behaves in the long term.

Event	transition	rate	Effect on I
Infection	$S \to I$	$R_0 I$	1
Recovery	$I \to R$	I	-1

TABLE 3. We specify a demographic model by describing the events that can occur; the way that the rates of these events depend on the state of the system; and the effect of these events on the variables that describe the state of our system.

We address the problem by constructing a "quasi-equilibrium". Consider the ensemble distribution confined to the subset of states where nothing is extinct. This system can be described as a *fully connected* (you can get anywhere from anywhere else, *open* (you can leave the set) flow. Intuition tells us that such a system has a unique, real, negative dominant eigenvalue, associated with a positive eigenvector. Linear algebra tells us this as well [**7**]. Thus, the system will converge to a stable *relative* distribution of probabilities of being in each non-extinct box – this relative distribution is called the quasi-equilibrium.

The quasi-equilibrium is the asymptotic probability of being in each system state with disease *given that the disease has not gone extinct.* The eigenvalue λ_q associated with the quasi-equilibrium distribution is the rate at which the probability of non-extinction decays (exponentially). The distribution of persistence times must be asymptotically exponential. The expected persistence time (looking forward) approaches $-1/\lambda_q$ as the system continues to persist.

The quasi-equilibrium perspective also gives us a useful tool for numerical investigations. Just as we modeled the ensemble distribution above (3.1), we can also model the *conditional* probability of being in a particular state given that extinction has not occurred. Since these probabilities converge in general to positive values (the quasi-equilibrium distribution), this approach tends to be computationally more stable than directly simulating the ensemble distribution. Since we can also keep track of the cumulative extinction probability, the information we obtain is equivalent. Define the conditional probabilities $q_S = p_S/(1 - p_N)$, where N is a 'null' state that we cannot escape from. Then we use the quotient rule to write equations for the conditional probabilities:

$$\dot{q}_S = \sum_{S'} q_{S'} r_{S' \to S} - q_S \sum_{S'} r_{S \to S'} - q_S r_{S \to N} + q_S \sum_{S'} q_{S'} r_{S' \to N}, \tag{4.1}$$

where the sums now go only over the states where the disease is not extinct.

4.3. Linear birth-death process. In deterministic systems, we study disease invasion by asking how the number of infectives behaves in the limit where we assume that virtually the whole population is susceptible. This is (typically) equivalent to linearizing about the disease-free equilibrium. We take an analogous approach with stochastic disease models. This corresponds to holding the number of susceptibles fixed at N; we are then left with a demographic model whose state is determined by the number of infectious individuals I. This system has only two events:

Surprisingly, the probability of eventual extinction in this system is not one. Our argument that the system must go extinct eventually breaks down, because the expected number of infectious individuals goes to ∞ in time. Thus, we can ask what is the extinction probability in this model.

This can be solved in a straightforward, and rather illuminating, fashion. Chains of infection are independent in this model: since the rate at which an infection spawns new infections never changes, infectious individuals have no effect on the number of cases that will be caused by another infectious individual. We can use this fact to solve directly for the probability of extinction when starting from I infections, E_I.

If we start with one infectious individual, the probability that the next event will be a recovery (and thus that the disease will go extinct immediately) is $1/(R_0+1)$. Otherwise, the next event will be an infection, and we will have two infectious individuals. Thus:

$$E_1 = \frac{1 + R_0 E_2}{1 + R_0}. \tag{4.2}$$

But, if our two new infectious individuals have independent chains of infection, the probability that they will both eventually go extinct is the product of the independent probabilities that each will go extinct: $E_2 = {E_1}^2$. Thus, we have a quadratic equation for E_1:

$$E_1 = \frac{1 + R_0 {E_1}^2}{1 + R_0}. \tag{4.3}$$

This has roots 1 and $1/R_0$, and it can be shown that the eventual extinction probability is $1/R_0$ when this quantity is < 1, and 1 otherwise. Making use of our independence observation, we conclude that the probability of eventual extinction starting from I infectious individuals is

$$E_I = R_0^{-I}, \text{when } R_0 > 1;\ 1, \text{otherwise}. \tag{4.4}$$

Going back to our anatomy of routes to extinction, we can use E_I as a working definition of fizzle probability: the probability that the disease would have gone extinct even without depleting any susceptibles is a good proxy for the probability of going extinct without causing an epidemic. So this calculation allows us to investigate quite broadly under what circumstances we might expect to see epidemics fizzle. Clearly, if neither R_0nor I is near 1, we expect E_I to be quite small. Thus, fizzles should be the result either of small introductions, or of very small R_0; and when $R_0$is not particularly small, we expect epidemics that fizzle to never grow very large.

We derived (4.4) by making use of the fact that (in our model) a single infectious individual will either cause a new, identical infection (increasing I to 2), or recover (decreasing I to 0). It is straightforward to generalize (4.4) to account for the possibility that a single infection will generate any given number of secondary infections, by writing:

$$E_1 = \sum_s P_s E_s = \sum_s P_s E_1^s, \tag{4.5}$$

where P_s is the probability of s secondary cases being generated by a given case, and solving the polynomial for E_1. We can interpret P_s as reflecting a discrete-time step, for models in discrete time [**3**], or as reflecting disease generations in either continuous or discrete time, allowing a broad framework that can include parametric heterogeneity [**13**].

Although this simple calculation provides a great deal of insight, we can in fact investigate our linearized invasion system Table 3 in even more detail, and in fact solve exactly for the ensemble distribution. One way to approach this is through moment methods.

4.4. Moment calculations. Moment methods seek to investigate systems by studying summary statistics called moments: e.g., means, variances, covariances, skewnesses and so on. In the case of our linearized system Table 3, we can simply ask: what is the behavior of the mean, variance, skewness, ..., of I over the ensemble? More complicated systems (such as Table 1) will also require 'cross'-moments (e.g., covariances).

We start by defining the ensemble mean $\mu = \sum_I I p_i$, and asking how this quantity changes through time. Since the set of possible values of I is fixed (the natural numbers), we can find the change in μ if we know how the p_I change:

$$\dot{\mu} = \sum_I I \dot{p}_I. \tag{4.6}$$

Plugging our event rates (Table 3) into (3.1), we see that we can enter each state two ways (by birth or death), and leave it by the same two ways, so:

$$\dot{p}_I = b_{I-1}p_{I-1} + m_{I+1}p_{I+1} - (b_I + m_I)p_I, \tag{4.7}$$

where $b_I = R_0 I$ is the 'birth' rate, and $m_I = I$ is the 'death' rate of infectious individuals.

Next, we plug (4.7) into (4.6)

$$\dot{\mu} = \sum_I I b_{I-1}p_{I-1} + \sum_I I m_{I+1}p_{I+1}(\sum_I I b_I + m_I)p_I. \tag{4.8}$$

Since m_0, the total death rate when there are no individuals in the population, and p_{-1}, the probability of having -1 individuals in the population, must both be zero, we can re-index our sums to run over p_I (as I runs from 0 to ∞):

$$\dot{\mu} = \sum_I (I+1)b_I p_I + \sum_I (I-1)m_I p_I(\sum_I I b_I + m_I)p_I, \tag{4.9}$$

which simplifies to

$$\dot{\mu} = \sum_I (b_I - m_I)p_I. \tag{4.10}$$

The result (4.10) is suspiciously simple, and in fact, we could have written it down from first principles: the rate of increase of the mean is equal to the expectation of the birth rate minus the death rate, with the expectation taken over the ensemble distribution. The exercise of formally deriving (4.10) from (3.1) is (I hope) illuminating in several ways, however. It helps shed insight into the ensemble-distribution equations, and gives some guidance for how we might develop moment equations for more complicated systems (or for higher moments).

Note that (4.10), while limited to simple birth-death systems, has not yet made use of our assumption of linearity. Plugging in the rates for our specific linearized birth-death system (Table 3), we find that the ensemble mean obeys:

$$\dot{\mu} = \sum_I (R_0 I - I)p_I = (R_0 - 1)\mu \tag{4.11}$$

We can solve this equation exactly: the expected value of μ (averaged over realizations) grows exponentially through time!

Similar expansions can be made for non-linear systems. In this case, however, we typically see a 'chain' of moment equations, where the equation for each moment depends on one or more higher moments. For example, in an SIS model, the per capita "birth" rate will decrease as the number of infectious individuals increases: $b_I = R_0 I(N - I)/N$. Since this model has linear *per capita* rates, we could write an equation for $\dot{\mu}$ that depends on the mean and the variance (i.e., the second moment). The dynamics of the second moment would depend on the third moment, and so on. There are a variety of techniques, broadly called "moment-closure" approximations for ending these chains and approximating the dynamics of such systems.

One approach that is worth mentioning briefly is that of moment-generating functions. This is a nice mathematical trick that involves describing the ensemble distribution as a function of a dummy variable x. In particular, we define $\phi = \sum_I p_I x^I$. If we know the function $\phi(x)$ at a given time, we know all of the probabilities p_I. We can then use our event-rate equations to write an expression for $\dot{\phi}$, which can be converted into a partial differential equation and analyzed, approximated, and (rarely) solved. For example, we can calculate the exact ensemble distribution through time of the linear birth-death process (Table 3). Starting from a fixed number of infectious individuals I_0, the ensemble distribution is given by a negative binomial distribution with mean $I_0 \exp((R_0 - 1)t)$ and parameter I_0.

To summarize: we understand the exact behavior of linearized invasion model (Table 3). This allows us to understand the properties of the SIR model, in the absence of effects due to depletion of susceptibles (ie., its behavior near the disease-free equilibrium). In particular, we can analytically calculate the relationship between model parameters and: the probability that an epidemic will fizzle; the size distribution of fizzled epidemics; and the mean and variance in the expected epidemic growth rate.

4.5. Diffusion approximations. We can approximate the discrete-valued demographic system with a real-valued system that reflects the mean *and variance* of the demographic system [**12**]. Thus we can incorporate demographic stochasticity in a continuous system. This gives an excellent approximation except when some values are very small. Such systems can be simulated as stochastic differential equations, but if we are going to simulate, we are usually better off simulating the full stochastic system; hybrid approaches also exist, which take advantage of the efficiency of approximating quantities which are not small.

The biggest strength of diffusion approximations is that they allow analytic understanding of demographic stochasticity. In a linear system, we can solve the equilibrium distribution of the continuous equations. We can therefore linearize around the disease-free equilibrium, and use a diffusion approximation to approximate the quasi-equilibrium distribution, and thus ask questions about whether the disease will persist, and how large we expect characteristic demographic fluctuations to be.

We linearize about the endemic equilibrium, in exact analogy to Jacobian methods for stability in deterministic models. A good explanation of the details can be found in [**14**]. Heuristically speaking, diffusion (and thus demographic stochasticity) is relatively unimportant when the square of the number infected is large compared to the demographic variance. We can ask roughly how we expect these numbers to scale.

$$\text{Number infected at equilibrium: } \mu = \frac{(R_0 - 1)\rho N}{R} \approx \rho N. \tag{4.12}$$
$$\text{Demographic variance: } \sigma^2 \approx N.$$

We can define a 'diffusion index' $U = \mu^2/\sigma^2 \approx \rho^2 N$ [**9**]. This gives a measure of the size of the infectious population relative to the amount of demographic variability expected. In the linear system, we expect the amount of time required to move a distance of μ from the equilibrium (and thus approach disease extinction), to be very roughly on the order of $\exp(U)$. Conversely, we expect U to give some insight into how large a human population must be to allow the disease to persist for many epidemic cycles (i.e., the critical community size [**5**])

This very crude calculation gives a major insight into the importance of demographic stochasticity in models of disease with acquired immunity. Recall that the quantity ρ is the ratio between the two key time scales in our system: the duration of infectiousness, and the duration of recalcitrance to infection after recovery. In acute human pathogens, the former is typically days to weeks, and the latter typically years to decades. Thus ρ can easily be as small as 10^{-3}, and demographic stochasticity may have important effects in populations of order $N = 10^6$ or larger. This is in sharp contrast to ecological (or SIS) models, where pure demographic stochasticity is not expected to have large effects in populations larger than a few dozen individual.

It is important to recall the limitations of the linear diffusion approximation in general, and our crude scaling quantity in particular. These methods depend on linearizing about the disease-free equilibrium. Linearization tells us the *local* behavior of system. We expect our diffusion approximation to give a good estimate of the size of small oscillations, but not necessarily of large ones. At parameter ranges of interest, disease extinction typically represents a rather large oscillation: thus, the diffusion approximation will not necessarily give a good estimate of the time to extinction (or of the critical community size).

Put another way, if our diffusion index is small, we expect local behavior, and persistence of the disease (in the sense that expected time to extinction from quasi-equilibrium is ridiculously long). However, if the diffusion index is large, we expect the behavior to become non-local, and thus the index itself is no longer expected to give a reliable guide of whether the disease is likely to go extinct. In particular, and unfortunately, numerical investigations show that the critical community size does not increase as quickly as $1/\rho^2$.

4.6. Conclusions. Treating individuals as individuals can have dramatic effects on models of disease transmission. Although this issue is fundamentally difficult to grapple with, we should give it at least some thought when analyzing, and fitting, models. It is important to recall that populations really are made of individuals, and that analytic results that are not robust to incorporating demographic stochasticity should be regarded with grave suspicion. Stochastic models are fundamentally hard to approach, and we usually combine techniques to understand them; available techniques include analytic approximation, simulating ensemble distributions, and simulating realizations.

Analytic consideration of simple models of disease transmission with demographic stochasticity has led to the development of several useful concepts [**2**]. In particular, we can distinguish the phenomena of fizzle, burnout and fadeout, and ask under what circumstances the first two are likely, and are what circumstances the third one is likely to happen within a non-ridiculous time frame. Simple calculations also lead to the conclusion that the relative duration of acquired immunity has extremely strong effects on the likelihood of persistence.

References

[1] L. J. S. Allen. *An Introduction to Stochastic Processes with Applications to Biology.* Prentice Hall, New Jersey, 2003.

[2] Roy M. Anderson and Robert M. May. *Infectious Diseases of Humans: Dynamics and Control.* Oxford Science Publications, Oxford, 1991.

[3] N. J. T. Bailey. *The Mathematical Theory of Infectious Diseases and its Application.* Griffin, London, 1975.

[4] S. Bansal, B. T. Grenfell, and L. A. Meyers. When individual behaviour matters: homogeneous and network models in epidemiology. *J. R. Soc. Interface*, 4:879–91, 2007.

[5] M. S. Bartlett. Measles periodicity and community size. *J. Roy. Stat. Soc.*, A120:48–70, 1957.

[6] M. S. Bartlett. Monte carlo studies in ecology and epidemiology. *Proc. Fourth Berkeley Symp. on Math. Statist. and Prob.*, 4:39–55, 1961.

[7] A. Berman and R. Plemmons. *Nonnnegative Matrices in the Mathematical Sciences.* Academic Press, New York, 1979.

[8] J. Dushoff. Host heterogeneity and disease endemicity: A moment-based approach. *Theor. Popul. Biol.*, 56:325–335, 1999.

[9] J. Dushoff. Carrying capacity and demographic stochasticity: Scaling behavior of the stochastic logistic model. *Theor. Popul. Biol.*, 57:59–65, 2000.

[10] D. T. Gillespie. A general method for numerically simulating the stochastic time evolution of coupled chemical reactions. *J. Comput. Phys.*, 22:403–434, 1976.

[11] H. W. Hethcote and J. A. Yorke. *Gonorrhea Transmission Dynamics and Control.* Springer-Verlag, Berlin, 1984.

[12] Egbert G. Leigh, Jr. The average lifetime of a population in a varying environment. *J. Theor. Biol.*, 90:213–239, 1981.

[13] J. O. Lloyd-Smith, S. J. Schreiber, P. E. Kopp, and W. M. Getz. Superspreading and the effect of individual variation on disease emergence. *Nature*, 438:355–359, 2005.

[14] I. Nasell. On the time to extinction in recurrent epidemics. *J. R. Stat. Soc. Ser. B-Stat. Methodol.*, 61:309–330, 1999.

[15] S. Riley. Large-scale spatial-transmission models of infectious disease. *Science*, 316:1298–301, 2007.

Department of Biology, McMaster University, Hamilton, Ontario L8S-4K1
E-mail address: dushoff@mcmaster.ca

DIMACS Series in Discrete Mathematics
and Theoretical Computer Science
Volume **75**, 2010

Using mathematical models to monitor and evaluate the impact of public health interventions on epidemics: the case of the TB/HIV co-pandemic in Africa

María S. Sánchez, James O. Lloyd-Smith, Brian G. Williams, and Wayne M. Getz

ABSTRACT. Curtailing the public health crises generated by the TB/HIV co-pandemic poses many challenges, including monitoring difficulties that complicate our ability to accurately predict the efficacy of public health interventions. Unfortunately, the dire and urgent need to inform policy makers on the individual and population benefits to be obtained from different disease control measures may result in our prioritizing predicting per se, over conducting in-depth system studies that can maximize our ability to properly address the question(s) posed. In this chapter we illustrate these difficulties and exemplify how analytical studies can be used not only as a powerful predictive tool that can help guide public health policy, but also as a means of gaining important insight into the system's functioning that, in turn, can help the monitoring of pandemics. We present in detail the mathematical, statistical and computational approach and methodology behind our recent research focused on evaluating the potential public health benefits to be derived from reducing TB treatment duration from the standard 6- to 8-month treatments to a 2-month treatment in areas of high HIV prevalence. Because of the considerable uncertainties and spatial and temporal heterogeneity in parameter values we conducted a calibration to historical TB/HIV trends that increased the validity of our predictive results for high HIV prevalence areas. Unexpectedly, our calibration unveiled incongruent epidemiological patterns between the two interacting diseases in Kenya, which led us to evaluate reported TB/HIV co-dynamics for the whole of Africa with a new statistic that quantifies the relative change in TB numbers as compared to HIV numbers. Our initial analysis of pan-African patterns placed Kenya as an outlier. However, Kenyan TB and HIV estimates have since been revised, and now the relative change in the co-dynamics of the two diseases place Kenya in a more intermediate position. We additionally conducted a sensitivity analysis to evaluate which parameters had a greater influence on the output variables of choice. In this chapter we briefly explain the results of our model predictions and of our sensitivity analysis–focusing on the general approach and methods–because many of the lessons learned related to the reasoning and steps we followed, and not exclusively to the results of our investigation. Thus, here our final conclusions and recommendations are geared towards the analytical process more than the public health implications of our studies. Most importantly, this study taught us the power of contrasting trends of interacting diseases in global disease monitoring and control. This is particularly so for such a complex co-pandemic as TB/HIV, where our analysis of the joint co-dynamics provided important insights into the individual epidemiology of each disease.

1. Introduction

Even though tuberculosis (TB) probably originated in Africa and from there spread worldwide, historical records of this devastating disease indicate that in this continent it did not reach the epidemic proportions it reached in other areas, including Western Europe and Asia (Gutiérrez et al. 2005; Wirth et al. 2008). Not surprisingly, Africa's human population was less densely distributed in recent history, and people spent less time indoors with suboptimal ventilation, in comparison to other areas of greater historical TB burden. However, HIV has managed to completely overturn this trend (Nunn et al. 2007; Rieder 2008). In 2007, of the 33 million people infected with HIV worldwide, 67% live in sub-Saharan Africa (for a total of 22 million persons), and 75% of all deaths due to AIDS occurred here (UNAIDS 2008). By incapacitating the immune system of those it infects, HIV has made it possible for many pathogens that were traditionally contained by otherwise healthy persons to reach epidemic proportions. In the case of TB, while HIV-uninfected persons have a 10% risk of developing TB over their entire lifetime, TB/HIV coinfected persons have a 15% yearly risk of developing TB. This increased relative risk of developing TB is not obliterated by treatment, because even though potent antiretroviral therapy (ARVT) has been shown to reduce the incidence of TB in HIV infected persons by more than 80%, TB is the most prevalent disease in people living with HIV/AIDS (PLWHA) that are taking ARVT (Badri et al. 2002; Girardi et al. 2000; Girardi et al. 2005). Moreover, as opposed to many other HIV-related opportunistic infections, TB manifests itself in PLWHA at all levels of their immune status functionality, as measured by a person's CD_4 lymphocyte count (World Health Organization 2004a). Regrettably, these factors have enabled the number of new TB cases (TB incidence) to triple in the last two decades in high-HIV prevalent countries. In 2006 85% of HIV positive TB patients lived in Africa, where TB is the leading cause of death among PLWHA. In addition, changing social and environmental conditions in Africa, mainly linked to poverty, are also important contributing factors to rising TB numbers, such as crowded living conditions and lack of proper nutrition (Eisenhut 2007; Muniyandi & Ramachandran 2008; Naidoo et al. 2008).

HIV-infected people are not only more susceptible to becoming infected and to develop TB than the HIV-uninfected (Middelkoop et al. 2008), they can also spread TB, including multi- and extremely-drug resistant TB (Escombe et al. 2008). This can lead to a spill-over effect in the HIV-uninfected subpopulation (Lawn & Wood 2006). In addition, TB is a disease with a high disseminating ability because people can be sick for long periods of time, while maintaining the ability to move while infectious (Ewald 1994). Modern traveling, particularly by airplane, has enabled aerially dispersed diseases such as TB to successfully spread in very short time frames vast distances, turning previously localized problems into major global issues (Abubakar & Fernández de la Hoz 2008; Al-Jahdali et al. 2003).

TB is a perfectly treatable and curable disease, with very high success rates when medications are taken as prescribed (Dye et al. 2007; World Health Organization 2008). However, typical treatments last for 6-8 months, regimens need to be completed in order to avoid the development of drug resistance (Chakaya et al. 2008; de Jong et al. 2004), and regrettably it can be difficult to adequately inform people of the necessity of getting, and staying, on treatment. Moreover, it can be very difficult for patients to complete an entire TB treatment regimen if they risk losing their jobs due to the fact that they need to go to the TB clinic on a daily basis to take their medication, and/or because their sickness affects their mobility. Traveling distances to and from home to a TB clinic can be considerable in rural Africa (Chakaya et al. 2005; Dowdy et al. 2006; Hopewell & Pai 2005; Mtei et al. 2005; Noor et al. 2006; Wilson et al. 2006). In addition, the social stigma associated with TB is very strong, such that persons may delay going into a clinic in order to avoid being shamed by family, friends, and fellow co-workers (Naidoo et al. 2008; Nnoaham et al. 2006; Van Rie et al. 2008). Because of the complexity of complying with such a lengthy treatment that has potentially serious side effects, the WHO developed a comprehensive TB control strategy in the mid-1990s. This strategy is called directly observed treatment, short-course (DOTS), that is officially recommended by this organization and implemented worldwide (Chakaya et al. 2005; De Cock & Chaisson 1999; Dye et al. 1998). The major features of this strategy are government commitment, diagnosis through microscopy, standardised and supervised treatment, uninterrupted drug supply, and regular monitoring (Raviglione & Uplekar 2006).

Because the market for TB drugs is in general an impoverished one, funding for TB drug research and development is scant (Spigelman 2007). No new effective medications against *Mycobacterium tuberculosis*, the bacterial agent causing TB, have been developed in over 40 years (Fujiwara et al. 2000). However, there are efforts targeted at developing medications with greater bactericidal activity that could treat TB in a shorter time frame (Andries et al. 2005; Combs et al. 1990; Ginsberg & Spigelman 2007; Salomon et al. 2006; Spigelman & Gillespie 2006). Reducing treatment time would simplify treatment from the individual and public health perspective, reducing the potential for serious side effects and the presence of negative interactions with HIV drugs. Moreover, reducing treatment duration would diminish the financial costs associated with treating patients on a daily basis for 6-8 months (de Jong et al. 2004). Concomitantly, this reduction is also expected to decrease the rates at which persons do not complete their treatment regimens (i.e., default from treatment) that ultimately can lead to uncured patients and the development of drug resistance (Shargie & Lindtjorn 2007; Spigelman & Gillespie 2006). Among the non-profit organizations leading the development of new TB drugs is the Global TB Alliance (Spigelman 2007). We were contacted by this organization to use a mathematical model to predict the impact of decreasing treatment duration for tuberculosis treatment in areas of high TB burden, both without a generalized HIV epidemic, and in areas of high HIV prevalence. The first part of the project was focused on conditions representative of the South-East Asia region (Salomon et al. 2006). The second part of the project was situated in sub-Saharan Africa, with particular focus on Kenya (Sánchez et al. 2008; Sánchez et al. 2009).

The biological complexity of TB and HIV epidemiology, together with the difficulties it presents from a surveillance point of view, made the predictive analysis requested by the TB Global Alliance an extremely interesting one (Sánchez et al. 2008), but laden with considerable challenges that unveiled unexpected incongruencies in reported TB and HIV trends in Kenya (Sánchez et al. 2009, Sánchez et al., 2010). As a result, many of the lessons learned were at the level of the overall approach and methods, and did not exclusively relate to the results of our investigation. However, these matters are too lengthy to present in the main text of a standard journal article focused on public health. In this chapter we present a more detailed explanation of the process involved in generating our quantitative predictions. Our goal is to clearly explain the reasoning behind why and how we conducted the analyses presented in Sánchez et al. (2008), and how it led us to the recommendations for further monitoring, evaluation, and predictions of TB/HIV trends in particular, and of infectious disease co-dynamics in general, presented in Sánchez et al. (2009) and Sánchez et al. (2010).

We begin by presenting the public health crisis created by the TB/HIV co-pandemics as relates to the issue of the lengthy treatment for TB, and proceed to discuss the use of predictive analytical analyses to guide public health policy. We then describe in detail our mathematical model, and its calibration to historical TB/HIV trends, a necessary step to validate our predictive results for high HIV prevalence areas. Unexpectedly, this calibration unveiled incongruent epidemiological patterns between the two interacting diseases in Kenya. We explain how HIV and TB trends in Kenya have since been revised, which provides strong support for the value of using analytical tools as a means not only for predicting trends–an essential process in public health–but for gaining knowledge on biological processes in general, and on disease dynamics in particular. We only briefly explain the results of our model predictions and of our sensitivity analyses, because these are presented in detail in Sánchez et al. (2008, 2009). Our final conclusions and recommendations are more oriented towards the analytical process than the public health implications of our studies, given that the latter was the focus in Sánchez et al. (2008, 2009, 2010).

2. Mathematical models and epidemics

The use of mathematical models to investigate epidemiological systems dates back to 1760, when Daniel Bernoulli advocated for universal inoculation against smallpox via a mathematical analysis (Blower & Bernoulli 2004). Mathematical models are widely used today as a predictive tool, in an effort to answer pressing questions about the efficacy of public health programs, and as a means to contrast potential benefits and risks of different interventions. In general, the medical/public health community needs to know how many lives and/or cases of a particular disease could be avoided by implementing particular public health interventions. This field has now flourished, and mathematical models are being used to determine public health policy worldwide. Studies predicting the different public health benefits to be obtained from different interventions are being conducted and published on a regular basis in journals of both specialized and general interest. These studies are particularly useful for evaluating the most efficacious measures to be taken against major deadly pandemics such as HIV and TB, where the morbidity and mortality tolls are extraordinarily high, but monitoring difficulties together with ethical considerations limit our ability to conduct studies that would enable us to know more accurately the present and future states of the epidemics, particularly when different and novel interventions are put in place.

The dire and urgent need to use models to inform policy makers on the individual and population benefits that can be obtained from applying different public health interventions may result in our prioritizing obtaining predictions per se over obtaining insights and understanding. Nevertheless, our ability to effectively use mathematical, computational, and statistical tools to accurately predict the benefits to be obtained from public health interventions is, in most cases, limited to our level of knowledge of the system we are working with. As such, *acquiring a level of knowledge of the system that is sufficiently adequate to properly address the question(s)* posed is essential for conducting proper science, for maximizing our ability to improve the lives of those afflicted by the epidemics, and for minimizing our potential negative impact if our predictions turn out to be inaccurate.

One of the main advantages mathematical modeling has over other forms of analysis is that it allows for the integration of information from a wide variety of sources. In the case of modeling major pandemics, information at the clinical, epidemiological, behavioral, social, public health, political, and financial levels can be incorporated. This synthetic aspect of modeling is a particularly valuable asset in the case of interacting epidemics, because it permits us to unravel factors through which each epidemic entrains the other. Here we demonstrate how mathematical models, beyond their application as purely predictive tools, can provide such insights into the current HIV-TB co-pandemic in Africa. Considerable funds, time, and energy are being spent purely on prediction, but unless our understanding of the system is sufficiently comprehensive, the models we build may be missing key structures or processes, and thus perform inadequately as a tool for developing effective interventions. Tracking pandemics is an extremely difficult task (García Calleja et al. 2005; Garnett et al. 2006; Ghys et al. 2006; Morgan et al. 2006; Walker et al. 2004), and as we will see below empirical data may be misleading if we do not interpret them carefully. We illustrate this point by presenting some of our recent research on controlling TB in areas of high HIV prevalence.

3. Our mathematical model

On behalf of the Global TB Alliance, we constructed a model to assess the population-level benefits of reducing TB treatment duration from the standard 6-8 months to a 2 month regimen in high HIV prevalence areas. Our model included both TB and HIV submodels under the assumption that persons could acquire either or both diseases. We did not model HIV transmission as a process, but included HIV incidence as an input. The health, general progression, infectiousness, and response to treatment of each TB infected person were determined by their TB and HIV statuses. Our model was an extension of that presented by Salomon et al. (2006), the major upgrade being the inclusion of the four recognized clinical disease categories and accepted progression rates to handle the HIV component. We conducted all our computational analyses using Matlab® and used Simlab® to generate the Latin Hypercube matrices for sensitivity and uncertainty analyses (Blower & Dowlatabadi 1994).

Our compartmental model (see Table 1 for a list of state variables and Fig. 1 for a flow diagram) comprised 42 TB infection and treatment categories and 5 HIV clinically recognized categories corresponding to HIV-uninfected and WHO HIV stages I-IV (Morgan et al. 2002). The transition steps characterizing the disease processes are given in mathematical terms in Table 2, and are represented graphically in Fig. 1. Because the impact of TB on the epidemiology of HIV is not as substantial as that of HIV on TB (Day et al. 2004; Kannangara et al. 2005; Lawn 2004; Williams & Dye 2003), we did not, as mentioned above, model HIV transmission dynamics explicitly, but rather incorporated the HIV epidemic into the model as an exogenous input. Accordingly, we assumed HIV affects TB infection, progression, and mortality rates; our approach implicitly assumes that TB only influences HIV dynamics indirectly, because TB does not alter the rates of HIV infection or progression.

3.1. Basic TB model. The TB model structure included elements from previous models used to investigate the response of the TB epidemic to alternative TB control strategies (Blower et al. 1996; Cohen & Murray 2004; Dye et al. 1998; Murray & Salomon 1998), and accounted for the most relevant complexities of TB aetiology, clinical presentations, sociology, and treatment options (Frieden et al. 2003; Maher et al. 2005; Reichman & Hershfield 2000). Moreover, the course of the disease could be vastly different in HIV-infected persons compared to non-immunocompromised individuals: in most persons TB remains a latent infection and has little effect on their health, but in immunocompromised persons TB infections are likely to become active, and potentially deadly (Fox et al. 2006; Keshinro & Diul 2006; Sonnenberg et al. 2001).

In Fig. 1A we depict the TB categories and flows of the model. Flows among the 42 TB categories reflected the most important processes determining TB incidence, prevalence, and mortality under different treatment regimens. We placed particular attention on the following TB processes: case detection, default, relapse and reinfection. Susceptible persons could become infected with TB upon contact with TB infected persons at a rate given by the force of infection $c_j\lambda$, which varied across HIV stages ($j = 1$ is HIV uninfected, $j = 2 - 5$ are HIV stages I-IV respectively). This force was calculated at each time step from the current number of persons in a TB infectious category (see below). We assumed the population mixed at random with density-independent contact rates, so that transmission was frequency-dependent. This assumption of density-independence is reasonable if we assume that the contact rate for TB related transmission is limited by household and work-related interactions that are only weakly dependent on changes in population density. Untreated persons with smear-positive active disease were the most likely to infect others (β_P), followed by the untreated smear-negative (β_N). Smear-positive persons that failed treatment were partially infectious (β_{PF}), and all of the other categories were not considered to transmit at measurable rates. Latent slow progressors and recovered individuals became reinfected at a reduced rate as compared to TB naïve persons ($b_j < 1$).

Upon becoming infected, a person entered a slow latent (with probability p_{Sj}) or a fast latent category (with probability $1 - p_{Sj}$). Persons in the fast latent stage progressed rapidly to active disease at rate ϕ_{Sj}, while those in the slow latent stage had a reduced endogenous reactivation rate ϕ_{Fj}. Upon development of active TB, a fraction s_{Pj} of persons presented smear positive symptoms, and a fraction $1 - s_{Pj}$ presented smear negative symptoms. Individuals infected with HIV, particularly in the advanced stages, were more likely to be smear-negative due to their reduced immunity (Corbett et al. 2004; Keshinro & Diul 2006). Smear-negative persons converted to smear-positive at rate σ_j. A fraction d of persons with active TB, regardless of their smear category, entered the detectable compartment, while a fraction $1 - d$ entered the non-detectable compartment. This partition represented all of the potentially possible impediments to initiating treatment. Pertinent impediments include subclinical symptoms, lack of access to health care due to long travelling distance from the home to a TB clinic, social stigma associated with TB

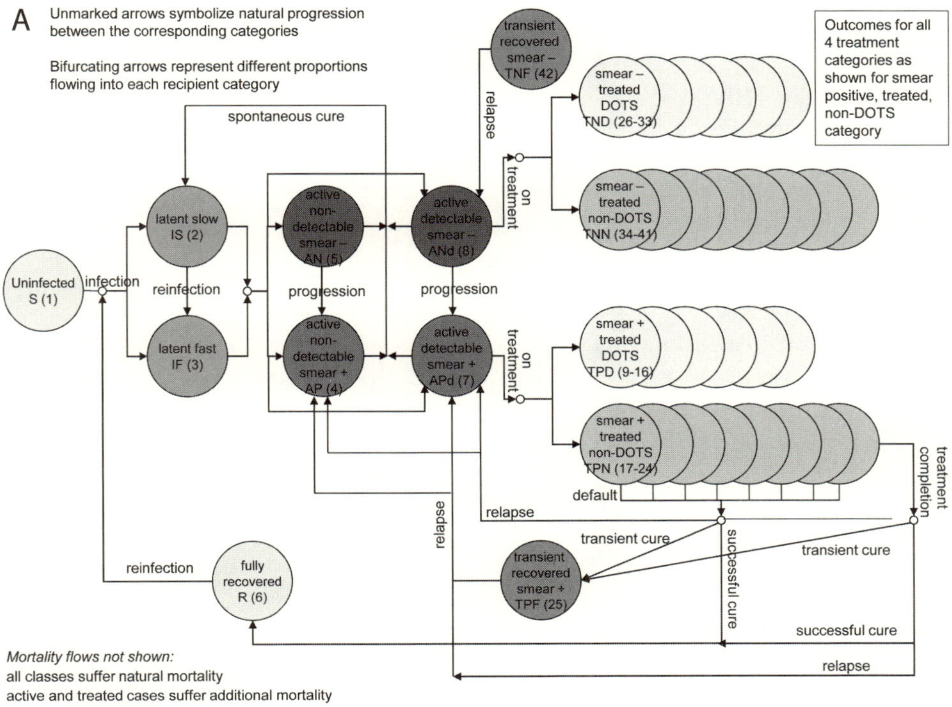

FIGURE 1. **(A) TB-HIV flow diagram.** TB transmission, treatment, and mortality in an HIV-free population were represented by progression through 42 categories.

infection that would deter people from seeking treatment, financial difficulties due to loss of work days while treated, inadequate case-finding efforts on behalf of any of the local health services, etc. (Chakaya et al. 2005; Dowdy et al. 2006; Hopewell & Pai 2005; Mtei et al. 2005; Noor et al. 2006). We retained the distinction between smear positive and smear negative cases throughout those compartments categorizing cases that were either active, on treatment, or partially cured. This approach provided flexibility in accounting for any differences in infectiousness, detectability, response to treatment, relapse, etc. Furthermore, we assumed active cases recovered spontaneously without treatment, and entered the slow latent compartment at rate π_j.

At each time step cases moved from the detectable category into treatment according to the case-detection rate (θ_j), and then started DOTS (with probability t_P for smear-positive and t_N for smear negative) or a non-DOTS program (with corresponding probabilities $1 - t_P$ and $1 - t_N$). Our model was flexible regarding treatment duration. In this particular study we were investigating treatment durations of 6 months for standard DOTS and 8 months for standard non-DOTS. We assumed patients defaulted at each time step with a certain probability δ_m, or took their medication throughout the entire course. Upon default or completion persons either (1) failed treatment and returned directly to the active category (with probabilities q_{PDj} for smear-positive persons on DOTS, q_{PNj} for smear-positive persons

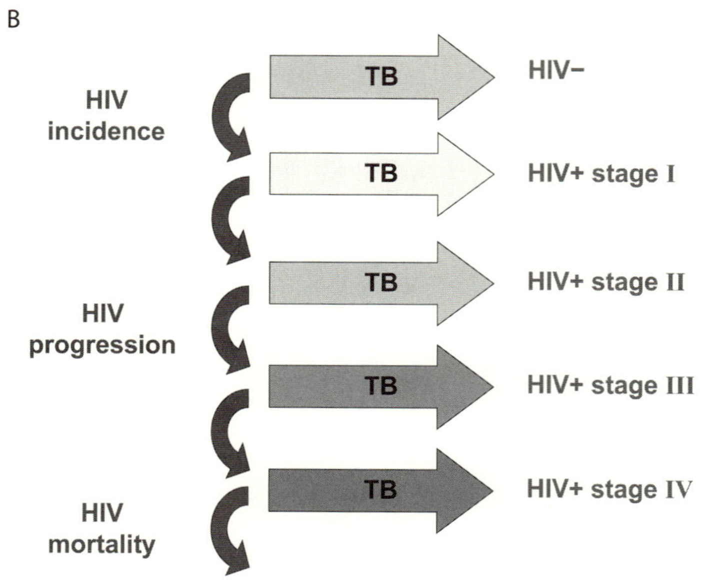

FIGURE 1. **(B) TB-HIV flow diagram.** In an HIV infected population, HIV incidence, progression, and mortality is accounted by 5 stages.

on non-DOTS, q_{NDj} for smear-negative persons on DOTS, q_{NNj} for smear-negative persons on non-DOTS, or $q_{complete,j}$), (2) entered a transiently recovered smear-positive (partially infectious) or smear-negative (non-infectious) category (with corresponding probabilities to (1) above $v_{kl,j}$ or $v_{complete,j}$), or (3) if finished treatment completely recovered in which case they were non-infectious (with probability $s_{complete,j} = 1 - v_{complete,j} - q_{complete,j}$). Transiently recovered persons relapsed back to active at rate ρ_j, and entered the detectable and non-detectable compartments corresponding to their smear status according to the same proportions as originally defined for those progressing to active from the latent stages. As in Salomon et al. (2006), we did not monitor treatment history explicitly or modeled particular retreatment regimens. We assumed that those persons that had recovered completely were partially immune to reinfection. All TB categories i (see Table 1) suffered the same natural background mortality (μ), and active untreated and treated cases suffered TB associated mortality to varying degrees across HIV stages (i.e. μ_{ij} for i =P, N, PD, PN, ND and NN, and $j = 1, \ldots 5$.).

3.2. Basic HIV model. HIV entered the system via a predefined incidence recruitment process that generated historical HIV prevalence patterns. As explained in greater detail below, our HIV incidence and prevalence trends emulated those most recently reported for Kenya by UNAIDS at the time we conducted our analysis (UNAIDS 2006). These data correspond to an increasing trend reaching a prevalence of 10-11% in 1997-98, followed by a decline to a level of approximately 7% in 2005 (Fig. 2 and Fig. 3 in Cheluget et al. 2006).

Upon infection with HIV, persons progressed through the 4 HIV disease stages ($j = 2, 3, 4, 5$ in Table 1) defined by the World Health Organization (Fig. 1B)

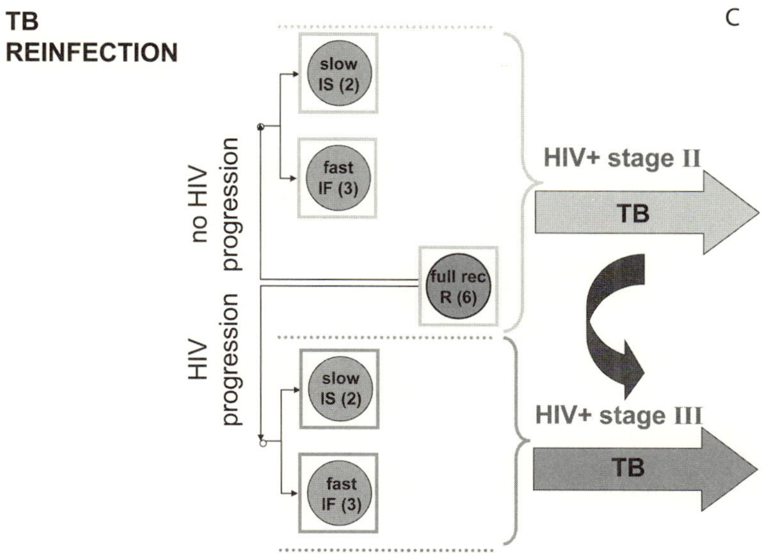

FIGURE 1. **(C) TB-HIV flow diagram.** Details of the TB reinfection flow from the 'fully recovered HIV+ stage III'. This pattern applies to all other HIV stages. Each HIV stage includes the 42 TB categories for a total of 210 combined TB/HIV categories (see Table 1).

according to the following time lines (Morgan et al. 2002): 24, 21, 66 and 9 months for HIV stages I, II, III and IV, respectively. The basic TB model was therefore replicated 5 times, once for HIV uninfected and once for each HIV infected stage, for a total of 42×5 different TB/HIV categories. At each monthly time step (Fig. 1C) HIV uninfected persons became HIV-positive and transitioned to HIV stage I according to the given incidence rate, progressed through the 4 disease stages, and ultimately died and exited the system. In the model, HIV induced death mimicked a TB process in that persons in HIV stage IV died of AIDS according to a fixed HIV mortality rate under the competing rates formulation. Accordingly, persons died of either TB or HIV, but not of both (Table 2).

3.3. Model formulation. The model consists of a set of discrete-time difference equations based on a competing rates formulation to approximate continuous processes of transmission and death. We used a discrete-time difference equation formulation (Getz & Lloyd-Smith 2006; Getz et al. 2006; Salomon et al. 2006) with a monthly time step, because the data itself is discrete and treatment is planned around monthly blocks of time. Further, in each time step we calculated HIV progression of stages I to IV as occurring concurrently with the progression through the various TB categories, under the assumption that each individual undergoes at most one of the three following disease processes in any given time step: any TB state transition including mortality from TB, HIV mortality, or natural mortality. More specifically, we assumed all TB processes and both the background and HIV mortality operate as competing rates, while HIV infection and progression occur independently from TB progression for those persons that do not die at each particular time step. Consequently, at each time step any given individual could progress in both its TB and HIV disease, in only one, or in neither (Table 2). This modeling scheme has the advantage that when a group of individuals is subject to multiple processes simultaneously (e.g. individuals in the latent fast-progressor, IF, class can either die or break down to active disease) their outcome at any time step is determined in such a way that an artificial order of processes does not have to be defined because all processes act contemporaneously. However, this approach does introduce the implicit assumption that each individual can only undergo one state transition per time step. Below we outline the steps we followed to determine, under this competing rates scheme, the specific rates at which individuals progressed through the different categories of the system when undergoing various multiple processes simultaneously.

Competing rates formulation. We first consider a pool of individuals C, subject to two possible competing processes: these individuals go to class A at per capita rate α, and to class G at per capita rate γ. Accordingly, the differential equation describing how persons in class C progress to the output classes A and G is given by the following equation:

$$\frac{dC}{dt} = -(\alpha + \gamma)C$$

That is,

$$\frac{1}{C}dC = -(\alpha + \gamma)dt.$$

This simple equation can be solved exactly, yielding:

$$C(t + \Delta t) = C(t) \exp\left[-(\alpha + \gamma)\Delta t\right]$$

If the time step $\Delta t = 1$, the proportion of individuals remaining in class C at the end of the time step is $\exp\left[-(\alpha + \gamma)\right]$. The proportion of individuals leaving class C is therefore what remains when we subtract those that stay from the total individuals in that class (since we are talking of proportions, the total is 1); that is, the proportion of persons exiting class C is $1 - \exp\left[-(\alpha + \gamma)\right]$. Of these individuals that exit, a fraction $\frac{\alpha}{\alpha+\gamma}$ go to class A and $\frac{\gamma}{\alpha+\gamma}$ go to class G. To update the system we use the following convention in order to facilitate the calculations. We first calculate the total leaving rate for each model class, a vector called '`exit_rates`'. In the case of the example above the value of `exit_rates` would be $\alpha + \gamma$. In each time step, beginning with a state vector $X_{\texttt{init}}$, we calculate the number of individuals that remain in class p, which we denominate $Z[p]$, as:

$$Z[p] = \exp\left(-\texttt{exit\_rates}[p]\right)X_{\texttt{init}}[p].$$

The total number of persons leaving class p is the product between the proportion leaving class p and the initial number of persons in class p, i.e.:
$\{1 - \exp\left(-\texttt{exit\_rates}[p]\right)X_{\texttt{init}}[p]$. The individuals that leave each class now distribute themselves into the different TB classes according to the rates determined by each process. For compactness of notation we introduce an intermediate vector Y with elements that are normalized by the total exit rate per state:

$$Y[p] = \left(\frac{1}{\texttt{exit\_rates}[p]}\right)\{1 - \exp\left(-\texttt{exit\_rates}[p]\right)\}X_{\texttt{init}}[p].$$

Now if the per capita transition rate from class p to class q is α_{pq} , the number of individuals making the transition from p to q is simply $\alpha_{pq}Y[p]$. In our example set forth above, this would be $\texttt{exit\_rates}[C] = \alpha+\gamma$, so $Z[C] = \exp[-(\alpha+\gamma)]X_{\texttt{init}}[C]$ and $Y[C] = \left\{\frac{1}{\alpha+\gamma}\right\}\{1-\exp[-(\alpha+\gamma)]\}\,X_{\texttt{init}}[C]$. The transition rate from class C to class A is α, so the number of individuals making that transition in one time step can be calculated with the equation $\alpha Y[C] = \left\{\frac{\alpha}{\alpha+\gamma}\right\}\{1-\exp[-(\alpha+\gamma)]\}\,X_{\texttt{init}}[C]$.

Model equations. The state vector X represents the number of individuals in each of the 210 TB/HIV states described in Table 1 and depicted in Fig. 1. The parameters used in the model are defined in Table 3. The total population of our model is $N = \displaystyle\sum_{i=1}^{42}\sum_{j=1}^{5} X[i,j]$, where i = TB category and j = HIV category. The force of infection $c_j\lambda$ describes the hazard rate of infection for each susceptible individual (where c_j is the factor corresponding to each HIV stage, Table 3), and can be calculated from the weighted sum of all infectious classes by the equation:

$$\lambda = \frac{1}{N}\sum_{j=1}^{5}\Bigg\{\beta_P(X[4,j]+X[7,j]) + \beta_N(X[5,j]+X[8,j]) + \beta_{PD}\sum_{m=9}^{16}X[m,j]$$
$$+\beta_{PN}\sum_{m=17}^{24}X[m,j] + \beta_{ND}\sum_{m=26}^{33}X[m,j]$$
$$+\beta_{NN}\sum_{m=34}^{41}X[m,j] + \beta_{PF}X[25,j] + \beta_{NF}X[42,j]\Bigg\}.$$

We now apply the competing rates formulation described above. The total exit rates for each state are defined in Table 2. We label the state vector at the beginning and end of the time steps as $X_{\texttt{init}}$ and $X_{\texttt{next}}$, respectively, and update their value from one time interval to the next by the relationship:

$$X_{\texttt{init}}[i,j]_{t+1} = X_{\texttt{next}}[i,j]_t,$$

where the subscript t refers to the interval under consideration. For simplicity we drop the time t subscript throughout. The number of individuals remaining in each class is then given by the vector Z with the following elements for the HIV categories 1-4:

$$Z[i,j] = \exp(-\texttt{exit\_rates}[i,j])X_{\texttt{init}}[i,j], \text{ for all } i \text{ and } j = 1,\ldots,4.$$

For the final HIV stage IV (category 5) there is an important difference as compared to the HIV categories 1-4, because now we also needed to account for the additional death rate from AIDS μ_H (Table 3). This additional outflow occurred simultaneously to the other TB processes, but because it implies permanent removal from the system we did not reincorporate into the inflows $\xi_{i,j}$ (see below):

$$Z[i,5] = \exp(-\texttt{exit\_rates}[i,5] - \mu H)X_{\texttt{init}}[i,5], \text{ for all } i.$$

The intermediate vector Y has the following elements for HIV categories 1-4:

$$Y[i,j] = \frac{1}{\texttt{exit\_rates}[i,j]}\{1-\exp(\texttt{exit\_rates}[i,j])\}\,X_{\texttt{init}}[i,j],$$
$$\text{for all } i \text{ and } j = 1,\ldots,4,$$

and for HIV category 5 they are

$$Y[i,5] = \frac{1}{\texttt{exit\_rates}[i,5] + \mu_H} \left\{1 - \exp\left(-\texttt{exit\_rates}[i,5] - \mu_H\right)\right\} X_{\texttt{init}}[i,5], \quad \text{for all } i.$$

We then proceeded to calculate the state vector $X_{\texttt{next}}$. For clarity purposes, we first describe the equations $\xi_{i,j}$ representing the inflows to each category due to TB infection and treatment. We would like to point out that all of these equations are identical for HIV stages $j = 1 \ldots 5$:

$$
\begin{aligned}
\xi_{i,j}[1,j] &= \nu N\\
\xi_{i,j}[2,j] &= p_S(\lambda Y[1,j] + b\lambda Y[6,j]) + \pi(Y[4,j] + Y[7,j] + Y[5,j] + Y[8,j])\\
\xi_{i,j}[3,j] &= (1-p_S)(\lambda Y[1,j] + b\lambda Y[2,j] + b\lambda Y[6,j])\\
\xi_{i,j}[4,j] &= s_P(1-d_P)(\phi_S Y[2,j] + \phi_F Y[3,j]) + \sigma Y[5,j] + (1-d_P)\rho Y[25,j]\\
\xi_{i,j}[5,j] &= (1-s_P)(1-d_N)(\phi_S Y[2,j] + \phi_F Y[3,j]) + (1-d_N)\rho Y[42,j]\\
\xi_{i,j}[6,j] &= \sum_{m=1}^{8} \{(1-\nu_D)K_D(Z[8+m,j] + Z[25+m,j])\\
&\qquad +(1-\nu_N)K_N(Z[16+m,j] + Z[33+m,j])\}\\
\xi_{i,j}[7,j] &= s_P d_P(\phi_S Y[2,j] + \phi_F Y[3,j]) + \sigma Y[8,j] + d_P\rho Y[25,j]\\
\xi_{i,j}[8,j] &= (1-s_P)d_N(\phi_S Y[2,j] + \phi_F Y[3,j]) + d_N\rho Y[42,j]\\
\xi_{i,j}[9,j] &= \theta t_P Y(7,j)\\
\xi_{i,j}[9+m,j] &= Z[9+m-1,j](1-K_D[m]), && m = 1,2,\ldots,7\\
\xi_{i,j}[17,j] &= \theta(1-t_P)Y(7,j)\\
\xi_{i,j}[17+m,j] &= Z[17+m-1,j](1-K_N[m]), && m = 1,2,\ldots,7\\
\xi_{i,j}[25,j] &= \sum_{m=1}^{8} \{\delta_D Y[8+m,j] + \delta_N Y[16+m,j]\\
&\qquad + \nu_D K_D[m] Z[8+m,j] + \nu_N K_N[m] Z[16+m,j]\}\\
\xi_{i,j}[26,j] &= \theta t_N Y(8,j)\\
\xi_{i,j}[26+m,j] &= Z[26+m-1,j](1-K_D[m]), && m = 1,2,\ldots,7\\
\xi_{i,j}[34,j] &= \theta(1-t_N)Y(8,j)\\
\xi_{i,j}[34+m,j] &= Z[34+m-1,j](1-K_N[m]), && m = 1,2,\ldots,7\\
\xi_{i,j}[42,j] &= \sum_{m=1}^{8} \{\delta_D Y[25+m,j] + \delta_N Y[33+m,j]\\
&\qquad + \nu_D K_D[m] Z[25+m,j] + \nu_N K_N[m] Z[33+m,j]\}
\end{aligned}
$$

To account for the simultaneous occurrence of HIV infection and progression, we introduced the parameter Ψ_j (Table 3). The first element of Ψ_j reflected HIV incidence values that generated reported HIV prevalence levels (Cheluget et al. 2006), as explained above. The next 3 elements represented progression of HIV stages I-III (Morgan et al. 2002), and, finally, the fifth element had a value of 0, since there is no transition beyond stage IV (only death, which was accounted for separately as a competing rate to TB process transitions, see above and Table 2). At each time step the new $X_{\texttt{next}}$ was calculated by the sum of the persons staying in the corresponding TB and HIV category, those progressing in only one disease, and those progressing in both. Accordingly, the HIV-uninfected category is updated with those persons that remain HIV uninfected $(1 - \Psi_1)$ and either do not progress in their TB category ($Z[i,1]$) or that do progress ($\sum_{i=1}^{42} \xi_{i,1}$):

$$X_{\texttt{next}}[i,1] = (1 - \Psi_1)(Z[i,1] + \sum_{i=1}^{42} \xi_{i,1}) \qquad \text{for } i = 1 - 42.$$

Likewise, the HIV infected categories are updated with persons that remain in that same HIV category ($1-\Psi_j$) and either do not progress in their TB category ($Z[i,j]$) or that do progress ($\sum_{i=1}^{42}\sum_{j=2}^{5} \xi_{i,j}$). The difference with the HIV uninfected category ($j = 1$ above) lies in that now we also have to account for those persons that either became infected or progressed from the previous HIV stage (Ψ_{j-1}) together with their TB dynamics, i.e., we need to include those persons that did not progress in their TB category ($Z[i, j-1]$), or that did progress ($\sum_{i=1}^{42}\sum_{j=2}^{5} \xi_{i,j-1}$):

$$X_{\texttt{next}}[i,j] = (1 - \Psi_j)(Z[i,j] + \sum_{i=1}^{42}\sum_{j=2}^{5} \xi_{i,j}) + \Psi_{j-1}(Z[i,j-1] + \sum_{i=1}^{42}\sum_{j=2}^{5} \xi_{i,j-1})$$
$$\text{for } i = 1 - 42, \text{ and } j = 2 - 5.$$

At any given time point, the number of persons in each HIV disease stage was determined by the year since the HIV epidemic began, by the average time spent in each HIV disease stage, and by the HIV prevalence. People become infected (i.e., move from the HIV uninfected stage into the HIV infected stage I, a process which corresponds to HIV incidence Ψ_1), progress through the subsequent HIV stages II-IV ($\Psi_2 - \Psi_4$) and ultimately die of HIV (μ_H) according to the time frames given by Morgan et al. (Morgan et al. 2002) for Africa. Our model formulation allows us to emulate the historical estimates of HIV prevalence (i.e., the sum of all the persons in HIV stages I through IV) as reported for Kenya (Cheluget et al. 2006) by altering the HIV incidence (Fig. 2).

In the equations referring to treatment states in the model, we include the "switch" variables K_D and K_N, which are vectors representing the monthly probabilities that a course of treatment ends. For conventional drug therapies, these vectors are:

$$K_D = [0\ 0\ 0\ 0\ 0\ 1\ 0\ 0] \qquad \text{for six-month DOTS treatment, and}$$
$$K_N = [0\ 0\ 0\ 0\ 0\ 0\ 0\ 1] \qquad \text{for eight-month non-DOTS treatment.}$$

For the two-month treatment achieved with novel drug technologies, they are:

$$K_D = K_N = [0\ 1\ 0\ 0\ 0\ 0\ 0\ 0].$$

In this formulation we assumed that shorter regimens, if available, would be used in both DOTS and non-DOTS treatment programs. New TB cases were computed as the sum of the flows from the latently infected, both slow and fast, and of the progressors from the failed treatment class, both smear-positive and smear-negative:

.

$$\text{New\_TBcases} = \sum_{j=1}^{5} (\phi_S Y_{2j} + \phi_F Y_{3j} + \rho_P Y_{25j} + \rho_N Y_{42j}).$$

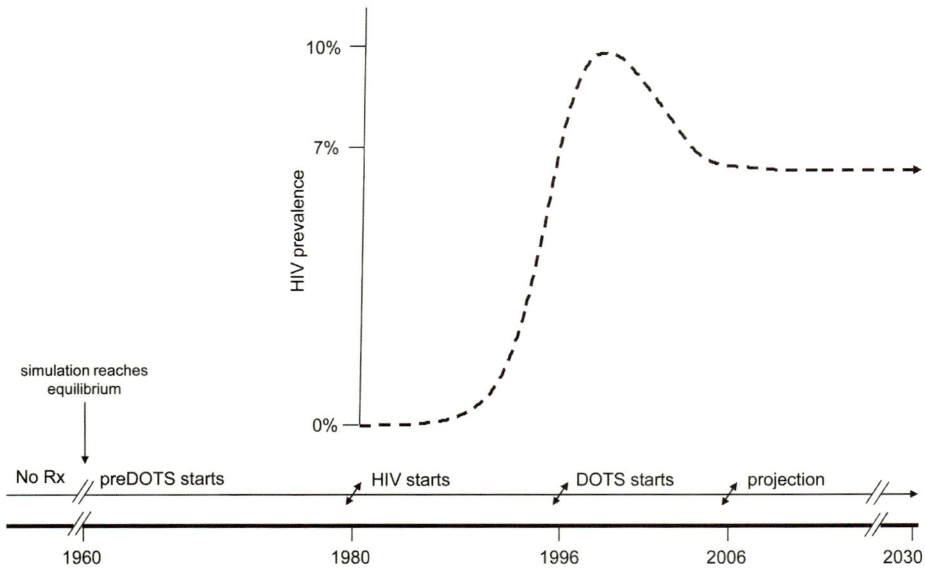

FIGURE 2. **Historical reconstruction of HIV prevalence following trends reported by Cheluget et al. (2006) and TB treatment options in Kenya.** Each simulation began as a virgin epidemic with only one infected person, which we ran until equilibrium. At this point we assumed conditions for the year 1960 were reached. After 2006 the projection period started and ran for 25 years, till 2030.

3.4. TB/HIV historical reconstruction. Each one of our individual simulations reconstructed the history of the TB and HIV epidemics in Kenya through a series of consecutive phases (Fig. 2). These phases represent historical periods in which distinct TB treatment programs were implemented in Kenya throughout the 20th century and beginning of the 21st century; they also include the beginning and future development of the HIV epidemic in this country. Accordingly, we initiated each simulation by generating an epidemic of TB with one infected person in a population of 10,000 susceptibles under conditions representative of a virgin epidemic where no TB treatment is available. This simulation was run to equilibrium, generating conditions corresponding to 1958. In this year, the first Kenyan national TB control program started (Odhiambo et al. 1999); we simulated this era of TB treatment prior to the advent of DOTS (pre-DOTS) assuming a partially-effective TB treatment was in place for a period of 20 years. We then introduced the HIV epidemic to match relevant increases in HIV prevalence beginning in the early 1980s (UNAIDS 2006). After 15 years we introduced DOTS, and gradually increased its coverage over the next 2 years; this was done in order to replicate the official start of the program in Kenya in 1993, and the achievement of nationwide coverage by 1996 (Hanson & Kibuga 2000). By 1996, 56% of smear positive and 71% of smear negative cases entered DOTS treatment programs, Annex 1a in (World Health Organization 2006a). We then proceeded to simulate conditions corresponding to the implementation of DOTS for 10 years, until we reached the year 2006 and our predictive scenario analysis began.

4. Model calibration

Once we had built the model we needed to establish the parameter values characterizing the forces represented in our model. This is one of the most difficult, if not the most difficult step in a process such as the one we are conducting. The medical and epidemiological literature for TB, HIV, and TB/HIV disease processes is quite vast, but not sufficiently refined as to provide precise estimates for most of our parameter values. Considerable uncertainty exists in the parameter values characterizing TB infection and progression, and HIV co-infection only deepens this uncertainty (Williams & Dye 2003). Many clinical trials have examined these issues, but differences in study design complicate the task of synthesizing their results. Moreover, results are in many cases inconclusive (Cruciani et al. 2001). We therefore cannot provide precise quantitative characterizations regarding the probability and/or speed at which many of the different processes occur. Moreover, because of the substantial heterogeneity in TB and HIV trends worldwide, we expect many of these parameter values to vary in space and time (Bates et al. 2004). In this regard, our model is relatively complex, with almost 600 parameter values. Fortunately, many of our parameters represent the same TB disease process partitioned across monthly treatment and across HIV disease stages, because we do expect many of the processes captured by our model to become more accentuated as a person progresses in their HIV infection. In any case, we would like to point out that each one of these parameter values deserves a meta-analysis unto itself (Cruciani et al. 2001) but for the most part the time and money available for TB research does not permit even a moderate meta-analysis of selected parameter values to take place.

Calibrating a model is an extremely useful tool to help us determine the most reliable parameter values for conducting the predictive exercise for which we had constructed our model. The ultimate goal of the calibration analysis is to identify the parameter set that generates the model trajectory with the closest fit to the epidemiological trends of interest. This computational tool is particularly valuable when the uncertainty in the numerical values of the parameters characterizing the different disease processes is large. Even though the calibration enables us to track reported epidemiological trends more precisely, it is also laden with assumptions because for many parameters we do not have a proper understanding of the minimum and maximum numerical values they can have (i.e., their valid ranges, see below). Moreover, there could be compensatory effects among the parameters that could lead us to choose a parameter set that does not correspond to the actual values characterizing the process in the field, but that tracks the reported trends (themselves potentially questionable) with high fidelity.

4.1. TB/HIV trends data for our model calibration. We first needed to decide which trends we were going to use in order to determine our parameter values. That is, we needed to identify the data set that we would make our model output match more closely. Our study entailed evaluating benefits of reducing treatment duration in high HIV prevalence areas, with a particular focus on sub-Saharan Africa. However, there is tremendous heterogeneity in disease monitoring infrastructure and overall TB and HIV prevalence levels in Africa. Accordingly, rather than calibrate our model at a wide regional level we opted for a smaller spatial scale calibration. We decided on the country level because it amounts to a monitoring unit where we can expect a certain degree of cohesiveness. Our goal with this approach was to limit any misinterpretations that non-congruent trends at broader spatial scales could generate in the quantitative characterization of the parameter values determining TB and HIV dynamics. Even though we do expect there to be substantial environmental, social, and public health heterogeneity within a country, on average countries tend to be sufficiently big that by using this relatively large spatial scale we anticipated avoiding using TB/HIV trends that would reflect odd local co-dynamics. Our country of choice was Kenya, because this country has one of the strongest surveillance systems for TB and HIV in sub-Saharan Africa, and the burden of both diseases is high. We used TB data presented in the WHO Global TB Database and the WHO 2001 through 2006 Global Reports (World Health Organization 2006a; World Health Organization 2006b). Our data set corresponds to a total of 106 data points representing different TB and TB/HIV measures spanning 1980-2004 in Kenya.

The different types of measures we used were:

1. TB incidence per 100,000 persons per year (per 100K/yr) for 1990, 1995-2004 (World Health Organization 2006a);
2. smear-positive TB incidence per 100K/yr for 1990, 1995-2004 (World Health Organization 2006a);
3. TB incidence excluding HIV-infected persons (HIV+) per 100K/yr for 1990 (World Health Organization 2006a);
4. TB incidence in HIV+ per 100K/yr for 1995-2004 (World Health Organization 2006a);
5. smear-positive TB incidence in HIV+ per 100K/yr for 1995-2004 (World Health Organization 2006a);
6. TB case notification rates per 100K/yr for 1980, 1981, 1983, 1985-2004 (World Health Organization 2006b);
7. smear-positive TB case notification rates per 100K/yr for 1993-2004 (World Health Organization 2006a);
8. TB deaths per 100K/yr for 1990, 1995-2004 (World Health Organization 2006a);
9. TB deaths excluding HIV+ per 100K/yr for 1990 (World Health Organization 2006a);
10. TB deaths in HIV+ per 100K/yr for 1995-2004 (World Health Organization 2006a);
11. proportion of cases that are HIV+ in 1999 (World Health Organization 2001), 2000 (World Health Organization 2002), 2001 (World Health Organization 2003), 2002 (World Health Organization 2004b), 2003 (World Health Organization 2005), and 2004 (World Health Organization 2006b).

Because our model operates on a monthly time step, we summed over our predicted 12-month model outputs to obtain the yearly estimates used to match the observed data points. We assigned an equal weight to all the 106 measures in order to minimize the assumptions we made throughout the study, although it is expected that certain measures and years may be more reliable than others. We originally included an additional 22 prevalence measures in our calibration. We opted to exclude them from the final calibration because these estimates require further assumptions in their calculation, and when included the resulting fit to the preferred measures of case notification, incidence and mortality became substantially worse. Our calibration and evaluation of benefits (see below) refers to the adult population because the HIV prevalence trends we follow refer to this segment of the population (Cheluget et al. 2006), the TB measures according to HIV status are also based on this age group, while the contribution of persons <15 years of age to the remaining TB measures (which are based on all age groups in the whole population) is minimal (World Health Organization 2002).

4.2. Parameters to vary in our calibration. Because the total number of parameters in our model was so large, it was not feasible to vary all parameters for computational reasons. Moreover, varying such a large number of parameters would most probably impede us from carrying out a sound interpretation of the resulting patterns. Therefore, the second step in our calibration process was to choose a subset of our parameters whose values we would vary in order to determine the optimal value for our particular analysis (as explained above, in our case this corresponds to the average parameter values that will characterize TB and HIV disease processes in sub-Saharan Africa most faithfully). We chose a total of 12 different parameter types (Table 4), of which nine were partitioned across HIV stage for a total of 47 parameters. In our selection we targeted those parameters that were most important in the sensitivity analysis of Salomon et al. (2006), and reflected core processes of TB natural history or the impact of TB control programs and HIV on TB dynamics.

4.3. Parameter ranges. The next step was to define reasonable ranges for the value of those parameters we selected to vary in our calibration, based on expert opinion, published literature (for details see Table 3), and preliminary investigations (see below). Because HIV infection results in increases in susceptibility to TB infection, progression through disease classes, display of symptoms, and mortality rates, we defined constraints for the relative magnitudes of specific parameters in order to address the impact of decreased immunity as a person advances in their HIV infection. Within a parameter type, those parameters representing HIV stages had to satisfy one of the following inequalities: either uninfected > (stage I and stage II) > stage III > stage IV, or the inverse uninfected < (stage I and stage II) < stage III < stage IV. We did not constrain the relative magnitudes of those HIV stage I and II parameters that we varied in the calibration, because of the uncertainty in the literature on how the immune system is affected by early stage HIV infection in regards to TB: the strong immune adjustments that occur during acute HIV infection (stage I) may potentially have a strong negative impact on TB infection and progression (Fox et al. 2006; Sonnenberg et al. 2005). As such, TB occurs in PLWHA at all CD_4 lymphocyte count levels (World Health Organization 2004a). By leaving the relative magnitudes of these HIV stage I and stage II parameters unconstrained, we wanted to establish what individual-level TB progression patterns would emerge from the calibration of our model to country-level data. The ranges we used are provided in Table 3.

4.4. Parameter sets. We then proceeded to generate candidate parameter sets using the Latin Hypercube Sampling method, LHS (Blower & Dowlatabadi 1994, Marino et al. 2008). Because of the large degree of uncertainty in values characterizing the disease processes of our model, we opted for a conservative approach that we hoped would least bias our results, and defined all parameter ranges to be uniform in favor, for example, of triangular distributions. In the latter, the sampling process selects values more often from the center of the predefined range as compared to the outer edges (Hogg & Craig 1995; Saltelli et al. 2000). All parameters had constant values throughout each run (i.e., throughout all the years corresponding to the historical reconstruction) except for two TB control parameters: the proportion of new cases entering the detectable pool d, and the proportion of cases entering DOTS programs, including both smear-positive cases t_p and smear-negative cases t_N.

4.5. Goodness-of-fit. Once we had generated a matrix of admissible parameter sets, we fed each individual set into the model and ran a separate simulation for all that started in the very initial virgin phase and progressed through the subsequent three phases characterizing the TB epidemic in Kenya, until 2006 (Fig. 2). We stored the model output in terms of the above mentioned reported trends data for each set, and we evaluated the outcome with several goodness-of-fit measures in order to determine which one of all of the parameter generated a model output that tracked reported TB and HIV trends in Kenya more closely. Given the problems we encountered when trying to fit the model output to the reported data (see below) for all of these different measures, we defined and used in our final calibration the following goodness-of-fit-like measure:

$$\text{GF} = \sum_{\text{over-all-values}} \frac{(\text{Obs} - \text{Exp})^2}{0.5(\text{Obs} + \text{Exp})^2},$$

where the observed data points (Obs) correspond to reported epidemiological data, and the expected data points (Exp) are the model output, which vary with each parameter set. The best-fit trajectory is the one with the smallest total GF value.

The reason why we used this measure and not the conventional goodness-of-fit measure that sums over (Obs - Exp)^2/Exp terms, is because the latter places greater weight on instances where observed values exceed expected values (Obs > Exp) than those where Obs < Exp. However, the empirically derived Obs values should not be given this privileged status since they appear to be subject to just as much uncertainty as the model derived Exp values: the Obs values incorporate numerous uncertainties related to disease surveillance, while the Exp values integrate numerous sources of knowledge via a mathematical model and hence contain a level of deductive coherency. The measure we defined is symmetric with respect to Obs and Exp values, and hence makes no *a priori* assumption about which is more reliable. The price we pay for this approach is the loss of the theoretical knowledge that GF is asymptotically chi-squared.

4.6. Model Calibration. Working in a gradual process with our candidate parameter sets, we evaluated the fit of the model outcome for each set to the TB and TB/HIV Kenyan measures spanning 1980 to 2004 through feedback and recalibration. Each parameter set was run as a separate simulation that started in the initial virgin phase, and progressed through the subsequent three phases characterizing the TB epidemic in Kenya during the last century and early part of the 21st century (i.e., until 2006). If any parameter values in the best GF set were at the margin of the pre-defined ranges, we shifted the range by 5% or 10%, depending on the breadth of the original range. Additionally, we restricted the original range if the 20 best GF parameter sets were in a close neighbourhood. We generated additional parameters sets with the LHS method, whose values fell within the constraints of the new parameter ranges, and ran further simulations. This approach permitted us to modify our designation of the parameter ranges characterizing the person-level processes according to the fit of the model to the 25-year country-level data. This iterative procedure involved >30,000 simulations. For the calibration with the final ranges, we ran >6,000 parameter sets. In our subsequent calibration conducted to match the model output to the full 1980-2004 TB and TB/HIV dataset, we used the same final parameter sets (and therefore the same parameter ranges and constraints) derived from our earlier fit to the reported HIV trends (Cheluget et al. 2006). However, in this last calibration we modified the HIV incidence such that HIV prevalence increased monotonically at different rates to a final 2004 value that ranged between 10%-25%, resulting in >37,000 runs.

4.7. Results of our model calibration. We then proceeded to evaluate the fit of our simulated trends to the full TB and TB/HIV datasets in Kenya (1980-2004, 106 measures, see above) under the background HIV prevalence series covering this same time period (Cheluget et al. 2006; UNAIDS 2006). However, none of the parameter sets generated under the parameter ranges defined were capable of tracking the reported TB and TB/HIV datasets adequately. If a given parameter set was capable of generating a model output that matched well the TB data points from the earlier part of the interval, invariably the model output would fall short of the reported TB numbers in the later years of our interval (Fig. 3). Only by allowing the initial model output to be much higher than that of reported TB numbers could we match the data points corresponding to the later years (approximately 1999 and beyond); that is, could we generate TB numbers as high as those officially reported by WHO. Table 3 provides the parameter values, together with the corresponding parameter ranges we used in our study.

In order to investigate further the potential reasons for why our model could not track the officially reported TB/HIV trends, we conducted an additional calibration to establish if our model could capture the rise in TB case notifications throughout the full dataset (1980-2004) given different assumptions regarding HIV trends. The main purpose of this calibration was not to determine the actual HIV prevalence in Kenya, which the model and the data are not sufficiently refined to do, but rather to establish whether our inability to track reported trends was due to some inherent limitation of our modeling exercise. The model was capable of tracking reported TB trends if we incorporated the HIV incidence into the system such that the HIV prevalence was increasing monotonically up to a 22.7% prevalence value (Fig. 4). Numerous reasons, elaborated further in Sánchez et al. (2009), do not support the assumption that HIV prevalence is anywhere close to such a high HIV prevalence value, and therefore this result if anything indicates that factors other than HIV prevalence were responsible, or were contributing, to the mismatch.

In our calibration of the model to this monotonically increasing HIV epidemic we focused on matching the TB case notifications. Accordingly, the fit to the TB case notifications improved substantially (0.42 vs. 0.08), while the overall fit to

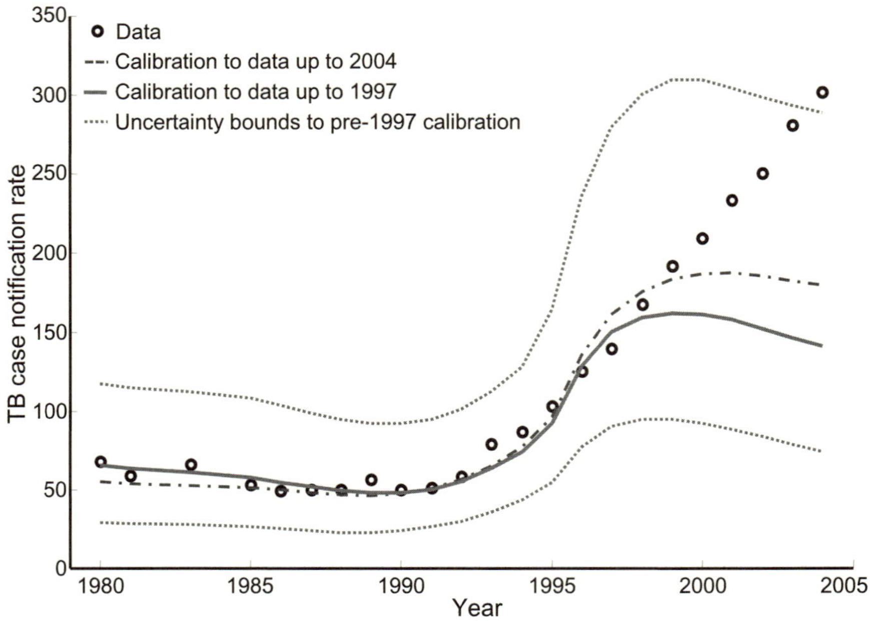

FIGURE 3. **TB case notifications per 100,000 persons in Kenya, including those officially reported at the time of our analysis, and those obtained by our model following reported HIV prevalence trends calibrated to various TB and joint TB-HIV measures for the two time periods spanning 1980-1997 and 1980-2004.** We present the uncertainty bounds, as determined by the 1000 runs with the best goodness-of-fit (GF, as defined in the text), for the calibration to data points up to 1997. We show TB case notifications because it is the measure with the longest time series, but similarly incongruent results were obtained for incidence and mortality. (Corresponds to Fig. 1 in Sánchez, M. S., Lloyd-Smith, J., Williams, B. G., Porco, T. C., Ryan, S. J., Borgdorff, M. W., Mansoer, J., Dye, C. & Getz, W. M. 2009 Incongruent HIV and tuberculosis co-dynamics in Kenya: Interacting epidemics monitor each other. *Epidemics* 1:14-20).

the full dataset worsened (from 6.2 to 7.4) in comparison with that of the best-fit parameter set under the calibration to reported HIV trends. The measures most responsible for the increase in the GF involved TB measures in HIV infected persons in the most recent years, particularly TB deaths in HIV infected and the proportion of TB cases that are HIV infected. When these two measures are not included in the calculation of the GF, then the overall fit to the full dataset under the monotonically increasing HIV epidemic is better than that under the reported HIV trends (4.9 vs. 5.5). Most significantly, the fit to the TB incidence in later years, and the fit to TB mortality in both early and later years, improved under the calibration to the monotonically increasing HIV epidemic.

Currie et al. (2003) had previously conducted a modeling investigation comparing the benefits to be derived from different TB control methods, namely prevention

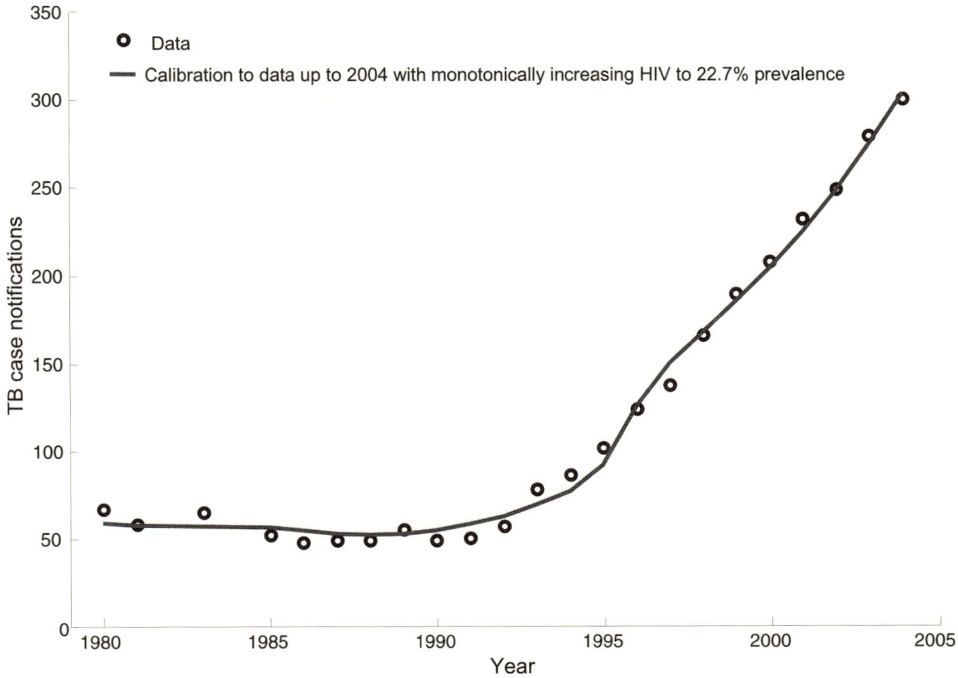

FIGURE 4. **Reported TB case notifications for Kenya and model output calibrated to various TB and joint TB-HIV measures reported for the period 1980-2004, following a monotonically increasing HIV epidemic that reaches a prevalence of 22.7% in 2005.**

of TB as compared to the treatment of active TB. Interestingly, these authors also obtain the critical result where a decrease in HIV trends is followed by a decrease in TB trends. However, our results are not identical with regards to when the decrease in TB numbers occurs as a consequence of the decrease in the HIV numbers. The reason for this is that we allowed for the potential increase in susceptibility to TB infection and progression to occur in earlier HIV stages (Fox et al. 2006; Sonnenberg et al. 2005) while Currie et al. (2003) grouped the uninfected and early HIV-infected (stages I and II) and assumed their epidemiological behaviour was equivalent. In consequence, the time lag between the HIV and TB declines in Currie et al. (2003) is longer than that predicted in our study.

In spite of all the difficulties we had encountered in fitting the model output to the post-1997 trends, we still needed to define adequate parameter values in order to generate our predictions regarding reducing TB treatment in high HIV prevalence areas. We decided that the most adequate approach entailed calibrating the model to the 'pre-1997' TB and TB/HIV dataset, which spanned 1980-1997 and comprised a total of 44 data points. Accordingly, we also used the HIV prevalence series only until 1997, which corresponds to the year in which HIV prevalence began to decrease (Table 3 and Fig. 2). This dual calibration process permitted us to compare the values of the parameter sets that provided the best fit to each of the time frames. Overall, these values were quite similar for both calibrations, a result that supports the robustness of the model and calibration process to the different time frames used in our analyses. The differences we observed between the two calibrations were: (*i*) susceptibility to becoming TB infected was higher in stage II, although smaller for the other 3 infection force values across HIV stages (λ_j) and, interestingly, this parameter had a greater impact on TB incidence changes in the full dataset vs. the pre-1997 dataset (Tables 3 and 4, see below); (*ii*) patients that transiently recovered were more infectious ($\beta_{TR} = 0.54$ vs. 0.26); and (*iii*) default rates were higher ($\delta_m = 0.027$ vs. 0.02). Otherwise the parameter estimates for the two calibrations were very similar for HIV uninfected and HIV stages I and II. Values were less similar for parameters characterizing HIV stage IV. This is partly due to these being parameters of lesser impact (Tables 3 and 4, see below), which is compounded by the inherent limitations of the calibration to country-level data.

We were also interested in understanding how the country-level calibration to the pre-1997 and the full datasets resolved the relative values of the parameters characterizing TB processes in HIV infected persons in stages I and II. With this process in essence we are deriving individual-level, clinical parameters for the different HIV stages from population-level data. It is interesting to note that although the relative magnitudes of the pertinent 8 parameter types across HIV stages I and II were not constrained in the calibration (λ_j,$p_{S,j}$,π_j,ρ_j,$s_{P,j}$,σ_j, θ_j,$q_{c,j}$, where j = 0 indicates HIV uninfected, and j = 1-4 indicates HIV stage I-IV, respectively, see Table 3 for ranges), when we calibrated the model to the pre-1997 (1980-1997) dataset all parameters ordered themselves in the expected increasing or decreasing relationships according to HIV stage. When we used the full dataset (1980-2004) only two parameters had their values inverted with respect to those expected under a progressive immune deterioration from the moment of HIV infection. Most importantly, the case-detection rates θ_1 and θ_2 had inverted values: $\theta_1 = 0.18 > \theta_2$ $= 0.16$ (in any case the ranges for θ_1 and θ_2 completely overlapped, while those of the other parameters did not, see Table 3). When we exchanged the values for θ_1 and θ_2, the GF became worse. Therefore, under this calibration the strikingly non-matching HIV and TB trends are best tracked by assuming that more TB infections are detected in persons in HIV stage I than in HIV stage II. In addition, the relapse rate from the failed treatment class to active disease in HIV stages I and II, ρ_1 and ρ_2, were also inverted in relative magnitude as compared to those expected under the general HIV progression scenario (0.119 and 0.112, respectively). In both cases, however, these two values have very similar magnitudes, and according to the sensitivity analysis these parameters do not have a great impact on TB incidence, so that small differences between them are not expected to have a large impact on the epidemic's course and therefore on their predictive value (Table 4). In addition, the GF score decreased when we exchanged the values.

In summary, under our detailed calibration scheme and with the Kenyan data officially reported in 2006, our mathematical model gave us sufficient insight to evaluate TB/HIV co-dynamics in Kenya and realize that officially reported trends were highly incongruent. To address the original question posed by the Global TB Alliance regarding expected reductions in TB numbers that a 2- month versus the current 6-8 month treatment regimen might yield, we decided to calibrate our model only until 1997, because the trends reported for this 1980-1997 period did follow the generally observed premise–both clinically and epidemiologically–by which increasing HIV trends lead to increasing TB trends in our model, and vice-versa

(Corbett et al. 2003; Lawn et al. 2006; Nunn et al. 2007; Sonnenberg et al. 2005; Williams & Dye 2003). But the question still remained regarding what factor(s) might be responsible for the observed incongruency in TB/HIV trends in Kenya of the beginning of the 21st century.

5. TB/HIV co-dynamics in Africa: Pan-African patterns

As with all models of biological systems, our model captures only a few of the processes involved, albeit we believe the dominant ones. Thus we cannot exclude the possibility that the mismatch between reported trends and model output arises because the model does not accurately reflect the epidemiological mechanisms at play. We note, however, that another model of TB/HIV co-dynamics (with a different structure from the model reported here) also failed to reconcile declining HIV prevalence with increasing TB incidence (Currie, pers. comm.). To further our understanding of TB/HIV co-dynamics in Kenya, and help establish if the inability of our model to track reported trends for the 1980-1997 period was due to a flawed approach in our analysis or rather to these pandemics behaving as outliers in this sub-Saharan country, we extended our investigation and compared TB/HIV trends across the whole of Africa. To facilitate this continental-scale comparison, we decided to define an indicator that would capture TB/HIV co-dynamics in a single number. After considering other potential indicators, we settled on a measure that would provide a quantitative comparison of the average change in TB numbers compared to the average change in HIV numbers. When we began our investigation, we were hoping to collect reliable data for an extended period of time (i.e., more than a decade) for a large number of countries. However, only in the case of Uganda could we obtain reasonable data for both TB and HIV over such a period because HIV estimates from earlier years for many countries had undergone substantial revisions (Sánchez et al. 2009). Because of these limitations on the availability of suitable TB and HIV data, we calculated the relative average annual change in TB case notifications between 1998 and 2004, and compared it to the relative average annual change in HIV prevalence between 2003 and 2005 for those African countries recently reported at the time by both WHO (World Health Organization 2006a) and UNAIDS (UNAIDS 2006). We subtracted 1 from this ratio to obtain a measure centered at 0:

$$relative\_change = \frac{1 + \left[\frac{\left(\frac{TB\_case\_notifications(2004)}{TB\_case\_notifications(1998)} - 1\right)}{6}\right]}{1 + \left[\frac{\left(\frac{HIV\_prevalence(2005)}{HIV\_prevalence(2003)} - 1\right)}{2}\right]} - 1$$

This formula was applied to all countries considered expect Zambia, because health officials in this country did not report a TB case notification estimate for 1998. Thus for Zambia we used the 1999 estimate and divided the ratio in the numerator by 5 instead of 6 (to accommodate for the 1-year shorter interval to 2004).

These officially reported numbers by WHO and UNAIDS at the time we conducted our analyses (UNAIDS 2006; World Health Organization 2006b) did not provide the ideal time frame for the comparison of TB and HIV trends across different countries in Africa because they did not capture the main drop in HIV prevalence occurring in Kenya in the late 90s. In spite of this, our continental-scale analysis of TB/HIV trends placed Kenya as a clear outlier in eastern and southern Africa (see Fig. 2 in Sánchez et al. 2009). Furthermore, our analysis exposed how the most worrisome TB trends are situated in western central Africa, where Cameroon and Nigeria are the two African countries with TB case notification rates growing at the fastest pace as compared to HIV prevalence.

In light of the results we obtained from our calibration analysis, we conducted a detailed review of the literature in an attempt to identify key factors affecting recent TB and HIV trends in Kenya. In principle, the mismatch could be due to faulty TB and HIV estimates: an unaccounted improvement in TB case detection could have occurred, or HIV is not actually declining as reported. The TB/HIV mismatch could be compounded by surveillance biases due to spatial heterogeneity in disease dynamics. Moreover, in recent years Kenya has undergone substantial demographic changes that include a rapid urbanization rate accompanied by poor living conditions, particularly in Nairobi. These processes could favor increased TB transmission rates, and accordingly contribute to the disproportionate increase in TB incidence. Other possible factors include immune reconstitution due to the recent delivery of antiretroviral therapy for HIV, and an increased presence of the virulent Beijing/W TB genotype. These causes are elaborated in greater detail in Sánchez et al. (2009).

6. Revisions of TB and HIV trends in Kenya

Since we conducted our study, the TB case detection rate in Kenya has been revised upwards from approximately 57% in 1996 to around 70% in 2006 (Mansoer et al. 2009). Because TB incidence rates are calculated from TB case notification rates and TB case detection rates using the formula (World Health Organization 2006b):

$$\text{incidence} = \frac{\text{case notifications}}{\text{proportion of cases detected}},$$

this implies that TB incidence has been revised downwards in Kenya–i.e., TB rates are not as high as estimated in 2006 (World Health Organization 2008). Furthermore, HIV estimates for Kenya are in the process of being revised upwards–i.e., HIV prevalence trends are most probably higher than those corresponding to values estimated in 2006 (UNAIDS 2008).

Furthermore, our model predicted that in 2004 the proportion of HIV infected persons among TB infected persons was 43% under the calibration to reported HIV trends, a substantially higher value than the 29% estimate provided for Kenya in 2006 (World Health Organization 2006b). In essence, this means that even though under our calibration to the declining HIV epidemic the model did not match up to the reported increase in TB case notifications, see Fig. 3, it still needed to account for the resulting lower-than-reported TB trends by having a greater-than-reported proportion of TB/HIV co-infected people. Recent surveillance efforts in Kenya also indicate that past surveys may have seriously underestimated the proportion of HIV infected among TB cases, and this number may actually be closer to 53% (World Health Organization 2008).

We have conducted an additional investigation of pan-African patterns with the most recently revised data (Sánchez et al. 2010), and results indicate that the incongruency in the TB/HIV data for Kenya is largely resolved. This analysis ranks the relative change in tuberculosis numbers as compared to HIV numbers for

Kenya in the 8th position out of 38 African countries, while in our earlier analysis Kenya ranked in 3rd position (Sánchez et al. 2009).

7. Model predictions

We set forth to establish our predictions regarding the potential benefits to be derived from implementing various TB control policies in different HIV settings (Sánchez et al. 2008) with the parameter set that provided the smallest GF under the calibration of the model to Kenyan TB/HIV data up to and including 1997. We used a population size of 33 million to derive our pertinent estimates, which corresponded to the population size of Kenya at the time of our investigation (World Health Organization 2006a). It must be borne in mind that our model results correspond to averages specific to a particular country at a particular time (i.e., Kenya). Different ecological and treatment histories may generate different dynamics within and between the twin epidemics (Currie et al. 2003; Lawn et al. 2006) that can impact the response of the TB epidemic to different TB control strategies. Below we outline the scenarios we considered in our investigation:

Baseline scenario: the first scenario mimicked present-day Kenyan conditions. We assumed patients entering a DOTS treatment program would take their medications for 6 months, while those entering a non-DOTS programs would be on medication for 8 months. We further assumed that default rates in months two and three were three times as great and twice as great, respectively, as the default rates in the first month. Patients in months four through six of DOTS programs, and four through eight of non-DOTS programs, defaulted at the same rate as those in the first month (Table 3). The pattern described follows those of reported default rates (Chan-Yeung et al. 2003; Chee et al. 2000; Combs et al. 1990). Please see above for how we introduced these aspects into the model formulation.

Alternative scenarios:

1) ***Reduced treatment duration.*** In the first alternative scenario, we assumed a novel drug that could cure TB patients in 2 months time became available. Accordingly, we reduced treatment duration to two months in both DOTS and non-DOTS regimens. This reduction in treatment time applied to both smear-positive and smear-negative TB cases. We further assumed there was a corresponding reduction in the rate at which patients stopped treatment before completing their regimen, such that default rates in the second month were equal to those in the first month. In this scenario the probability of cure at the end of two months was assumed equal to the probability of cure at the end of treatment (six or eight months) in the status quo.

2) ***Reduced treatment duration and increased detection rate.*** Scenario 2 differed from scenario 1 only with respect to doubling the case detection rate across all HIV categories.

3) ***Reduced treatment duration and increased cure rate.*** Scenario 3 differed from scenario 1 only in the sense that we now directed 80% of those patients that were previously susceptible to relapse (i.e., transiently recovered) into the completely cured category upon completion of both DOTS and non-DOTS treatment. This occurred across all 5 HIV categories.

4) ***Reduced treatment duration, increased detection rate, and increased cure rate.*** Scenario 4 is scenario 1 with both the modifications of scenarios 2 and 3 (i.e., interventions in all three scenarios combined).

7.1. HIV prevalence levels. In order to be able to apply our findings to other HIV-affected settings, we evaluated the benefits obtained from implementing the alternative TB control measures described above under the following 5 different HIV prevalence levels: 3%, 7%, 15%, 20% and 35%. We introduced the alternative scenarios in 2006, at the end of our dataset, and projected the data forward until 2030, which corresponds to a projection period of 25 years (Fig. 2). During this 25-year period we assumed HIV prevalence remained approximately constant for the five different levels considered. Additionally, for each HIV setting, the HIV trends prior to the year 2006 were scaled to those reported in Cheluget et al. (2006). These conditions lead to the HIV epidemic peaking at ~51% in 1997-1998, in the setting that had defined a 35% prevalence in the year 2006. We investigated TB dynamics at such an elevated HIV prevalence because there are populations that have reported similarly appallingly high HIV levels (UNAIDS 2006).

7.2. Benefits. We measured benefits as 'new TB cases' and 'TB deaths' avoided under each alternative scenario (1-4) as compared to the baseline case scenario. In our analysis we calculated both the absolute benefits in terms of the total number of cases avoided:

$$TBcases\_avoided = New\_TBcases\_baseline - New\_TBcases\_alternative,$$

and the relative benefits in terms of the proportional change in TB cases:

$$TBcases\_avoided = \frac{New\_TBcases\_baseline}{New\_TBcases\_alternative}.$$

Under this definition a relative benefit of 3 corresponds to a three-fold decrease in new TB cases under the alternative as compared to the baseline scenario. The same reasoning was applied to obtain absolute and relative benefits in terms of TB deaths avoided.

Our results indicated that reducing TB treatment duration, whether it be alone or combined with other control strategies, has the potential to generate vast benefits in terms of TB control in those populations where HIV prevalence is high. As such, at an HIV prevalence of approximately 3-20% and compared to present-day strategies, we can attain a decrease in TB incidence and mortality of 6-20% in a 25 year period when implementing a TB control program that has the same features as the present control program, but where a complete TB regimen lasts for 2 months instead of 6 to 8 months. These benefits are expected to gradually increase when, in addition, we increase detection or cure, and to exceed 300% when we increase both detection and cure. Moreover, our results also provided strong support for the claim that TB control policies need to account for HIV population levels (Borgdorff et al. 2001; Daley et al. 1998; De Cock & Chaisson 1999; Gouws et al. 2006; Lawn et al. 2006) because the efficacy of the different interventions we considered in our scenario analysis (see above) varied substantially with HIV prevalence. Moreover, when subdividing the population according to HIV status, we observed that benefits varied substantially in the HIV-positive subpopulation compared with the HIV-negative subpopulation. In absolute terms the number of TB cases and deaths increased dramatically as HIV prevalence increased. On the other hand, the relative efficacy of the TB control program scenarios we considered displayed a non-linear pattern whereby they became less effective on a per-capita-basis at HIV prevalence levels >15%. This effect was so strong, that our model predicted that the benefits of reducing treatment duration may even be reversed at extreme HIV prevalence levels–according to our model results, at an HIV prevalence of approximately 35% we could potentially generate a greater number of TB cases when reducing treatment duration due to the accelerated dynamics of the TB epidemic in HIV infected persons. HIV further impacted the system by altering the relative benefits to be obtained from the different TB control strategies, such that the benefits of increasing cure versus detection increased as HIV prevalence increased. For greater detail on the results obtained in this analysis please refer to (Sánchez et al. 2008).

Benefits derived from increasing detection and/or cure without reducing treatment duration. Other authors have investigated the impact of increasing cure versus detection under various conditions (Currie et al. 2003; Dye et al. 1998), and in our analysis we focused on the impact of reducing treatment duration alone or in combination with these other TB control measures. However, we did observe that compared with scenarios 2-4 presented in (Sánchez et al. 2008) both the absolute and relative benefits of the interventions considered are smaller when increasing detection and/or cure rate under the same specifications as scenarios 2-4, but without reducing treatment duration. This reduction is approximately additive, such that the relative magnitudes of the effects are similar. In consequence, the overall trends regarding absolute and relative cases and deaths avoided when increasing detection and/or cure rate under the same specifications as scenarios 2-4, but without reducing treatment duration, were analogous to when we did reduce treatment to 2 months. The only substantial difference in trends we detected between the 2- and the 6-month regimens was in regards to the relative benefits obtained when increasing detection vs. increasing cure: when treatment lasts for 6 months, increasing detection provides greater absolute and relative benefits than increasing cure as compared to when treatment lasts for 2 months. However, as in the main analysis, this general trend is reversed at very high HIV levels, because increasing cure becomes progressively more beneficial as HIV prevalence increases, particularly in terms of TB cases avoided.

8. Sensitivity analysis

Sensitivity analyses is a computational tool that allows us to quantify the impact of the model parameters on the model output (Blower & Dowlatabadi 1994; Saltelli et al. 2000, Marino et al. 2009). That is, in our case we can get a sense of the relative importance of the different disease processes in determining TB epidemiology. Moreover, because in our model we have TB disease processes categorized according to HIV stage, we can also use the sensitivity analysis to identify the HIV stage at which we can intervene to cause a greater reduction in TB numbers. And, very importantly, these processes should represent those measures most crucial to determine accurately from the data.

In our study we determined which parameters cause greater changes in TB incidence over the 25-year projection period (2006-2030) at a stable 6.7% HIV prevalence level. Different measures can be calculated: we chose to calculate the partial rank correlation coefficients (PRCC) with respect to TB incidence at the very beginning and end of this 25-year time period for the 47 parameters we varied in the model calibration. Because of the problems in matching the reported TB/HIV data, we had undergone two independent calibrations, one to the 1980-2004 dataset, and the other one to the 1980-1997 dataset (see above). This process had opened up new questions. In particular, we were interested in furthering our understanding on how the partition in the calibration period impacted the value of our parameters. Of all the parameter sets we had generated with LHS (see above, sections 4.4-4.6) we used those 1000 parameter sets that matched reported Kenyan trends more closely, i.e., that provided the 1000 smallest GF values (Fig. 3) for the two independent calibrations, and obtained that–with minor exceptions–parameters with PRCC>0.2 in magnitude were the same and had similar magnitudes for the two calibrations. For greater detail on the results of this analysis please refer to Sánchez et al. (2009).

When interpreting the results of the sensitivity analysis we must keep in mind that it offers information not only on the biological processes and public health control measures with the greatest potential to impact our measure of choice (e.g., TB incidence), but also on how our uncertainty in the parameter estimates impacts the uncertainty in the model outcome (Blower & Dowlatabadi 1994; Currie et al. 2003; Saltelli et al. 2000). Consequently, given our large degree of uncertainty regarding both the most suitable parameter ranges characterizing TB/HIV processes, and the reliability of nationwide epidemiological trends, our results should be interpreted with caution. Moreover, as with any sampling method, the sampling strategy for the parameters will impact the distribution of outcomes (see above). As we refine our knowledge on TB and HIV interactions we will limit our sources of uncertainty regarding the co-dynamics of the two pathogens. Accordingly, the parameter ranges should then reflect to a lesser degree our lack of understanding of the system, and more the actual temporal and spatial variation characterizing TB/HIV co-dynamics. More precise knowledge of parameter values will enable more robust policy recommendations to be derived from sensitivity analyses of epidemic models.

9. Conclusions and recommendations

The process of calibrating a model in order to make a prediction on the impact of novel therapies for TB control led us to uncover how at odds TB and HIV trends are in Kenya. That is, the original intent with which we built our model was not to address whether HIV and TB co-dynamics in Kenya follow a pattern that is consistent with our general understanding of the temporal co-epidemiology of these two diseases. Rather, our original goal was to investigate the potential impact of shortening TB treatment duration, alone or combined with enhanced case detection and/or cure, in areas of high HIV prevalence. Our results sparked the realization that a re-evaluation of TB trends was needed (Fig. 5), and consequently TB numbers have undergone a major revision in this sub-Saharan country. New numbers indicate TB had not increased as much as originally estimated (Mansoer et al. 2009; World Health Organization 2008). HIV trends are now in the process of being revised, and preliminary estimates indicate HIV numbers are most probably higher than previous estimates (UNAIDS 2008). This process exemplifies the value and the power of mathematical modeling as an epidemiological tool for proper monitoring of pandemics, and can provide enormous insight into the system's functioning. This is particularly the case for complex co-pandemics such as TB/HIV. It is in the best interest for TB and HIV control to analyze the available data in different ways in order to maximize the information we can derive from it. Mathematical modeling can help us expand our understanding of a biological system by unraveling the way epidemics interact, particularly so because integrating the data from the two separate epidemics is a much more insightful process than simply investigating the

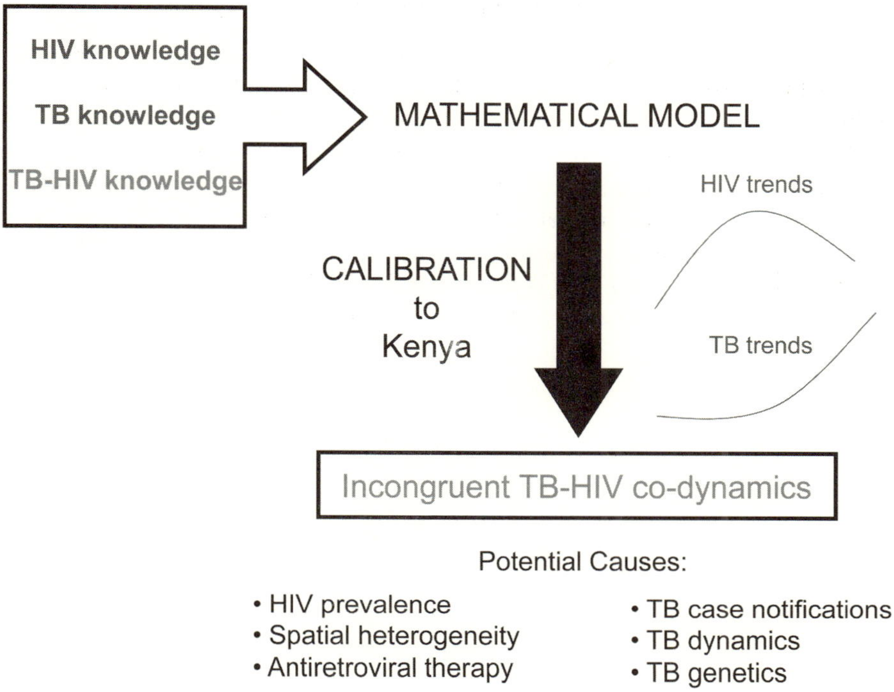

FIGURE 5. **Study schematic.** We contrasted HIV and TB trends reported for Kenya by integrating person-level information for both diseases in a mathematical model and calibrating the model to country-level TB and TB-HIV measures spanning the period 1980-2004. The model cannot reconcile the substantial rise in TB numbers in light of the decreasing HIV numbers. We discuss potential causes for the reported discrepancies.

performance of one of the diseases. The interaction between the diseases holds much information, and trends in joint estimates (e.g., indicators such as HIV prevalence among TB patients) are an extremely powerful tool that can help us unravel past trends and predict future trends much more accurately. Investigating the system in depth permitted us to add another layer of understanding by integrating the two data sets in a novel way, which resulted in greater confidence regarding our predictions on the impact of decreasing TB treatment duration in high HIV prevalence areas. In our case, this was particularly valuable because results were not obviously intuitive at very high HIV prevalence levels, given that when prevalence is in the order of 35% in the general adult population the reduction in treatment time may not provide the benefits desired, and expected. Our results, however, did corroborate that important benefits can be obtained from reducing TB treatment duration when HIV prevalence is below 35%, and fortunately this is the case for most of Africa and the rest of the world today.

Acknowledgements:

We thank anonymous reviewers and David Bangsberg, Jason Barbour, Frank Cobelens, Kathryn DeRiemer, Judy Hahn, John Hargrove, Philip Hopewell, Gwynne Oosterbaan, Perry de Valpine, Francois Venter, Suzanne Verver, and members of Wayne Getz's lab, for their help and orientation. We would especially like to thank the Kenyan public health authorities and all persons participating in the data collection. This research was supported by NIH-NIDA (MSS and WMG), the James S. McDonnell Foundation 21st Century Science Initiative (WMG), the Global Alliance for TB Drug Development (WMG), and SACEMA, the South African Center for Epidemiological Modeling and Analysis (WMG).

TABLE 1. **State variables for the combined TB and HIV models.**

TB State (i)	**Abbrev.**	**Definition**
1	S	TB susceptible
2	IS	TB infection, slow progressor (latent)
3	IF	TB infection, fast progressor
4	AP	Smear-positive active TB, not detectable
5	AN	Smear-negative active TB, not detectable
6	R	TB recovered
7	APd	Smear-positive active TB, detectable
8	ANd	Smear-negative active TB, detectable
9-16	TPD	Smear-positive TB case undergoing DOTS treatment, months 1-8
17-24	TPN	Smear-positive TB case undergoing non-DOTS treatment, months 1-8
25	TPF	TB treatment failure, smear-positive case
26-33	TND	Smear-negative TB case undergoing DOTS treatment, months 1-8

34-41	TNN	Smear-negative TB case undergoing non-DOTS treatment, months 1-8
42	TNF	TB treatment failure, smear-negative case

HIV State (j)	**Abbrev.**	**Definition**
1	U	HIV uninfected
2	I	HIV infected stage I
3	II	HIV infected stage II
4	III	HIV infected stage III
5	IV	HIV infected stage IV

The distribution of the population across different TB states is presented as a 42-element vector, while that of HIV as a 5-element vector, for a total of 42×5 combined TB-HIV categories.

TABLE 2. **Exit rates at which persons progress from each individual TB and HIV state in the model.**

TB State	TB exit rates	HIV State	HIV exit rates
1	$\lambda + \mu$	1	Ψ_1
2	$\lambda b(1 - p_S) + \phi_S + \mu$	2	Ψ_2
3	$\phi_F + \mu$	3	Ψ_3
4	$\pi + \mu_P + \mu$	4	Ψ_4
5	$\pi + \sigma + \mu_N + \mu$	5	μ_H $(\Psi_5 = 0)$
6	$\lambda b + \mu$		
7	$\theta + \pi + \mu_P + \mu$		
8	$\theta + \pi + \sigma + \mu_N + \mu$		
9-16	$\delta + \mu_{PD} + \mu$		
17-24	$\delta + \mu_{PN} + \mu$		
25	$\rho + \mu$		
26-33	$\delta + \mu_{ND} + \mu$		
34-41	$\delta + \mu_{NN} + \mu$		
42	$\rho + \mu$		

TABLE 3. **Model parameters, grouped by category: population, HIV, TB infection, TB natural history, and TB treatment parameters.**

	Definition and units when applicable♠	HIV- ($j = 1$)	HIV+ stage I ($j = 2$)	HIV+ stage II ($j = 3$)	HIV+ stage III ($j = 4$)	HIV+ stage IV ($j = 5$)	Source
Population parameters							
ν	total population growth (persons per 1000 individuals per year)			64 (computed to achieve reported population growth rate)			NA
μ	natural mortality rate per year			0.016			(CIA 2003)

HIV parameters

Ψ_j	HIV incidence Ψ_1 (rate at which persons become newly infected with HIV) progression Ψ_{2-4} (rate of progression to next HIV stage)	calibration to trends in (Cheluget et al. 2006)	0.0417	0.0476	0.0152	0*	(Jaffar et al. 2004; Morgan et al. 2002)
μ_H	HIV mortality rate per year	NA	NA	NA	NA	0.1111	(Jaffar et al. 2004; Morgan et al. 2002)

TB infection parameters

$c_j\lambda$	force of infection – computed** (rate at which persons become newly infected with TB)	1λ	1.26λ $\{1.19\lambda\}$ $(1\lambda - 1.4\lambda)$	1.34λ $\{1.4\lambda\}$ $(1.2\lambda - 1.6\lambda)$	1.67λ $\{1.62\lambda\}$ $(1.6\lambda - 2.3\lambda)$	4.21λ $\{3.72\lambda\}$ $(2.5\lambda - 5\lambda)$	calibration
β_P	number of new infections per untreated SS+ case			0.78 {0.79} (0.7 – 1.05)			[a]
β_N	number of new infections per untreated SS- case			$0.15\beta_P$			[b]
β_{PD} β_{ND} β_{PN} β_{NN} β_{NF}	number of new infections per treated case and per SS- case that has failed treatment			0			(Salomon et al. 2006)
β_{PF}	number of new infections per SS+ case that failed treatment			0.26 {0.54} (0.15 – 0.92)			(Salomon et al. 2006), a and calibration

b	relative susceptibility to reinfection for latent slow progressors and recovered	0.35	0.5	0.6	0.7	0.8	[a]
TB natural history parameters							
p_S	proportion of new TB infections entering latent slow-progressor pool	0.82 {0.84} (0.8 – 0.95)	0.59 {0.6} (0.55 – 0.85)	0.58 {0.57} (0.45 – 0.75)	0.43 {0.36} (0.25 – 0.45)	0.28 {0.05} (0.0 – 0.3)	[a] and calibration
ϕ_S	breakdown rate for slow progressors (endogenous reactivation)	.00013/12	0.0002/12	0.001/12	.06/12	.1/12	(Currie et al. 2003) and a
ϕ_F	breakdown rate for fast progressors	0.88/12	0.9/12	1/12	2/12	4/12	[a] and calibration
s_P	proportion of new active cases with SS+ disease	0.51 {0.52} (0.45 – 0.57)	0.48 {0.48} (0.425 – 0.525)	0.48 {0.48} (0.40 – 0.50)	0.40 {0.42} (0.20 – 0.45)	0.20 {0.11} (0.0 – 0.20)	[a],[b] and calibration

d	proportion of new cases entering detectable pool (a) preDOTS, no HIV (1960-1979) (b) preDOTS, HIV (1980-1994) (c) DOTS, HIV (1995-2004)			0 – 0.5 0.5 – 0.6 0.6 – 0.8			calibration
σ	rate of conversion from SS- to SS+ disease	0.0019 {0.0019} (0.0016 – 0.0021)	0.0014 {0.0015} (0.0013 – 0.0018)	0.0012 {0.0015} (0.0011 – 0.0016)	0.001 {0.0009} (0.0007 – 0.0011)	0.0004 {0.0005} (0.0 – 0.0007)	calibration
π	rate of spontaneous recovery to latency	0.032 {0.032} (0.017 – 0.033)	0.017 {0.015} (0.012 – 0.020)	0.008 {0.012} (0.007 – 0.016)	0.005 {0.006} (0.0025 – 0.0065)	0.001 {0.0001} (0.0 – 0.0011)	[a] and calibration
μ_P	TB mortality rate, untreated SS+	0.3/12	0.3/12	0.32/12	0.8/12	1/12	[a] and (Currie et al. 2003)
μ_N	TB mortality rate, untreated SS-	0.2/12	0.2/12	0.21/12	0.8/12	1/12	calibration

TB treatment parameters

θ	case-detection rate	0.12 {0.09} (0.08 – 0.15)	0.14 {0.18} (0.10 – 0.20)	0.17 {0.16} (0.10 – 0.20)	0.3 {0.25} (0.20 – 0.40)	0.75 {0.45} (0.40 – 0.80)	calibration
t_P	proportion of SS+ treated cases entering DOTS programs a) preDOTS, no HIV b) preDOTS, HIV c) DOTS, HIV			0 0 0-0.56			(World Health Organization 2006b)
t_N	proportion of SS- treated cases entering DOTS programs a) preDOTS, no HIV b) preDOTS, HIV c) DOTS, HIV			0 0 0-0.71			(World Health Organization 2006b)
δ_6	default rate for 6- and 8-month programs, month m	δ_6 = monthlyFactor·baseDefault, where monthlyFactor*** $m(1) = 1$ $m(2) = 3$ $m(3) = 2$ $m(4-8) = 1$ baseDefault $D = 0.02$ {0.027} (0.01 – 0.03)					(Salomon et al. 2006) and calibration

δ_2	default rate for 2-month programs, month m		δ_2 = monthlyFactor·baseDefault, where monthlyFactor***					(Salomon et al. 2006) and calibration
					$m(1) = 1$			
					$m(2) = 1$			
				baseDefault	$D = 0.02\ \{0.027\}\ (0.01 - 0.03)$			
q_{PD} q_{PN} $[m = 1:8]$	proportion of SS+ cases defaulting from month m of treatment that return to active disease							(Salomon et al. 2006; World Health Organization 2006b) and calibration
		$m = 1$	0.8	0.8	0.85	0.95	1	
		$m = 2$	0.5	0.6	0.75	0.9	1	
		$m = 3$	0.3	0.5	0.7	0.875	1	
		$m = 4$	0.2	0.4	0.65	0.85	1	
		$m = 5$	0.1	0.35	0.6	0.825	1	
		$m = 6$	0.01	0.3	0.5	0.8	1	
		$m = 7$	0.01	0.3	0.5	0.8	1	
		$m = 8$	0.01	0.3	0.5	0.8	1	
q_{ND} q_{NN} $[m = 1:8]$	proportion of SS- cases defaulting from month m of treatment that return to active disease		$q_{N1} = 0.9q_{P1}$	$q_{N2} = 0.9q_{P2}$	$q_{N3} = 0.9q_{P3}$	$q_{N4} = 0.9q_{P4}$	$q_{N5} = 0.9q_{P5}$ =	(Salomon et al. 2006; World Health Organization 2006b) and calibration

ν_{kl} $[m = 1:8]$	proportion of SS+ and SS- cases defaulting from month m of treatment that enter failed treatment class	$\nu_{kl} = 1 - q_{kl}$, where $k = P$ represents SS+, $k = N$ represents SS-, $l = D$ represents DOTS, $l = N$ represents non-DOTS					(Salomon et al. 2006; World Health Organization 2006b) and calibration
$q_{complete}$	proportion of cases that return to active disease after completing treatment	0.12 {0.14} (0.05 – 0.15)	0.18 {0.19} (0.10 – 0.20)	0.21 {0.25} (0.15 – 0.25)	0.26 {0.31} (0.25 – 0.35)	0.43 {0.35} (0.35 – 0.50)	(Salomon et al. 2006; World Health Organization 2006b) and calibration
$\nu_{complete}$	proportion of cases that enter failed treatment class after completing treatment	0.14 {0.13} (0.05 – 0.20)	0.10 {0.21} (0.10 – 0.23)	0.21 {0.17} (0.15 – 0.25)	0.33 {0.33} (0.20 – 0.35)	0.34 {0.32} (0.30 – 0.50)	(Salomon et al. 2006; World Health Organization 2006b) and calibration
$s_{complete}$	proportion of cases cured after completing treatment	$s_{complete} = 1 - \nu_{complete} - q_{complete}$					

ρ	relapse rate from failed treatment class to active disease	0.088 {0.083} (0.06 – 0.10)	0.118 {0.119} (0.097 – 0.127)	0.126 {0.112} (0.105 – 0.135)	0.172 {0.141} (0.135 – 0.175)	0.176 {0.222} (0.175 – 0.325)	(Salomon et al. 2006) and calibration
μ_{PD}	TB mortality, SS+ cases on DOTS treatment						calibration
	$m = 1$	0.320/12	0.320/12	0.424/12	0.536/12	0.800/12	
	$m = 2$	0.160/12	0.160/12	0.216/12	0.264/12	0.480/12	
	$m = 3 - 8$	0.040/12	0.040/12	0.040/12	0.048/12	0.056/12	
μ_{ND}	TB mortality, SS- cases on DOTS treatment						calibration
	$m = 1$	0.160/12	0.160/12	0.320/12	0.480/12	0.800/12	
	$m = 2$	0.080/12	0.080/12	0.160/12	0.240/12	0.480/12	
	$m = 3 - 8$	0.040/12	0.040/12	0.040/12	0.048/12	0.056/12	
μ_{PN}	TB mortality, SS+ cases on non-DOTS treatment			$\mu_{PN} = 3\mu_{PD}$			calibration
μ_{NN}	TB mortality, SS- cases on non-DOTS treatment			$\mu_{NN} = 3\mu_{ND}$			calibration

Throughout this study we used: a) parameters of fixed value, b) the best-fit parameter values in the 1980-1997 calibration, c) the best-fit parameter values in the full dataset (1980-2004) calibration in brackets { }, and d) the ranges for those parameters whose values were allowed to vary in the calibrations in parenthesis ( ). Greek symbols represent rates, lower case Roman symbols represent proportions. Vectors indices are shown in square brackets [ ]. All rates are monthly unless specified otherwise. Constraints for the calibration ranges are given below. Abbreviations used are NA: not applicable, SS-: smear-negative TB, SS+: smear-positive TB, HIV-: HIV uninfected, HIV+: HIV infected.

♠ for parameters representing rates or proportions, we multiply the parameter value by the total number of persons in the category from which the corresponding process is exiting, in order to obtain the total number of persons at each time step that exits that category due to that particular process

* a value of 0 was given to nullify the impact of the last element of this vector, because persons die from AIDS and exit the system once they reach HIV stage IV, see Model Formulation

** $\lambda =$ the force of infection, was computed at each monthly time step, see Model Formulation

*** $m =$ month of treatment, which ranges from 8 months for non-DOTS programs, 6 months for present-day DOTS programs, and 2 months for DOTS and non-DOTS programs that implement the new 2-month drug regimen

[a] parameter values and ranges adapted from Dye and Williams, 2000 and Dye et al., 1998

[b] parameter values and ranges adapted from Murray and Salomon, 1998

Calibration constraints in relation to HIV stages:

- HIV stage I, HIV stage II $<$ HIV stage III $<$ HIV stage IV for $c_j\lambda$
- HIV uninfected $>$ HIV stage I, HIV stage II $>$ HIV stage III $>$ HIV stage IV for parameters $p_S, \pi, \rho, \theta, q_{complete}, s_{complete}$
- HIV uninfected $<$ HIV stage I, HIV stage II $<$ HIV stage III $<$ HIV stage IV for parameters for s_P, σ
- $\beta_{TR} < \beta_P$

These constraints were applied to all the pertinent parameters allowed to vary in the calibration, except for $v_{complete}$ (see above) which was unconstrained given that its value is calculated from $s_{complete} + v_{complete} + q_{complete} = 1$, and both $s_{complete}$ and $q_{complete}$ (see above) were constrained as described here. In our analysis we only used those parameter sets generated by the Latin Hypercube Sampling that conformed to these constraints.

TABLE 4. **Results of our sensitivity analysis in terms of partial rank correlation coefficients (PRCC).**

		PRCC (a) 1997	PRCC (b) 2004
force of infection			
1	λ_1	0.179	0.207 (18)
2	λ_2	0.128	0.163
3	λ_3	0.533 (9)	0.531 (9)
4	λ_4	0.025	0.032
number of new infections per untreated SS+ case			
5	β_P	0.848 (1)	0.830 (3)
number of new infections per SS+ case that failed treatment			
6	B_{PF}	0.802 (4)	0.805 (4)
proportion of new TB infections entering latent slow-progressor pool			
7	p_{S0}	-0.711 (7)	-0.697 (7)
8	p_{S1}	-0.374 (11)	-0.341 (13)
9	p_{S2}	-0.272 (16)	-0.318 (15)
10	p_{S3}	-0.327 (15)	-0.310 (16)
11	p_{S4}	0.018	0.009
rate of spontaneous recovery to latency			
12	π_0	-0.143	-0.039
13	π_1	-0.042	-0.026
14	π_2	-0.017	-0.0003
15	π_3	-0.139	-0.125
16	π_4	-0.020	-0.067

relapse rate from failed treatment class to active disease			
17	ρ_0	-0.330 (14)	-0.323 (14)
18	ρ_1	-0.044	-0.073
19	ρ_2	-0.011	-0.021
20	ρ_3	-0.041	-0.041
21	ρ_4	-0.032	-0.029
proportion of new active cases with SS+ disease			
22	s_{P0}	0.565 (8)	0.545 (8)
23	s_{P1}	0.035	0.031
24	s_{P2}	0.072	0.137
25	s_{P3}	0.845 (2)	0.844 (1)
26	s_{P4}	0.180	0.177
rate of conversion from SS- to SS+ disease			
27	σ_0	0.007	-0.014
28	σ_1	0.040	0.032
29	σ_2	-0.009	0.001
30	σ_3	0.047	0.012
31	σ_4	-0.016	0.005
base default rate for DOTS and non-DOTS programs			
32	D	0.741 (5)	0.754 (5)
case-detection rate			
33	θ_0	-0.833 (3)	-0.833 (2)
34	θ_1	-0.109	-0.145
35	θ_2	-0.024	-0.070
36	θ_3	-0.405 (10)	-0.443 (10)
37	θ_4	-0.027	0.005

proportion of cases that return to active disease after completing treatment			
38	$q_{complete,0}$	0.356 (13)	0.394 (11)
39	$q_{complete,1}$	0.003	0.050
40	$q_{complete,2}$	0.0004	-0.015
41	$q_{complete,3}$	0.224 (17)	0.219 (17)
42	$q_{complete,4}$	0.004	-0.031
proportion of cases that enter failed treatment class after completing treatment			
43	$\nu_{complete,0}$	0.715 (6)	0.731 (6)
44	$\nu_{complete,1}$	0.040	0.110
45	$\nu_{complete,2}$	0.069	0.043
46	$\nu_{complete,3}$	0.374 (12)	0.353 (12)
47	$\nu_{complete,4}$	0.015	0.003

Note: This table provides the PRCC values for key variables with respect to reductions in incidence when we projected the runs to 2030, relative to 2005, at a stable HIV prevalence of 6.7%. We used the 1,000 parameter sets that provided the best goodness-of-fit (GF) scores (Fig. 3) when the model was calibrated to fit TB and HIV data in Kenya spanning the time periods: (a) 1980-1997, and (b) 1980-2004. Numerical subindices indicate the HIV infection status (0 corresponding to the HIV-uninfected, and numbers 1-4 corresponding to the WHO HIV disease stages I-IV). We include the relative ranking of the PRCCs in parenthesis, with only those with absolute values >0.2 ranked.

REFERENCES:

Abubakar, I. & Fernández de la Hoz, K. 2008 WHO publishes the third edition of guidelines for the prevention and control of air-travel-associated tuberculosis. *Euro Surveill* **13**.

Al-Jahdali, H., Memish, Z. A. & Menzies, D. 2003 Tuberculosis in association with travel. *Int J Antimicrob Agents* **21**, 125-30.

Andries, K., Verhasselt, P., Guillemont, J., Gohlmann, H. W. H., Neefs, J. M., Winkler, H., Van Gestel, J., Timmerman, P., Zhu, M., Lee, E., Williams, P., de Chaffoy, D., Huitric, E., Hoffner, S., Cambau, E., Truffot-Pernot, C., Lounis, N. & Jarlier, V. 2005 A diarylquinoline drug active on the ATP synthase of *Mycobacterium tuberculosis*. *Science* **307**, 223-227.

Badri, M., Wilson, D. & Wood, R. 2002 Effect of highly active antiretroviral therapy on incidence of tuberculosis in South Africa: a cohort study. *Lancet* **359**, 2059-64.

Bates, I., Fenton, C., Gruber, J., Lalloo, D., Lara, A. M., Squire, S. B., Theobald, S., Thomson, R. & Tolhurst, R. 2004 Vulnerability to malaria, tuberculosis, and HIV/AIDS infection and disease. Part II: Determinants operating at

environmental and institutional level. *Lancet Infect Dis* **4**, 368-75.
Blower, S. & Bernoulli, D. 2004 An attempt at a new analysis of the mortality caused by smallpox and of the advantages of inoculation to prevent it. 1766. *Rev Med Virol* **14**, 275-88.
Blower, S. M. & Dowlatabadi, H. 1994 Sensitivity and Uncertainty Analysis of Complex-Models of Disease Transmission – an HIV Model, as an Example. *International Statistical Review* **62**, 229-243.
Blower, S. M., Small, P. M. & Hopewell, P. C. 1996 Control strategies for tuberculosis epidemics: New models for old problems. *Science* **273**, 497-500.
Borgdorff, M. W., Nagelkerke, N. J. D., de Haas, P. E. W. & van Soolingen, D. 2001 Transmission of *Mycobacterium tuberculosis* depending on the age and sex of source cases. *American Journal of Epidemiology* **154**, 934-943.
Chakaya, J., Getahun, H., Granich, R. & Havlir, D. 2008 Confronting TB/HIV in the era of increasing anti-TB drug resistance. *J Int AIDS Soc* **11**, 6.
Chakaya, J. M., Meme, H., Kwamanga, D., Githui, W. A., Onyango-Ouma, W. O., Gicheha, C., Karimi, F., Mansoer, J. & Kutwa, A. 2005 Planning for PPM-DOTS implementation in urban slums in Kenya: knowledge, attitude and practices of private health care providers in Kibera slum, Nairobi. *Int J Tuberc Lung Dis* **9**, 403-8.
Chan-Yeung, M., Noertjojo, K., Leung, C. C., Chan, S. L. & Tam, C. M. 2003 Prevalence and predictors of default from tuberculosis treatment in Hong Kong. *Hong Kong Med J* **9**, 263-8.
Chee, C. B., Boudville, I. C., Chan, S. P., Zee, Y. K. & Wang, Y. T. 2000 Patient and disease characteristics, and outcome of treatment defaulters from the Singapore TB control unit- -a one-year retrospective survey. *Int J Tuberc Lung Dis* **4**, 496-503.
Cheluget, B., Baltazar, G., Orege, P., Ibrahim, M., Marum, L. H. & Stover, J. 2006 Evidence for population level declines in adult HIV prevalence in Kenya. *Sexually Transmitted Infections* **82**, I21-I26.
CIA. 2003 World Factbook. Available from: https://www.cia.gov/cia/publications/factbook/geos/ke.html; 2003.
Cohen, T. & Murray, M. 2004 Modeling epidemics of multidrug-resistant *M. tuberculosis* of heterogeneous fitness. *Nat Med* **10**, 1117-21.
Combs, D. L., O'Brien, R. J. & Geiter, L. J. 1990 USPHS Tuberculosis Short-Course Chemotherapy Trial 21: effectiveness, toxicity, and acceptability. The report of final results. *Ann Intern Med* **112**, 397-406.
Corbett, E. L., Charalambous, S., Moloi, V. M., Fielding, K., Grant, A. D., Dye, C., De Cock, K. M., Hayes, R. J., Williams, B. G. & Churchyard, G. J. 2004 Human Immunodeficiency Virus and the Prevalence of Undiagnosed Tuberculosis in African Gold Miners. *Am J Respir Crit Care Med.*
Corbett, E. L., Watt, C. J., Walker, N., Maher, D., Williams, B. G., Raviglione, M. C. & Dye, C. 2003 The growing burden of tuberculosis: global trends and interactions with the HIV epidemic. *Arch Intern Med* **163**, 1009-21.
Cruciani, M., Malena, M., Bosco, O., Gatti, G. & Serpelloni, G. 2001 The impact of human immunodeficiency virus type 1 on infectiousness of tuberculosis: a meta-analysis. *Clin Infect Dis* **33**, 1922-30.
Currie, C. S., Williams, B. G., Cheng, R. C. & Dye, C. 2003 Tuberculosis epidemics driven by HIV: is prevention better than cure? *AIDS* **17**, 2501-8.

Daley, C. L., Hahn, J. A., Moss, A. R., Hopewell, P. C. & Schecter, G. F. 1998 Incidence of tuberculosis in injection drug users in San Francisco - Impact of anergy. *American Journal of Respiratory and Critical Care Medicine* **157**, 19-22.

Day, J. H., Grant, A. D., Fielding, K. L., Morris, L., Moloi, V., Charalambous, S., Puren, A. J., Chaisson, R. E., De Cock, K. M., Hayes, R. J. & Churchyard, G. J. 2004 Does tuberculosis increase HIV load? *J Infect Dis* **190**, 1677-84.

De Cock, K. M. & Chaisson, R. E. 1999 Will DOTS do it? A reappraisal of tuberculosis control in countries with high rates of HIV infection. *Int J Tuberc Lung Dis* **3**, 457-65.

de Jong, B. C., Israelski, D. M., Corbett, E. L. & Small, P. M. 2004 Clinical management of tuberculosis in the context of HIV infection. *Annual Review of Medicine* **55**, 283-301.

Dowdy, D. W., Chaisson, R. E., Moulton, L. H. & Dorman, S. E. 2006 The potential impact of enhanced diagnostic techniques for tuberculosis driven by HIV: a mathematical model. *AIDS* **20**, 751-62.

Dye, C., Garnett, G. P., Sleeman, K. & Williams, B. G. 1998 Prospects for worldwide tuberculosis control under the WHO DOTS strategy. Directly observed short-course therapy. *Lancet* **352**, 1886-91.

Dye, C., Hosseini, M. & Watt, C. 2007 Did we reach the 2005 targets for tuberculosis control? *Bull World Health Organ* **85**, 364-9.

Dye, C. & Williams, B. G. 2000 Criteria for the control of drug-resistant tuberculosis. *Proc Natl Acad Sci USA* **97**, 8180-5.

Eisenhut, M. 2007 Malnutrition and variability in CD4+ cell counts in African populations. *J Infect Dis* **195**, 1550; author reply 1550-1.

Escombe, A. R., Moore, D. A., Gilman, R. H., Pan, W., Navincopa, M., Ticona, E., Martinez, C., Caviedes, L., Sheen, P., Gonzalez, A., Noakes, C. J., Friedland, J. S. & Evans, C. A. 2008 The Infectiousness of Tuberculosis Patients Coinfected with HIV. *PLoS Med* **5**, e188.

Ewald, P. W. 1994 *Evolution of Infectious Diseases.* New York: Oxford University Press.

Fox, J., Weber, J. & Fidler, S. 2006 Primary HIV. *Sexually Transmitted Infections* **82**, 267-268.

Frieden, T. R., Sterling, T. R., Munsiff, S. S., Watt, C. J. & Dye, C. 2003 Tuberculosis. *Lancet* **362**, 887-99.

Fujiwara, P. I., Munsiff, S. S. & Simone, P. M. 2000 Treatment of Tuberculosis. In *Tuberculosis. A Comprehensive International Approach,*, vol. 144 (ed. L. B. Reichman & E. S. Hershfield), pp. 401-446. New York: Marcel Dekker, Inc.

García Calleja, J. M., Marum, L. H., Carcamo, C. P., Kaetano, L., Muttunga, J. & Way, A. 2005 Lessons learned in the conduct, validation, and interpretation of national population based HIV surveys. *AIDS* **19 Suppl 2**, S9-S17.

Garnett, G. P., Garcia-Calleja, J. M., Rehle, T. & Gregson, S. 2006 Behavioural data as an adjunct to HIV surveillance data. *Sexually Transmitted Infections* **82**, I57-I62.

Getz, W. M. & Lloyd-Smith, J. O. 2006 Basic methods for modeling the invasion and spread of contagious diseases. In *Disease Evolution: Models, Concepts and Data Analyses.* (ed. Z. Fenge, U. Dieckmann & S. A. Levin): AMS-DIMACS Series.

Getz, W. M., Lloyd-Smith, J. O., Cross, P. C., Bar-David, S., Johnson, P. L., Porco, T. C. & Sánchez, M. S. 2006 Modeling the Invasion and Spread of Contagious Diseases in Heterogeneous Populations. In *Disease Evolution: Models, Concepts and Data Analyses.* (ed. Z. Fenge, U. Dieckmann & S. A. Levin): AMS-DIMACS Series.

Ghys, P. D., Kufa, E. & George, M. V. 2006 Measuring trends in prevalence and incidence of HIV infection in countries with generalised epidemics. *Sexually Transmitted Infections* **82**, I52-I56.

Ginsberg, A. M. & Spigelman, M. 2007 Challenges in tuberculosis drug research and development. *Nat Med* **13**, 290-4.

Girardi, E., Antonucci, G., Vanacore, P., Libanore, M., Errante, I., Matteelli, A. & Ippolito, G. 2000 Impact of combination antiretroviral therapy on the risk of tuberculosis among persons with HIV infection. *AIDS* **14**, 1985-91.

Girardi, E., Sabin, C. A., d'Arminio Monforte, A., Hogg, B., Phillips, A. N., Gill, M. J., Dabis, F., Reiss, P., Kirk, O., Bernasconi, E., Grabar, S., Justice, A., Staszewski, S., Fatkenheuer, G. & Sterne, J. A. 2005 Incidence of Tuberculosis among HIV-infected patients receiving highly active antiretroviral therapy in Europe and North America. *Clin Infect Dis* **41**, 1772-82.

Gouws, E., White, P. J., Stover, J. & Brown, T. 2006 Short term estimates of adult HIV incidence by mode of transmission: Kenya and Thailand as examples. *Sex Transm Infect* **82 Suppl 3**, iii51-55.

Gutiérrez, M. C., Brisse, S., Brosch, R., Fabre, M., Omais, B., Marmiesse, M., Supply, P. & Vincent, V. 2005 Ancient origin and gene mosaicism of the progenitor of *Mycobacterium tuberculosis. PLoS Pathog* **1**, e5.

Hanson, C. & Kibuga, D. 2000 Effective tuberculosis control and health sector reforms in Kenya: challenges of an increasing tuberculosis burden and opportunities through reform. *International Journal of Tuberculosis and Lung Disease* **4**, 627-632.

Hogg, R. V. & Craig, A. T. 1995 *Introduction to Mathematical Statistics.* Englewood Cliffs, NJ, USA: Prentice Hall.

Hopewell, P. C. & Pai, M. 2005 Tuberculosis, vulnerability, and access to quality care. *JAMA-Journal of the American Medical Association* **293**, 2790-2793.

Jaffar, S., Grant, A. D., Whitworth, J., Smith, P. G. & Whittle, H. 2004 The natural history of HIV-1 and HIV-2 infections in adults in Africa: a literature review. *Bulletin of the World Health Organization* **82**, 462-469.

Kannangara, S., DeSimone, J. A. & Pomerantz, R. J. 2005 Attenuation of HIV-1 infection by other microbial agents. *J Infect Dis* **192**, 1003-9.

Keshinro, B. & Diul, M. Y. 2006 HIV-TB: epidemiology, clinical features and diagnosis of smear-negative TB. *Trop Doct* **36**, 68-71.

Lawn, S. D. 2004 AIDS in Africa: the impact of coinfections on the pathogenesis of HIV-1 infection. *J Infect* **48**, 1-12.

Lawn, S. D., Bekker, L. G., Middelkoop, K., Myer, L. & Wood, R. 2006 Impact of HIV infection on the epidemiology of tuberculosis in a peri-urban community in South Africa: the need for age-specific interventions. *Clin Infect Dis* **42**, 1040-7.

Lawn, S. D. & Wood, R. 2006 The epidemic of HIV-associated tuberculosis in sub-Saharan Africa: does this also impact non-HIV-infected individuals? *AIDS* **20**, 1787-1788.

Maher, D., Harries, A. & Getahun, H. 2005 Tuberculosis and HIV interaction in sub-Saharan Africa: impact on patients and programmes; implications for policies. *Trop Med Int Health* **10**, 734-42.

Mansoer, J., Scheele, S., Floyd, K., Dye, C., Sitienei, J. & Williams, B. G. 2009 New methods for estimating the tuberculosis case detection rate in high-HIV prevalence countries: the example of Kenya. *Bull World Health Organ* **87**, 186-92, 192A-B.

Marino S, Hogue IB, Ray CJ, Kirschner DE. 2008 A methodology for performing global uncertainty and sensitivity analysis in systems biology. *J Theor Biol* **254**, 178-96.

Middelkoop, K., Bekker, L. G., Myer, L., Dawson, R. & Wood, R. 2008 Rates of tuberculosis transmission to children and adolescents in a community with a high prevalence of HIV infection among adults. *Clin Infect Dis* **47**, 349-55.

Morgan, D., Mahe, C., Mayanja, B., Okongo, J. M., Lubega, R. & Whitworth, J. A. G. 2002 HIV-1 infection in rural Africa: is there a difference in median time to AIDS and survival compared with that in industrialized countries? *AIDS* **16**, 597-603.

Morgan, M., Walker, N., Gouws, E., Stanecki, K. A. & Stover, J. 2006 Improved plausibility bounds about the 2005 HIV and AIDS estimates. *Sexually Transmitted Infections* **82**, III71-III77.

Mtei, L., Matee, M., Herfort, O., Bakari, M., Horsburgh, C. R., Waddell, R., Cole, B. F., Vuola, J. M., Tvaroha, S., Kreiswirth, B., Pallangyo, K. & von Reyn, C. F. 2005 High rates of clinical and subclinical tuberculosis among HIV-infected ambulatory subjects in Tanzania. *Clin Infect Dis* **40**, 1500-7.

Muniyandi, M. & Ramachandran, R. 2008 Socioeconomic inequalities of tuberculosis in India. *Expert Opin Pharmacother* **9**, 1623-8.

Murray, C. J. & Salomon, J. A. 1998 Modeling the impact of global tuberculosis control strategies. *Proc Natl Acad Sci USA* **95**, 13881-6.

Naidoo, P., Dick, J. & Cooper, D. 2008 Exploring Tuberculosis Patients' Adherence to Treatment Regimens and Prevention Programs at a Public Health Site. *Qual Health Res.*

Nnoaham, K. E., Pool, R., Bothamley, G. & Grant, A. D. 2006 Perceptions and experiences of tuberculosis among African patients attending a tuberculosis clinic in London. *Int J Tuberc Lung Dis* **10**, 1013-7.

Noor, A. M., Amin, A. A., Gething, P. W., Atkinson, P. M., Hay, S. I. & Snow, R. W. 2006 Modelling distances travelled to government health services in Kenya. *Trop Med Int Health* **11**, 188-96.

Nunn, P., Reid, A. & De Cock, K. M. 2007 Tuberculosis and HIV infection: the global setting. *J Infect Dis* **196** Suppl 1, S5-14.

Odhiambo, J. A., Borgdorff, M. W., Kiambih, F. M., Kibuga, D. K., Kwamanga, D. O., Ng'ang'a, L., Agwanda, R., Kalisvaart, N. A., Misljenovic, O., Nagelkerke, N. J. & Bosman, M. 1999 Tuberculosis and the HIV epidemic: increasing annual risk of tuberculous infection in Kenya, 1986-1996. *Am J Public Health* **89**, 1078-82.

Raviglione, M. C. & Uplekar, M. W. 2006 WHO's new Stop TB Strategy. *Lancet* **367**, 952-5.

Reichman, L. B. & Hershfield, E. S. 2000 *Tuberculosis. A comprehensive international approach.* Lung Biology in Health and Disease. New York:

Marcel Dekker, Inc.

Rieder, H. L. 2008 Editorial commentary: on the risk of being and becoming infected with *Mycobacterium tuberculosis. Clin Infect Dis* **47**, 356-7.

Salomon, J. A., Lloyd-Smith, J. O., Getz, W. M., Resch, S., Sánchez, M. S., Porco, T. C. & Borgdorff, M. W. 2006 Prospects for advancing tuberculosis control efforts through novel therapies. *PLoS Med* **3**, e273.

Saltelli, A., Chan, K. & Scott, E. M. 2000 *Sensitivity Analysis.* Wiley Series in Probability and Statistics. West Sussex, England: Wiley.

Sánchez, M. S., Lloyd-Smith, J. O., Getz, W. M. 2010 Monitoring linked epidemics: the case of tuberculosis and HIV. *PLoS One* **5**: e8796.

Sánchez, M. S., Lloyd-Smith, J., Williams, B. G., Porco, T. C., Ryan, S. J., Borgdorff, M. W., Mansoer, J., Dye, C. & Getz, W. M. 2009 Incongruent HIV and tuberculosis co-dynamics in Kenya: Interacting epidemics monitor each other. *Epidemics* 1:14-20.

Sánchez, M. S., Lloyd-Smith, J. O., Porco, T. C., Williams, B. G., Borgdorff, M. W., Mansoer, J., Salomon, J. A. & Getz, W. M. 2008 Impact of HIV on novel therapies for tuberculosis control. *AIDS* **22**, 963-72.

Shargie, E. B. & Lindtjorn, B. 2007 Determinants of Treatment Adherence Among Smear-Positive Pulmonary Tuberculosis Patients in Southern Ethiopia. *PLoS Med* **4**, e37.

Sonnenberg, P., Glynn, J. R., Fielding, K., Murray, J., Godfrey-Faussett, P. & Shearer, S. 2005 How soon after infection with HIV does the risk of tuberculosis start to increase? A retrospective cohort study in South African gold miners. *J Infect Dis* **191**, 150-8.

Sonnenberg, P., Murray, J., Glynn, J. R., Shearer, S., Kambashi, B. & Godfrey-Faussett, P. 2001 HIV-1 and recurrence, relapse, and reinfection of tuberculosis after cure: a cohort study in South African mineworkers. *Lancet* **358**, 1687-93.

Spigelman, M. & Gillespie, S. 2006 Tuberculosis drug development pipeline: progress and hope. *Lancet* **367**, 945-947.

Spigelman, M. K. 2007 New tuberculosis therapeutics: a growing pipeline. *J Infect Dis* **196 Suppl 1**, S28-34.

UNAIDS. 2006 UNAIDS Annual Report: 2006 Report on the global AIDS epidemic: A UNAIDS 10th anniversary special edition. Geneva.

UNAIDS. 2008 UNAIDS Annual Report: 2008 Report on the global AIDS epidemic. Geneva.

Van Rie, A., Sengupta, S., Pungrassami, P., Balthip, Q., Choonuan, S., Kasetjaroen, Y., Strauss, R. P. & Chongsuvivatwong, V. 2008 Measuring stigma associated with tuberculosis and HIV/AIDS in southern Thailand: exploratory and confirmatory factor analyses of two new scales. *Trop Med Int Health* **13**, 21-30.

Walker, N., Grassly, N. C., Garnett, G. P., Stanecki, K. A. & Ghys, P. D. 2004 Estimating the global burden of HIV/AIDS: what do we really know about the HIV pandemic? *Lancet* **363**, 2180-5.

Williams, B. G. & Dye, C. 2003 Antiretroviral drugs for tuberculosis control in the era of HIV/AIDS. *Science* **301**, 1535-7.

Wilson, D. P., Kahn, J. & Blower, S. M. 2006 Predicting the epidemiological impact of antiretroviral allocation strategies in KwaZulu-Natal: The effect of the urban-rural divide. *Proc Natl Acad Sci U S A.*

Wirth, T., Hildebrand, F., Allix-Beguec, C., Wolbeling, F., Kubica, T., Kremer, K., van Soolingen, D., Rusch-Gerdes, S., Locht, C., Brisse, S., Meyer, A., Supply, P. & Niemann, S. 2008 Origin, spread and demography of the *Mycobacterium tuberculosis* complex. *PLoS Pathog* **4**, e1000160.

World Health Organization. 2001 Global Tuberculosis Control. WHO Report 2001. Geneva.

World Health Organization. 2002 Global Tuberculosis Control. Surveillance, planning, financing. WHO report 2002. Geneva.

World Health Organization. 2003 Global Tuberculosis Control. Surveillance, planning, financing. WHO report 2003. Geneva.

World Health Organization. 2004a Interim policy on collaborative TB/HIV activities. Geneva.

World Health Organization. 2004b Global Tuberculosis Control: surveillance, planning, financing. WHO report 2004. Geneva.

World Health Organization. 2005 Global Tuberculosis Control: surveillance, planning, financing. WHO report 2005. Geneva.

World Health Organization. 2006a WHO Global TB Database. Available from: http://www.who.int/tb/country/global_tb_database/en/index.html.

World Health Organization. 2006b Global Tuberculosis Control: surveillance, planning, financing. WHO report 2006. Geneva.

World Health Organization. 2008 Global tuberculosis control: surveillance, planning, financing: WHO report 2008. Geneva.

Department of Environmental Science, Policy and Management, University of California, Berkeley, CA 94720, USA

Center for Infectious Disease Dynamics, Pennsylvania State University, University Park, PA 16802, USA

World Health Organization, Stop TB Department, 1211 Geneva 27, Switzerland

Department of Environmental Science, Policy and Management, University of California, Berkeley, CA 94720, USA

DIMACS Series in Discrete Mathematics
and Theoretical Computer Science
Volume **75**, 2010

Modelling the epidemiological and economic impact of HIV/AIDS with particular reference to Zimbabwe

Senelani D. Hove-Musekwa, Vengai Runyowa, and Zindoga Mukandavire

ABSTRACT. HIV/AIDS is a major concern in Zimbabwe, not just in terms of disease spread but also in terms of its impact on society and economic development. The paper presents the epidemiological and economic impact of HIV/AIDS which is analysed using a conventional epidemiological model which captures the dynamics of the epidemic with multi-intervention strategies and a total cost function which analyzes the fiscal economic impact of the pandemic to Zimbabwe. The model assesses the effects of treating using anti-retroviral (ARVs) drugs (based on efficacy and adherence), condom use (based on efficacy and compliance), voluntary testing and counselling and the epidemiological impact on the country. The model shows that reduction in effective sexual contacts by increasing condom use and avoidance of multiple sexual partners has a significant impact in reducing the transmission of the disease. It is shown that without behavioral change, effective treatment of the infected individuals re! sults in more spread of the epidemic. Increasing the incubation by treatment tends to benefit the infected individuals as this increases the number of years lived but the total annual cost maybe too high to be sustained by the government. On the other hand the cost of doing "nothing" as represented by an incubation period of less than 9 years appears to be costly as well. Treatment and caring for those who have developed clinical AIDS constitute a major part of our cost function followed by treatment of those who are infected but have not yet developed clinical AIDS. In Zimbabwe, where the pandemic has reached epidemic proportions, combating the disease and its economic effects successfully will require a large and determined fiscal effort. This study therefore sheds light on the economic consequences of decisions taken in the prevention, treatment and care of HIV/AIDS individuals.

1. Introduction

The HIV/AIDS pandemic is growing in all areas of the world, with worrisome signs of resurgence in some countries that were trumpeted as successes in combating the disease. At the same time, the prevalence of HIV, the virus that causes AIDS, among young people has declined in eight countries in Africa, showing that

2000 *Mathematics Subject Classification.* Primary .
Key words and phrases. Epidemiological impact, Economic impact, Equilibria, Reproduction number, Stability.

prevention efforts can work. Limited resources can give high returns when investments are focused on reaching people most at risk and adapted to changing national epidemics. The World Health Organization and the UNAIDS report [**14**] indicated that prevention efforts have reached far too few people at risk, like gay men, prostitutes, injecting drug users and members of minority groups. An estimated 39.5 million people are now living with HIV, of that total 4.3 million became infected in 2006 alone [**15**], [**16**]. The report indicates that there has been 2.9 million AIDS deaths in 2006, the highest number reported in any previous year. The comparable figures in 2004 were 36.9 million living with HIV, 3.9 million new infections and 2.7 million deaths. In Eastern Europe and Asia, infection rates have risen by more than 50 % since 2004. The global death total would be even higher without efforts undertaken in recent years to provide preventive and treatment measures, such as educational campaigns and antiretroviral therapy respectively, to hundreds of thousands of AIDS patients in poor countries. However measures such as drug therapy have not reached enough poor people to match the degree of decline in wealthy countries.

The first reported case of AIDS in Zimbabwe occurred in 1985. By the end of the 1980's around 10% of the adult population were thought to be infected with HIV. This figure rose dramatically in the first half of the 1990s, peaking and stabilizing at 29% between 1995 and 1997. But since this point, HIV/AIDS prevalence is thought to have declined, making Zimbabwe one of the first Sub-Saharan African countries to witness such a trend. The adult prevalence in 2005 was 20.1% according to government figures [**16**] and has since declined to 15.6% [**16**]. There is evidence that Zimbabwe's HIV/AIDS prevalence has genuinely fallen as a result of an increase in awareness of HIV/AIDS. Prevention schemes have been significantly expanded since the turn of the millennium, but remain critically under-funded. Changes in sexual behaviour have played a role in achieving this. The increase in condom use, late sexual debut and a reduction in the number of sexual partners by many people [**16**] have all contributed to this decline.

HIV/AIDS has the potential to create severe economic impacts in many African countries, including Zimbabwe, because it is different from most other diseases since it strikes people in the most productive age groups and is essentially 100 % fatal. The effects will vary according to the severity of the HIV/AIDS epidemic and the structure of the national economies. Reduction in the labour supply and increased costs are the two major economic effects. The direct costs of AIDS include expenditures for medical care, drugs, and funeral expenses. Indirect costs include lost time due to illness, recruitment and training costs to replace workers and care of orphans. If costs are financed out of savings, then the reduction in investment could lead to a significant reduction in economic growth. The economic effects of HIV/AIDS will be felt first by individuals and their families, then ripple outwards to firms and businesses and the macro-economy [**2**].

In terms of the economic policy, HIV/AIDS has particularly two important implications. The first is fiscal in nature. By killing off mainly young adults, HIV/AIDS also seriously weakens the tax base, and so reduces the resources available to meet the demands for public expenditures, including those aimed at accumulating human capital, such as education and health services not related to HIV/AIDS. As a result, the state's finances will come under increasing pressure. Slower growth of the economy means slower growth of the tax base, an effect that will be reinforced if there are growing expenditures on treating the sick and caring for orphans. The other effect is to exacerbate inequality. If the children left orphaned are not given the care and education enjoyed by those whose parents remain uninfected, the weakening of the inter-generational transmission mechanism will express itself in increasing inequality among the next generation of adults and the families they form. Under this background the government is likely to experience increasing fiscal difficulties, and so lack the resources to assume this additional burden in full.

2. Model development and analysis

In this section we formulate an HIV/AIDS model using ordinary differential equations that explicitly take account of epidemiology, demography and account for the economic impact with regards to cost and resource allocation. The HIV/AIDS model subdivided the total sexually active population into the following sub-populations, Susceptibles $S(t)$, Infectives $I(t)$, Treated $T(t)$ individuals and AIDS $A(t)$ individuals. Those who are not sexually active are the treated who responded to treatment and pre- and post-counselling $T_c(t)$ and $A_c(t)$ which consists of infected individuals and displaying symptoms of AIDS where treatment failed, but are counselled and those who cannot afford treatment. Treated individuals will be offered post-treatment counselling and they join a class $T_c(t)$ and those where treatment has failed join the AIDS class $A(t)$. The AIDS class will also be offered treatment and they join a class of treated individuals $T(t)$ if they respond well to treatment.

The major parameters of the model are the probability of HIV transmission β, the number of sexual contacts per unit time, c and intervention parameters. Probability of infection β, is probability of transmission from an infected individual to a susceptible individual which can be said to be a conditional probability. It consists of the likelihood of close contacts between two individuals such that HIV transmission can occur (dependent upon the pattern of mixing in the population) and the probability that HIV transmission will occur as a result of sexual contact. There is a vulnerability constant $r_i, i = 1, 2$ which is a factor by which the probability of HIV transmission is raised in the case of the AIDS cases and treated individuals having sexual contact with the susceptible group. The rate of acquiring HIV infection λ is given by,

$$\lambda = \frac{c\beta[I(t) + r_1 A(t) + r_2 T(t)]}{N(t)}.$$

Here, the total sexually active population is given by $N(t) = S(t) + I(t) + A(t) + T(t)$. The rate of acquisition of new partners c, depends largely on social and environmental factors that determine the living conditions, resources and social opportunities. Culture and religion also have an influence on the number of partners one can acquire. In some cultural settings men are allowed to have as many partners as they wish and this definitely has significant impact on the value of c. Poverty, the need to get financial support, revenge for having been innocently infected and lack of knowledge of reinfection are some of the factors which may push individuals to indulge in risky behaviors. Risk behavior change can be measured by measuring the trends of the value of c indicating an increase in behavioral change.

We assume that the sexually active population, that is, the susceptibles, the infectives, the treated infectives and the clinical AIDS, are exposed to education on prevention using condoms and sticking to one partner. The proportion of people who will use condoms consistently and correctly is α_1 (compliance rate) with condom efficacy of ϵ_1 such that $0 \leq (\alpha_1, \epsilon_1) \leq 1$ and the level of protection against HIV by condom use is measured by the product $\omega = \alpha_1\epsilon_1$ which is the condom induced preventability [**8**], [**9**]. We need to distinguish between condom efficacy and condom effectiveness. Efficacy of condom is the protection that the user would get when using the condom correctly and consistently. The protection depends on a number of factors such as breakages, slippage and leak rates [**8**]. Condom effectiveness is the proportionate reduction in disease transmission due to the use of the condom. Compliance in condom use is a critical factor in preventing HIV transmission and does not offer 100% protection. This factor is defined as the proportion of the sexually-active population that uses condoms consistently and correctly. Consistent use is defined as using a condom for all acts of penetrative vaginal intercourse or anal sex. This implies that $(1 - \omega)$ measures the condom induced preventability failure. The proportion of people who will seek treatment, ! after counselling during voluntary testing, is ν_1 and this will largely depends on an individual being aware of his or her status and this will also measure the success of the voluntary testing campaigns being advocated by the increase in the value of ν_1. The rate at which those infected will seek treatment is ρ_i and the rate of adhering to treatment is α_2 with a drug efficacy ϵ_2 so that $p = \epsilon_2\alpha_2$, is the drug induced preventability of progression to AIDS, thus measuring the level of reduction in the severity of HIV when an individual is taking treatment. We also assume that a proportion $(1 - \nu_1) = \nu$ will develop AIDS without knowing their status at a rate σ. Treated individuals, from the classes $T(t)$ and $A(t)$, are offered post-treatment counselling at a rate $\psi_i, i = 1, 2$.

It is assumed that some individuals will progress from the infective class $I(t)$ at a rate $\sigma_1 = \nu_1\rho_1$ to the treated class $T(t)$, and at a rate $\nu\sigma$ to the AIDS class (σ is the rate of developing AIDS). It is common to have non-adherence to treatment due to forgetting, non-availability of the drug, non-affordability of the drug, absence from home or even the feeling that one is fine. As a result some treated individuals will progress to the AIDS class $A(t)$ at a rate $\sigma_2 = \gamma(1 - p)$, where $1 - p$ is treatment failure and γ is the rate of developing clinical AIDS. The rest of the treated individuals join a class of counselled individuals $T_c(t)$ and later join the class $A_c(t)$ as the disease progresses at a rate η and are assumed not to spread the disease.

Recruitment, either by immigration or maturity, Π is in terms of the number of susceptible individuals admitted into the community per unit time. Rate of recruitment also covers children who become sexually active adults. We assume that the natural death rate for all individuals is constant μ in all classes, and proportional to the number of individuals in the class. We also assume that the AIDS individuals suffer a disease-induced mortality at a constant rate $\delta_i, i = 1, 2$ and that it is proportional to the number of individuals in the AIDS classes. The parameters used in the model are given in Table 1.

TABLE 1. Table of Parameters used in the model.

Parameter	Symbol	Parameter	Symbol
Recruitment rate	Π	Natural death rate	μ
Probability of transmission	β	Partner acquisition rate	c
Probability of infection	β	Vulnerability constant	$r_i, i = 1, 2$
Condom induced preventability	ω	Condom compliance	α_1
Condom efficacy	ϵ_1	Rate of voluntary testing	ν_1
Rate of seeking treatment	ρ_1	Treatment adherence	α_2
Drug efficacy	ϵ_2	Drug induced preventability	p
Post-treatment counselling rate	$\psi_i, i = 1, 2$	Disease progression	σ_1
Disease progression	γ	Disease progression	η
Disease progression	σ	Disease progression	σ_2
Natural death rate	$\mu, i = 1, 2$	Death induced rate	$\delta_i, i = 1, 2$

The assumptions result in the following model flow diagram.

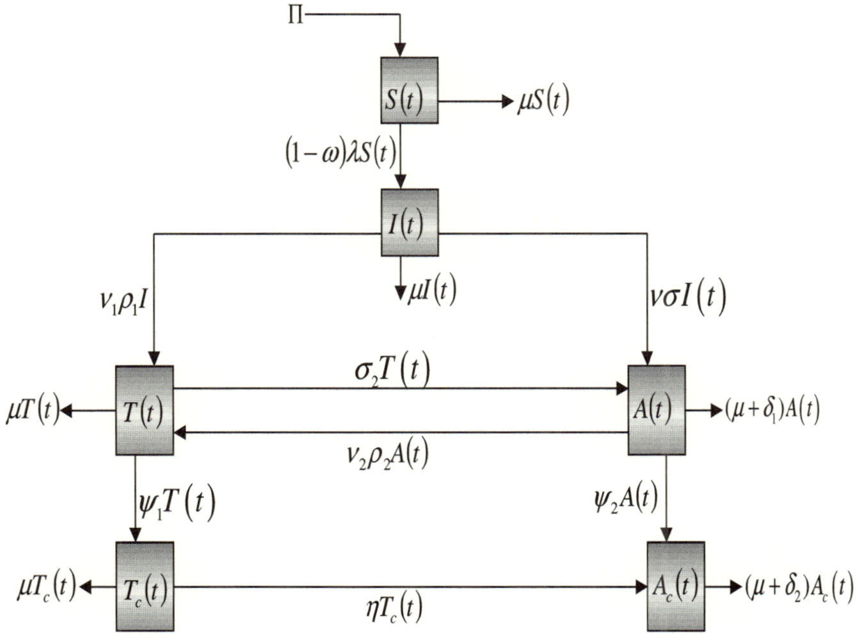

FIGURE 1. Model flow diagram

The model equations are as follows,

$$
\begin{aligned}
\frac{dS}{dt} &= \Pi - (1-\omega)\lambda S - \mu S \\
\frac{dI}{dt} &= (1-\omega)\lambda S - (\nu_1\rho_1 + \nu\sigma + \mu)I \\
\frac{dT}{dt} &= \nu_1\rho_1 I + \nu_2\rho_2 A - [\sigma_2 + \psi_1 + \mu]T \\
\frac{dT_c}{dt} &= \psi_1 T - (\eta + \mu)T_c \\
\frac{dA}{dt} &= \nu\sigma I + \sigma_2 T - (\delta_1 + \nu_2\rho_2 + \psi_2 + \mu)A \\
\frac{dA_c}{dt} &= \eta T_c + \psi_2 A - (\delta_2 + \mu)A_c.
\end{aligned} \tag{1}
$$

where $\sigma_2 = \gamma(1-p)$ and $\lambda = \dfrac{c\beta[I(t) + r_1 A(t) + r_2 T(t)]}{N(t)}$. All parameters and state variables for model system (1) are assumed to be non-negative for $t \geq 0$ and the total population size is given by,

$$N_T(t) = S(t) + I(t) + T(t) + T_c(t) + A(t) + A_c(t).$$

Next we consider the invariant regions.

2.1. Invariant regions. The model system (1) will be analysed in a suitable feasible region Γ, which is the region of biological interest as follows.

LEMMA 1. *The region $\Gamma \in \mathbb{R}^6_+$ is positively invariant and attracting with respect to model system (1).*

PROOF. Let $\{S(t), I(t), T(t), T_c(t), A(t), A_c(t)\}$ be any solution of the system with non-negative initial conditions. We use a theorem on differential inequality [**1**], that says

$$\limsup_{t\to\infty} S(t) \leq \frac{\Pi}{\mu}.$$

Taking the time derivative of our total population along the solution path gives,

$$N_T' = \Pi - \mu N_T - \delta_1 A - \delta_2 A_c.$$

Let

$$\alpha = \min(\delta_1, \delta_2),$$

then

$$
\begin{aligned}
N_T' &\leq \Pi - \mu N_T - \delta_1 A - \delta_2 A_c \\
&\leq \Pi - \mu N_T - \alpha(A + A_c) \\
&< \Pi - \mu N_T.
\end{aligned}
$$

Applying Rota and Birhoff's Theorem on differential inequality results in

$$0 \leq N_T \leq \frac{\Pi}{\mu} + N_T(0)e^{-\frac{\Pi}{\mu}t}$$

where $N_T(0)$ represents the initial values of the respective variables. Thus, as $t \to \infty$,

$$0 \leq N_T \leq \frac{\Pi}{\mu}.$$

Therefore, all feasible solutions of the system enter the region,

$$\Gamma = \Big\{(S, I, T, T_c, A, A_c) \in \mathbb{R}^6_+ : N_T \leq \frac{\Pi}{\mu}\Big\}.$$

Hence, the region of biological interest Γ is positively invariant under the flow induced by system (1). Further it can be shown, using the theory of permanence Hutson and Schmitt, [**5**] that all solutions on the boundary of Γ eventually enter the interior of Γ. Furthermore, in Γ, the usual existence, uniqueness and continuation results hold for model system (1), making the model system well-posed mathematically and epidemiologically. Hence, it is sufficient to consider the dynamics of the flow generated by the model (1) in Γ. □

2.2. Disease-free equilibrium. The model has a disease-free equilibrium, P_0, which is given by

$$P_0 \;=\; \Big(S^*, I^*, T^*, T_c^*, A^*, A_c^*\Big) \;=\; \Big(\frac{\Pi}{\mu}, 0, 0, 0, 0, 0\Big).$$

We need the threshold quantity R_e, which is known as the effective reproduction number for model system (1). This is defined as the number of new infected individuals generated by a single infected individual introduced in a population where multiple strategies are used as control strategies. This provides the necessary condition for the eradication of an epidemic. If $R_e < 1$ the disease can be eradicated otherwise it will persist within the population. Using the method in [**12**], the reproduction number R_e, is

$$\begin{aligned} R_e \;=\; & R_{0I} + \Big[\frac{\rho_1\nu_1}{\nu_1\rho_1 + \nu\sigma + \mu} + \Big(\frac{\nu\sigma}{\nu\sigma + \rho_1\nu_1 + \mu}\Big)\Big(\frac{\nu_2\rho_2}{\nu_2\rho_2 + \psi_2 + \delta_1 + \mu}\Big)\Big] R_{0T} \\ & + \Big[\frac{\nu\sigma}{\nu_1\rho_1 + \nu\sigma + \mu} + \Big(\frac{\nu_1\rho_1}{\nu_1\rho_1 + \nu\sigma + \mu}\Big)\Big(\frac{\sigma_2}{\sigma_2 + \psi_1 + \mu}\Big)\Big] R_{0A} \end{aligned} \tag{2}$$

where

$$R_{0I} = \frac{c\beta(1-\omega)}{\nu_1\rho_1 + \nu\sigma + \mu}, \qquad R_{0T} = \frac{cr_2\beta(1-\omega)}{(\sigma_2 + \psi_1 + \mu)(1 - R_p)},$$

$$R_{0A} = \frac{cr_1\beta(1-\omega)}{(\rho_2\nu_2 + \psi_2 + \mu + \delta_1)(1 - R_p)}$$

and

$$R_p = \Big(\frac{\sigma_2}{\sigma_2 + \psi_1 + \mu}\Big)\Big(\frac{\rho_2\nu_2}{\rho_2\nu_2 + \psi_2 + \mu + \delta_1}\Big) < 1.$$

We explain the different terms in expression (2).

- R_{0I}, R_{0T} and R_{0A} are the contributions of the infected I, the treated T and the AIDS individuals A to the reproduction number respectively.
- $\dfrac{1}{\nu_1\rho_1 + \nu\sigma + \mu}$ is the average time an individual spends in the infected class or the average death adjusted infective period.
- $\dfrac{1}{\psi_1 + \sigma_2 + \mu)}$ is the death adjusted infective period of individuals being treated.
- $\dfrac{\nu_1\rho_1}{\nu_1\rho_1 + \nu\sigma + \mu}$ is the proportion of individuals who are infected that progress to the treated class T.
- $\Big(\dfrac{\nu_1\rho_1}{\nu_1\rho_1 + \nu\sigma + \mu}\Big)\Big(\dfrac{\sigma_2}{\psi_1 + \sigma_2 + \mu}\Big)$ is the fraction of individuals who are infected and treated who progress to the AIDS class.

- $\dfrac{\nu\sigma}{\nu_1\rho_1+\nu\sigma+\mu}$ is the proportion of individuals from the infected class who progress to AIDS without any form of intervention
- $\dfrac{1}{\rho_2\nu_2+\psi_2+\delta_1+\mu}$ is the death adjusted infective period of individuals with AIDS.
- $\dfrac{\sigma_2}{\sigma_2+\psi_1+\mu}$ is the fraction of individuals who are infected and treated who progress to the AIDS class.
- $\Big(\dfrac{\nu\sigma}{\nu\sigma+\rho_1\nu_1+\mu}\Big)\Big(\dfrac{\nu_2\rho_2}{\nu_2\rho_2+\psi_2+\delta_1+\mu}\Big)$ is the fraction of individuals who are infected and treated AIDS individuals who progress to the treated class.

2.3. Discussion on R_e. Here, we consider different cases when different strategies are being implemented using the reproduction number R_e.

Case 1: No intervention - Basic model

This implies that $\omega=\rho_1=\rho_2=\nu_1=p=\psi_1=\psi_2=\sigma_2=\sigma_3=0,\Rightarrow\nu=1$. Therefore the basic reproduction number for the basic model is

$$R_0=c\beta\Big[\frac{1}{\mu+\nu\sigma}+\frac{r_1\nu\sigma}{(\mu+\nu\sigma)(\delta_1+\mu)}\Big].$$

It can be shown that $R_e<R_0$ showing the effect of intervention because the reproduction number when there is intervention reduces the number of people who will be infected by one single individual introduced into a whole susceptible population.

Case 2: Condom use only: No counselling and treatment

We have only condom use as a single strategy of controlling the epidemic, that is $\rho_1=\rho_2=\nu_1=p=\psi_1=\psi_2=\sigma_2=\sigma=0,\Rightarrow\nu=1$. This is a situation which is common in Zimbabwe especially among the poor. The reproduction number becomes

$$R_c=c\beta(1-\omega)\Big[\frac{1}{\mu+\nu\sigma}+\frac{r_1\nu\sigma}{(\mu+\nu\sigma)(\mu+\delta_1)}\Big]=(1-\omega)R_0.$$

Clearly $R_c<R_0$ since $0<\omega<1$. We obtain the critical threshold value for ω as

$$\omega^*=1-\frac{1}{R_0}.$$

Using the same analysis used by Moghadas *et al.* [**8**] we conclude that HIV can be eradicated from the community if

$$\omega=\alpha_1\epsilon_1>\omega^*.$$

Case 3: Pre-treatment counselling and treatment, that is $\omega=0$

For a case without condom use except counselling and treatment, we have

$$\begin{aligned}R_{c'} &= R_{0Ic'}+\Big[\frac{\rho_1\nu_1}{\nu_1\rho_1+\nu\sigma+\mu}+\Big(\frac{\nu\sigma}{\nu\sigma+\rho_1\nu_1+\mu}\Big)\Big(\frac{\nu_2\rho_2}{\nu_2\rho_2+\psi_2+\delta_1+\mu}\Big)\Big]R_{0Tc'}\\ &\quad+\Big[\frac{\nu\sigma}{\nu_1\rho_1+\nu\sigma+\mu}+\Big(\frac{\nu_1\rho_1}{\nu_1\rho_1+\nu\sigma+\mu}\Big)\Big(\frac{\sigma_2}{\sigma_2+\psi_1+\mu}\Big)\Big]R_{0Ac'} \qquad (3)\end{aligned}$$

where $R_{0Ic'}=\dfrac{c\beta}{\nu_1\rho_1+\nu\sigma+\mu}$, $R_{0Tc'}=\dfrac{cr_2\beta}{(\sigma_2+\psi_1+\mu)(1-R_p)}$,

$R_{0Ac'}=\dfrac{cr_1\beta}{(\rho_2\nu_2+\psi_2+\mu+\delta_1)(1-R_p)}$

and $R_p = \left(\frac{\sigma_2}{\sigma_2+\psi_1+\mu}\right)\left(\frac{\rho_2\nu_2}{\rho_2\nu_2+\psi_2+\mu+\delta_1}\right) < 1$. It can be shown that $R_0 > R_{c'}$.

Case 4: No condom and post-treatment counselling except pre-treatment counselling and treatment, that is $p_1 = \psi_1 = \psi_2 = 0$.
We have

$$R_t = \frac{c_1\beta_1}{\nu_1\rho_1+\nu\sigma+\mu} + \frac{c_2\beta_2\nu_1\rho_1)}{[\mu+\gamma(1-p_2)]}. \tag{4}$$

Case 5: No post-counselling after treatment
Treatment and condom use only, that is, $\psi_1 = \psi_2 = 0$. The reproduction number becomes

$$\begin{aligned} R_{(pc)'} = \quad & R_{0I(pc)'} + \left[\frac{\rho_1\nu_1}{\nu_1\rho_1+\nu\sigma+\mu} + \left(\frac{\nu\sigma}{\nu\sigma+\rho_1\nu_1+\mu}\right)\left(\frac{\nu_2\rho_2}{\nu_2\rho_2+\delta_1+\mu}\right)\right]R_{0T(pc)'} \\ & + \left[\frac{\nu\sigma}{\nu_1\rho_1+\nu\sigma+\mu} + \left(\frac{\nu_1\rho_1}{\nu_1\rho_1+\nu\sigma+\mu}\right)\left(\frac{\sigma_2}{\sigma_2+\mu}\right)\right]R_{0A(pc)'} \end{aligned} \tag{5}$$

where $R_{0I(pc)'} = \frac{c\beta(1-\omega)}{\nu_1\rho_1+\nu\sigma+\mu}$, $R_{0T(pc)'} = \frac{cr_2\beta(1-\omega)}{(\sigma_2+\mu)(1-R_p)}$,
$R_{0A(pc)'} = \frac{cr_1\beta(1-\omega)}{(\rho_2\nu_2+\mu+\delta_1)(1-R_p)}$ and $R_p = \left(\frac{\sigma_2}{\sigma_2+\mu}\right)\left(\frac{\rho_2\nu_2}{\rho_2\nu_2+\mu+\delta_1}\right) < 1$. It can be shown that $R_e < R_{0(pc)'}$.

Since it is not easy to find the relationship between the various reproduction numbers, we will use sensitivity and uncertainty analysis in Section 4 to find the relationship between the various reproduction numbers. In addition numerical simulations for some of these different cases with different strategies will be carried out to determine the dynamics of the epidemic model.

2.4. Stability analysis of the disease-free equilibrium. We analyse the stability of the model equations by using R_e as the bifurcation parameter. The model equations depend on parameters and therefore the qualitative structure of the flow can change as parameters are varied. The qualitative changes in the dynamics of a system are called bifurcations and the parameter values at which they occur are called bifurcation points. In epidemiology, bifurcation phenomena is associated with threshold parameters, and R_0, the basic reproduction number or R_e, the effective reproduction number, are the most common. Scientifically, bifurcations are important because they provide models of transitions and stabilities as some control parameters are varied in the model equations.

Using Theorem 2 of [**12**] the following result is established.

THEOREM 1. *The disease-free equilibrium is locally asymptotically stable if $R_e < 1$ and unstable if $R_e > 1$.*

The local stability of the disease-free equilibrium stated above, shows that every solution of (1) with an initial condition close to P_0 eventually approaches P_0. The theorem shows that if the sizes of the subpopulations are close enough to the values of the components of the disease-free equilibrium, then the epidemic can be eradicated from the population whenever $R_e < 1$.

2.5. Global stability of the disease-free equilibrium. We define the following Lyapunov functional, $V = b_1 I + b_2 A + b_3 T$ with

$$\begin{aligned} b_1 &= k_3(\psi_2+\delta_1+\mu)+r_1\nu\sigma k_3+r_1\sigma_2\nu_1\rho_1+r_2\nu\sigma\nu_2\rho_2+r_2k_2\nu_1\rho_1 \\ b_2 &= k_1(r_1k_3+r_2\nu_2\rho_2),\ b_3=k_1(r_1\sigma_2+r_2k_2),\ k_1=\nu_1\rho_1+\nu\sigma+\mu, \\ k_2 &= \nu_2\rho_2+\psi_2+\delta_1+\mu,\ k_3=\sigma_2+\psi_1+\mu. \end{aligned}$$

Letting $a = 1-\omega$, we have,

$$\begin{aligned} \dot V &= b_1\dot I + b_2\dot A + b_3\dot T \\ &= b_1(a\lambda S - k_1 I) + b_2(\nu\sigma I + \sigma_2 T - k_2 A) + b_3(\nu_1\rho_1 I + \nu_2\rho_2 - k_3 T), \\ &= b_1 a\lambda S - k_1k_2k_3 I - r_1k_1k_2k_3 A - r_2k_1k_2k_3 T + \sigma_2\nu_2\rho_2k_1 I + r_1\sigma_2\nu_2\rho_2k_1 A \\ &\quad + r_2\sigma_2\nu_2\rho_2k_1 T \\ &= b_1 a\lambda S - k_1k_2k_3(I+r_1A+r_2T) + (I+r_1A+r_2T)\sigma_2\nu_2\rho_2k_1 \\ &= b_1 a\lambda S - k_1(k_2k_3-\sigma_2\nu_2\rho_2)(I+r_1A+r_2T) \\ &= b_1 a\lambda S - k_1(k_2k_3-\sigma_2\nu_2\rho_2)\lambda N, \quad (I+r_1A+r_2T=\lambda N) \\ &= k_1(k_2k_3-\sigma_2\nu_2\rho_2)\lambda N\Big[\frac{b_1 a\lambda S}{k_1(k_2k_3-\sigma_2\nu_2\rho_2)\lambda N}-1\Big] \\ &\le k_1(k_2k_3-\sigma_2\nu_2\rho_2)\lambda N(R_e-1) \ \text{ for } \ S\le N \\ &= k_1k_2k_3\Big(1-\frac{\sigma_2\nu_2\rho_2}{k_2k_3}\Big)\lambda N(R_e-1) \\ &= k_1k_2k_3(1-R_p)\lambda N(R_e-1) \\ &\le 0 \quad \text{if } R_e\le 1 \text{ since } R_p<1. \end{aligned}$$

Since all the model parameters are nonnegative, it follows that $\dot V \le 0$ for $R_e \le 1$ with $\dot V = 0$ only if $I = T = A = 0$. Hence, V is a Lyapunov function on Γ. Since Γ is invariant and attracting, it follows that the largest compact invariant set in $\{(S, I, T, T_c, A, A_c) \in \Gamma : \dot V = 0\}$ is the singleton $\{P_0\}$. It follows from LaSalle Invariance Principle [**6**] that every solution to model system (1) with initial conditions in Γ converge to P_0 as $t \to \infty$. That is, $((I(t), T(t), A(t)) \to (0,0,0))$ at $t \to \infty$. Substituting $I = T = A = 0$ in model system (1) gives $S \to \Pi/\mu$ as $t \to \infty$. Thus, $(S(t), I(t), T(t), T_c(t), A(t), A_c(t)) \to (\Pi/\mu, 0, 0, 0, 0, 0)$ as $t \to \infty$ for $R_e < 1$ so that P_0 is globally asymptotically stable in Γ if $R_e < 1$. We summarize the result in the following theorem.

THEOREM 2. *The disease-free equilibrium, P_0 is globally asymptotically stable for the model (1) provided $R_e < 1$ and unstable if $R_e > 1$.*

2.6. Endemic equilibrium. The endemic equilibrium for model system (1) is given by $P_e = (S^*, I^*, T^*, T_c^*, A^*, A_c^*)$, where

$$\begin{aligned}
S^* &= \frac{N^*}{R_e},\ I^* = \frac{\Pi}{R_e(\nu_1\rho_1 + \nu\sigma + \mu)}(R_e - 1) \\
T^* &= \frac{\Pi[\nu_1\rho_1\Delta + \rho_2\nu_2\nu\sigma]}{(1 - R_p)\Delta(\sigma_2 + \mu + \psi)(\nu_1\rho_1 + \nu\sigma + \mu)}(R_e - 1) \\
T_c^* &= \frac{\Pi\psi_1[\nu_1\rho_1\Delta + \rho_2\nu_2\nu\sigma]}{(1 - R_p)\Delta(\sigma_3 + \mu)(\nu_1\rho_1 + \nu\sigma + \mu)(\sigma_2 + \mu + \psi)}(R_e - 1) \\
A^* &= \frac{\Pi[\nu_1\rho_1\sigma_2\nu_2 + \nu\sigma(\sigma_2 + \psi_1 + \mu)]}{(1 - R_p)\Delta(\sigma_2 + \mu + \psi)(\nu_1\rho_1 + \nu\sigma + \mu)}(R_e - 1) \\
A_c^* &= \frac{\Pi[\psi_2\{\nu_1\rho_1\sigma_2\nu_2 + \nu\sigma(\sigma_2 + \psi_1 + \mu)\} + \sigma_3\{\nu_1\rho_1\Delta + \rho_2\nu_2\nu\sigma\}]}{(1 - R_p)\Delta(\delta_2 + \mu)(\sigma_2 + \mu + \psi)(\nu_1\rho_1 + \nu\sigma + \mu)}(R_e - 1),
\end{aligned}$$

where $\Delta = \rho_2\nu_2 + \psi_2 + \mu + \delta_1$. We have therefore established the following Lemma from the coordinates of P_e expressed in terms of R_e.

LEMMA 2. *If $R_e > 1$, then model system (1) has a unique positive endemic equilibrium P_e.*

Numerical simulations of model system (1) using a program coded in C^{++} indicate that there is transcritical bifurcation at $R_e = 1$, where stability changes from the disease-free equilibrium to endemic-equilibrium. The bifurcation diagram is illustrated in Figure 2.

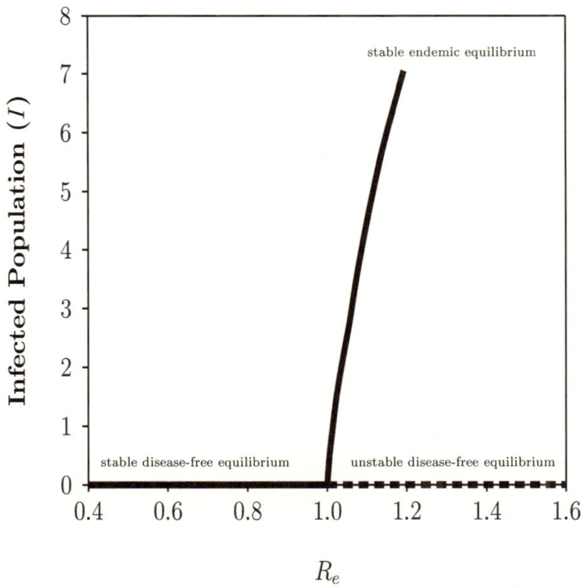

FIGURE 2. Bifurcation diagram for the model system (1) obtained from numerical simulations, which show that the disease-free and endemic equilibria exchange stability when R_e is 1 for an arbitrary set of parameter values. The bold lines show stability and dashed lines show instability.

3. Measuring the economic cost of HIV/AIDS

We explore the economic cost of HIV/AIDS in Zimbabwe based on the direct monetary values that are incurred as the epidemic runs its course. We will base all our analysis on model system (1), where prevention and treatment have been used to track the epidemiological progress of the disease. The purpose of economic evaluation is to identify, measure, value and compare the costs and consequences of alternate interventions, strategies or policies. Cost analysis (CA) is the measurement or estimation of the resources consumed by a particular HIV/AIDS prevention and treatment program [**11**]. This is essential for policy makers to decide whether they have sufficient resources to afford a particular type of intervention.

Costs involved affects the patient, the worker and the government. The cost of condoms C_c, is proportional to the total number of sexual active individuals at any given time. The cost of screening C_s, is the sum of the proportion of the infected who have chosen to be screened and the proportion of the individuals with clinical AIDS who have chosen to be screened. The costs C_{TI}, of fighting opportunistic infections like Tuberculosis, pneumonia, is the cost of the different prophylaxis drugs on the said population and the cost of CD4 cell counts, viral load done by NGOs, MSF-doctors without borders and this is important where there is drug resistant or treatment failure. The cost C_{TA}, of treating those who have developed clinical AIDS is determined by the proportion of the treated who go on to develop clinical AIDS. Costs such as home based care, hospitalization, supply of structured ARV treatment, home nursing which is about Z\$2m a month per patient paying Z\$50, are not included. The cost C_{PC}, of post infection counseling, includes the cost of training peer educators, printing booklets and other related material. The cost C_R, is the cost of running the clinic and other related administrative issues such as follow up of defaulters. Therefore the total cost rate function $C(t)$, (in dollars per unit time) at time t, is defined as

$$\begin{aligned} C(t) &= C_c[(S(t)+I(t)+T(t)+A(t)]+C_s[\nu_1\rho_1 I(t)+\nu_2\rho_2 A(t)]+C_{TI}I(t) \\ &\quad +C_{TA}\sigma_2 T(t)+C_{PC}[\psi_1 T(t)+\psi_2 A(t)]+C_R. \qquad (6) \end{aligned}$$

The total cost C_{TC}, of running the prevention and treatment programs over a planning period of n years, is given by

$$C_{TC}=\int_0^n C(t)dt.$$

4. Numerical simulations

Mathematical models often include parameters, estimated from experiments, for which their actual values are not known precisely [**13**]. This will be accomplished by sensitivity and uncertainty analysis using the proposed ranges of the model parameters given below. Such analysis can be used for various purposes, such as ranking the parameters in order of their relative importance to the results and for assessing changes in the results due to variability in the parameter ranges. Numerical simulations will also help in bringing out the relationship of the theoretical results from the different scenarios which were discussed in Section 2. The simulation analysis will also help to properly identify those parameters that have the most effect in changing the reproduction number, R_e. We used a fourth order Runge-Kutta numerical scheme coded in C^{++} programming language for the numerical simulations to solve the system of differential equations describing the dynamics ! of the model and the cost function. Runge-Kutta solutions obtained were then substituted per given time into the cost function (6). Graphs of the different population groups with time and the resulting values from the cost function were plotted and analysed using parameter values in Table 2 and Table 3.The simulations for the model dynamics are conducted using absolute numbers and then converted back to proportions for the figures.

We will use parameter values from the range that was used elsewhere in [**10**], as shown in Table 2.

TABLE 2. Table of Range of Parameters used in the model.

Parameter	Symbol	Value	Source
β	$0.01 \leq \beta \leq 0.15$	σ	$0.1 \leq \sigma \leq 0.6$
c	$1 \leq c \leq 20$	r_1	$1 \leq r_1 \leq 1.5$
r_2	$0.2 \leq r_2 \leq 1$	ψ_1	$0 \leq \psi_1 \leq 1$
p	$0 \leq p \leq 1$	ρ_2	$0 \leq \rho_2 \leq 1$
γ	$0.06 \leq \gamma \leq 0.02$	ψ_2	$0 \leq \psi_2 \leq 1$
ν_1	$0 \leq \nu_1 \leq 1$	ν_2	$0 \leq \nu_2 \leq 1$
η	$0.01 \leq \eta \leq 0.05$	ρ_1	$0.07 \leq \rho_1 \leq 0.4$
α_1	$0. \leq \alpha_1 \leq 1$	α_2	$0 \leq \alpha_2 \leq 1$
ϵ_1	$0 \leq \epsilon_1 \leq 1$	ϵ_2	$0 \leq \epsilon_2 \leq 1$
ω	$0 \leq \omega \leq 1$	μ	$0.015 \leq \mu \leq 0.025$
δ_1	$0.025 \leq \delta_1 \leq 0.35$	δ_2	$0.05 \leq \delta_2 \leq 0.2$

The other specific parameter values which were used are indicated in Table 3.

TABLE 3. Table of Parameters used in the model.

Parameter	Symbol	Value	Source
Recruitment rate	Π	0.029	Central Statistics Office
Natural death rate	μ	0.02	Central Statistics Office
Probability of transmission	β	0.1035	Central Statistics Office
Partner acquisition rate	c	5	Central Statistics Office
Clinical Trial Cost	C_R	\$50 000 per year	Estimated
HIV screening	C_s	\$10 per test	Estimated
Treatment	C_{TI}	\$200 per person	Estimated
Treatment	C_{TA}	\$10000	Estimated
Counseling	C_{CP}	\$200 per person	Estimated
Condom Subsidies	C_c	\$0.25 per person	Estimated

4.1. Sensitivity Analysis: Trends of reproduction numbers. We accomplish the effects of parameter uncertainties on the model predictions of the basic reproduction number of the infection by sensitivity and uncertainty analysis using the proposed ranges of the model parameters.

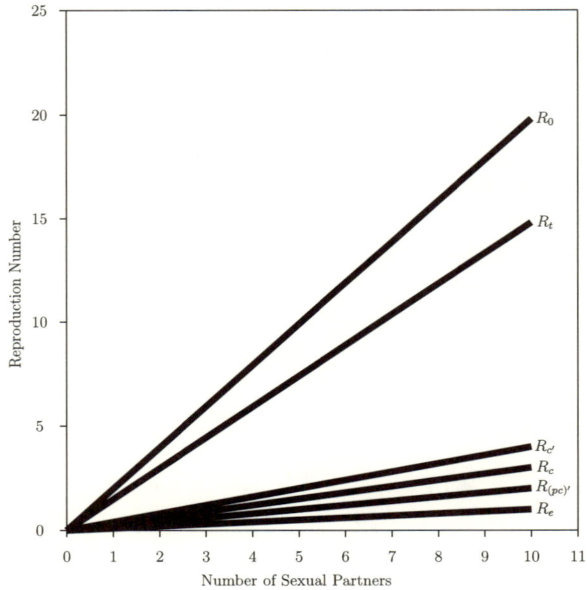

FIGURE 3. Trend of reproduction numbers with $\beta = 0.104, \nu_1 = 0.7, \nu_2 = 0.5, r_1 = 0.6, r_2 = 1.2, \rho_1 = 0.3, \rho_2 = 0.5, \sigma_1 = 0.4, \sigma_2 = 0.04, \sigma_3 = 0.08, \psi_1 = 0.6, \psi_2 = 0.7, \mu = 0.02, \delta_1 = 0.333, \delta_2 = 0.15$

The simulations show that

$$R_e < R_{(pc)'} < R_c < R_{c'} < R_t < R_0.$$

It can be seen that while treatment alone reduces the epidemic ($R_t < R_0$), condom use alone and treatment with pre- and post-treatment counselling are better strategies than treatment alone ($R_c < R_{c'} < R_t$). The use of condoms alone is even better than treatment with pre- and post-treatment counselling ($R_c < R_{c'}$). While post-treatment counselling together with the other strategies is the best strategy to reduce the epidemic, it can be seen that leaving post-treatment counselling is the next best option ($R_e < R_{(pc)'}$).

4.2. Effects of pre-treatment counselling and treatment without other strategies. This is similar to Case 4 in section 2.3. In this simulation, we vary the proportion of the infectives who receive treatment to study the effect of treating HIV-infected individuals on the spread of the epidemic and the results are illustrated in Figure 4.

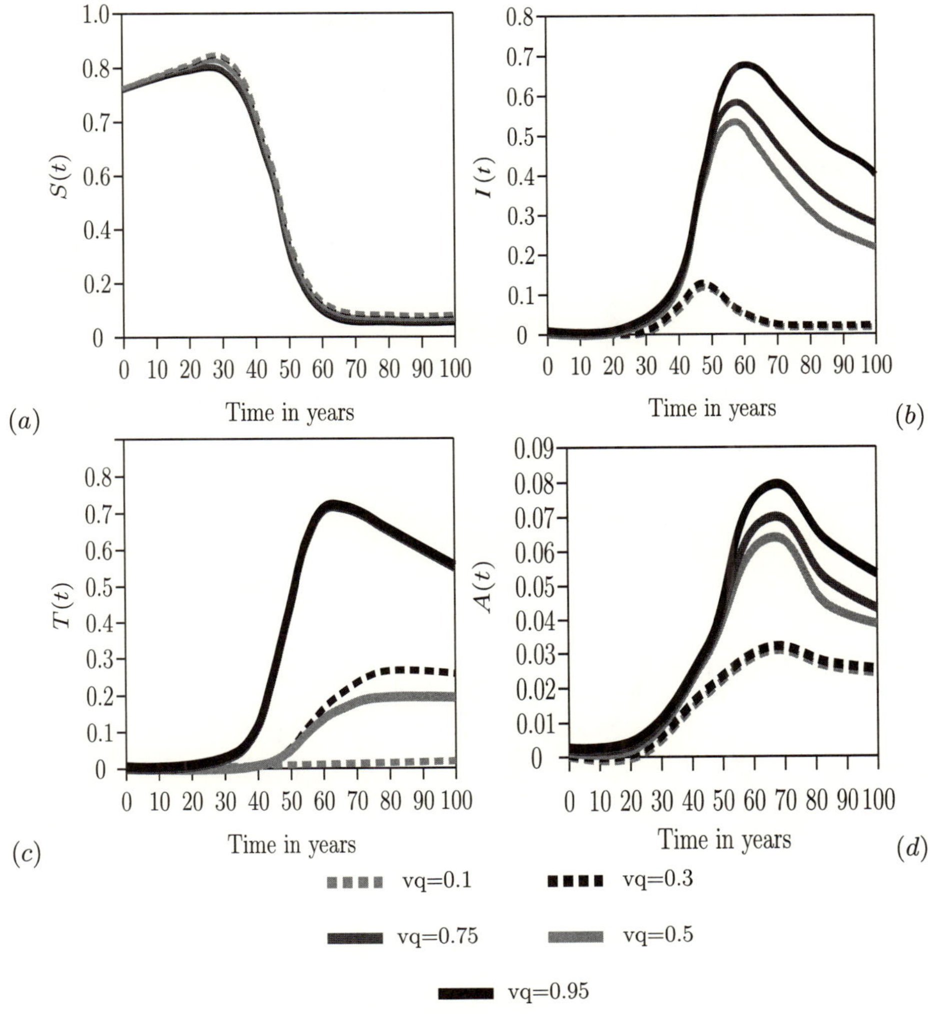

FIGURE 4. Simulation results showing the effect of treatment: (*a*) Susceptible population, (*b*) Infected individuals, (*c*) Treated population, and (*d*) AIDS cases. vq is the proportion of individuals receiving treatment with initial conditions $s = 0.8725, i = 0.1275, t = t_c = a = a_c = 0$. Parameter values used $\beta = 0.104, \nu_1 = 0.7, \nu_2 = 0.5 r_1 = 0.6, r_2 = 1.2, \rho_1 = 0.3, \rho_2 = 0.5, \sigma_1 = 0.4, \sigma_2 = 0.04, \sigma_3 = 0.08, \psi_1 = 0.6, \psi_2 = 0.7, \mu = 0.02, \delta_1 = 0.333, \delta_2 = 0.15$.

The increase in the number of HIV infectives with increased treatment is due to the fact that treatment lengthens the lives of the infectives and as a result those who would have developed clinical AIDS become more healthy and continue to be sexually active. Although the simulation shows insignificant difference in the susceptible populations, it is clear from Figure 4 (a) that the susceptible population will be reduced and stabilise to very low levels. We also observe an increased number of AIDS cases in the population with increased treatment as is shown in Figure 4 (d). This is in agreement with Gupta and Anderson [**4**] in which they noted that therapy lengthens the incubation period thereby reducing on the AIDS incidence rate and increasing the infectious period. More people will be treated as a result. We also note that the epidemic will reach a peak after about 60 years and all the infected individuals will start to decrease.

4.3. Effects of the incubation period. Treatment of HIV infectives prolongs the incubation period (the length of time that an infected person takes to develop clinical AIDS symptoms). We look at the effect of lengthening the average incubation period (due to treatment) on the susceptible, infected, AIDS and treated populations. The following values of the average incubation periods, 9, 13, 15, and 16 years are used in the model system (1), with an assumption that a large proportion of the infected are taking treatment. It is also assumed that at this stage there is very little behavioral change, that is, pre-treatment counselling and treatment alone.

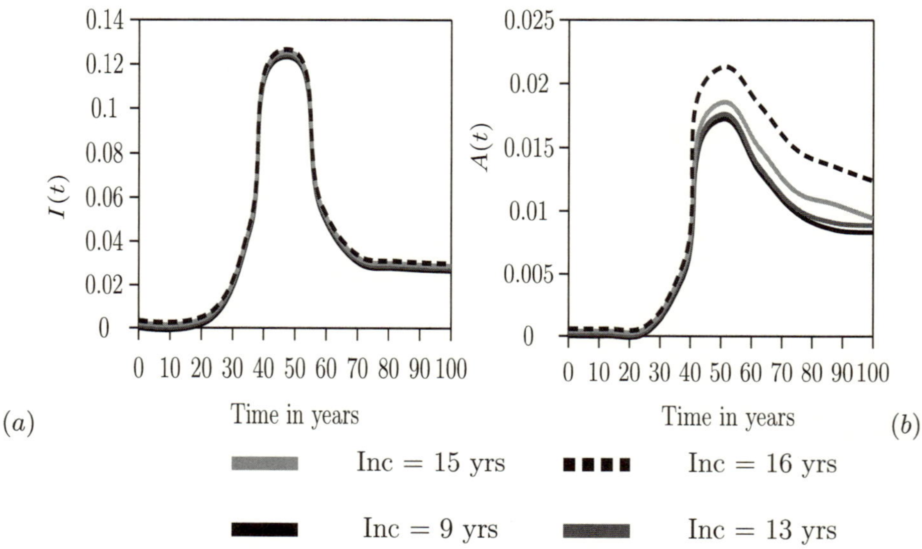

FIGURE 5. Effects of incubation period and effective treatment of: (a) infectives, and (b) AIDS individuals. *Inc*: is the incubation period (average time an individual spends in the infected class before clinical AIDS with initial conditions $s = 0.95, i = 0.05, t = t_c = a = a_c = 0$. Parameter values used $\beta = 0.104, \nu_1 = 0.7, \nu_2 = 0.5 r_1 = 0.6, r_2 = 1.2, \rho_1 = 0.3, \rho_2 = 0.5, \sigma_1 = 0.4, \sigma_2 = 0.04, \sigma_3 = 0.08, \psi_1 = 0.6, \psi_2 = 0.7, \mu = 0.02, \delta_1 = 0.333, \delta_2 = 0.15$

4.4. Effects of treatment with counseling. In this section, we study the trend of the spread of the epidemic, in relation to effective treatment that is accompanied by all strategies. In model system (1), c is the average rate at which individuals change or acquire new sexual partners. Control measures such as condom use, abstinence from sex and sticking to one partner can reduce β. The combination of these leads to smaller values of β and the force of infection in general. Since treatment lengthens incubation period we take 14 years as an average incubation period of the treated. Taking the values of $\beta c = 0.01, 0.22, 0.33, 0.4$ (with smaller values taken to mean positive behavioral change and larger values to mean little or no change in one's social behavior). We simulate the susceptibles, infectives, the treated and the AIDS individuals as shown in Figures 6 (a), (b), (c) and (d) respectively.

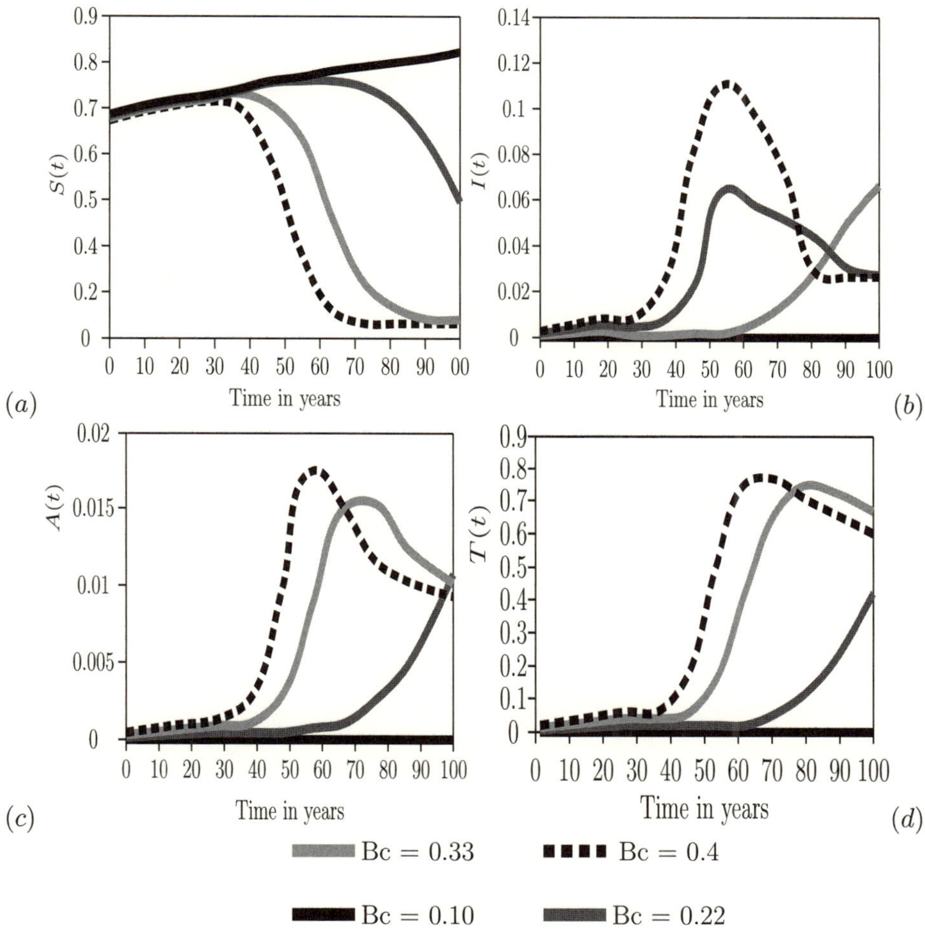

FIGURE 6. Effective treatment and effect of change in social behavior: The distribution of: (a) susceptible adults, (b) infected individuals, (c) treated individuals and (d) AIDS cases. βc, the change in social behavior, smaller values of βc indicate positive change i.e. less partners per individual while large values indicate the converse. Initial conditions: $s = 0.795, i = 0.205, t = t_c = a = a_c = 0$. Parameter values used $\beta = 0.104, \nu_1 = 0.7, \nu_2 = 0.5 r_1 = 0.6, r_2 = 1.2, \rho_1 = 0.3, \rho_2 = 0.5, \sigma_1 = 0.4, \sigma_2 = 0.04, \sigma_3 = 0.08, \psi_1 = 0.6, \psi_2 = 0.7, \mu = 0.02, \delta_1 = 0.333, \delta_2 = 0.15$

Effective treatment of HIV-infected individuals whereby a large proportion of the infected population seek medical treatment coupled with a positive change in one's social behavior, increases the number of the susceptible population, as shown in Figure 6 (a). But with less change in one's social behavior, we note that there is a notable early decrease in the susceptible population. This then implies that making βc as small as possible, we note from Figure 6 (a) that the susceptible population grows without a decline. This shows that treatment accompanied with measures such as counseling the treated HIV patients to refrain from unprotected sexual activities will eventually reduce and/or control the epidemic in the long run.

As noted in Figure 4 (a), effective treatment of the infected population does not have much significance on the number of the susceptible population. As previously stated, this is because treatment of HIV-infected is not curing them from the disease. The significant increase in the number of infected individuals and the AIDS cases consequently is attributed to the prolonged incubation periods as shown in Figure 5 (a) and (b). This is an indication that without behavioral change, effective treatment of adult infectives results in more spread of the epidemic. We note that with little or no change in one's social behavior, the number of infectives in the population start to grow rapidly earlier than when there is a positive change. As a result of this we also note an immediate rise in AIDS cases.

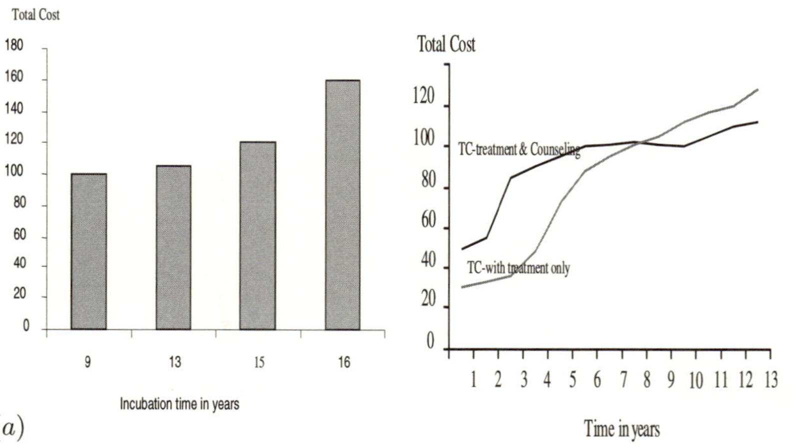

(a) (b)

FIGURE 7. Simulation results for: (a) total cost with increasing incubation period (b) a comparison of total cost (TC) (US\$000) for the case with treatment only and treatment with counselling.

4.5. Simulating Total Cost: Varying incubation period with no counseling. In Figure 7 (a) we present a histogram of the total cost with increasing incubation period. We deduce that increasing the incubation by treatment tends to benefit the infected individual as we increase the number of years lived but the total annual cost maybe too high to be sustained by the government. On the other hand, the cost of doing "nothing" as represented by an incubation period of less than 9 years appears to be costly as well. Treatment and caring for those who have developed clinical AIDS constitute a major part of our cost function followed by treatment of those who are infected but have not yet developed clinical AIDS. Increasing the incubation time tends to shorten the AIDS incubation period thereby reducing the major cost, however from Figure 5 (a) and (b), this tends to increase the number of the infective population and the period over which medication will be administered to them, thereby eroding the initial gains and thus raising the annual cost per person to USD 160 000.

The rise in cost at an incubation period of 16 years can be explained in terms of C_{TI}, the cost of treating the infected (i.e. the longer the period one is under treatment the higher the costs incurred). The elongated incubation period coupled by the large rising numbers of the infected individuals will certainly rise costs as depicted in Figure 7 (a). The total cost incurred in treating the infected population over time is in two scenarios, that is, Treatment coupled by preventive measures and Treatment only. Figure 7 (b) show that at the initiation of the programs the all encompassing approach (treatment coupled with prevention) has a high costs compared to offering treatment alone to patients. As time progress the costs incurred in the former case tend to stabilize while in the latter case costs continue to sore. This can be explained in terms of the increasing number of new infections when treatment is not coupled by counseling. A large proportion of the susceptible population becomes infected, hence more patients will need to be catered for and thus raising the total costs incurred in combating the pandemic over time.

4.6. Discussion. Treatment increases the length of the incubation period of HIV without significantly reducing the infectiousness; this will necessarily increase the prevalence of the infection as observed by Gupta and Anderson, [**4**]. Unless accompanied by appropriate levels of behavioral change treatment would only bring short relief to the sick individual but catastrophic results in the long run to communities. However, if treatment coverage and efficacy are high coupled by a high positive change in social behavior there is a big chance that the epidemic would even be controlled.

The robustness of the pandemic within the affected individuals makes it difficult to forecast the exact economic impact per given time in monetary value terms. It is however possible to make adjustments to budgets in line with policies that we would have chosen in the fight against the pandemic. For example, if Zimbabwe were to concentrate more on prevention policies and put small subsidies on treatment, this would translate to a relatively small constant expenditure over time (in present value terms) coupled by a low number of "premature" deaths of the infected.

5. Summary and concluding remarks

We have presented an HIV/AIDS model with multiple classes of infectives for assessing the effects of multi-strategies on the transmission dynamics and economic impact of HIV/AIDS in Zimbabwe. The model incorporate prevention strategies for behavior change and we numerically analysed the model with therapy in two scenarios that are treatment with positive change in sexual behaviour and treatment with no change in sexual behavior. Reproduction numbers and equilibria for the model were determined and stabilities were analysed. The cost function was constructed taking into account all the interventions which have been suggested.

The results from the study show that prolonged incubation period of HIV/AIDS enlarge the epidemic. Positive changes in sexual behavior by reducing the number of sexual partners reduces HIV/AIDS prevalence. Treatment of AIDS patients only speed up the development of the epidemic if not accompanied by a positive change in sexual behavior in a community. From the analysis of the threshold parameter, the effective reproduction number R_e, it is shown that multi strategies are better than pre-treatment counselling and treatment alone and the cost of using multi strategies has been shown to be lower, in the long run, than the cost of the latter strategy. The cost can be further cut if post-treatment counselling is left out since it is the second best option to reduce the disease. Therefore the reproduction number can be used to evaluate the cost effectiveness of particular strategies. In Zimbabwe, where the pandemic has reached epidemic proportions, combating the disease and! its economic effects successfully will require a large and determined fiscal effort. Most parameters on our Total Cost function are complementary. In our case where fiscal resources are scarce some trade-offs will be unavoidable, requiring the concentration of resources on some programs or groups at the expense of others. While there is rise in cost after increasing the incubation period, this will benefit the government and the families affected since the infected individuals might be able to come back to work and earn more money to meet the costs. The hope is that our epidemiological knowledge of HIV/AIDS in this regard will be distilled into a form where it reveals how to formulate combined programs of interventions that will ward off the threat of an economic collapse.

We conclude that a major breakthrough in the management of HIV/AIDS will come as a result of multiple strategies in combating the epidemic. There is need to expand HIV/AIDS awareness and education programmes, accelerated training of public health workers, developing nutritional guidelines for children and adults living and working with HIV/AIDS, expand prevention program

Drug efficacy and adherence to treatment are of paramount importance since HIV treatment requires strict dosage taking adherence. The investigation of the impact of these therapies on the spread of HIV/AIDS was measured by the use of the parameter p. Numerical results have shown that increasing the values of p without increasing the values of ω has no significant impact on the dynamics of the disease, demonstrating the importance of primary intervention as observed in another study by [**10**]. We can see that more interventions reduce the basic reproduction number which in turn shows that the disease is under control. Antiretroviral drugs can significantly prolong HIV patient's life span [**3**] and the individual may become more active, that is, have more sexual partners per unit time after being treated or vaccinated [**7**]. The implication of our findings are that if treatment program prolongs an individual's sexually active lifetime more than it reduces the individual's infectivity, it can never reduce R_e to below 1. The negative effect of the treatment program may be that partially recovered patients become carriers and hence undermine the effectiveness of the drug program over the whole population. However, this will provide a tangible and economic benefit as lives improved or prolonged will add productivity and income to the government in general and the affected family in particular. Resources allowing, it will be therefore be prudent on the part of policy makers to initiate an all encompassing approach.

However, there are some limitations in our analysis. We acknowledge that the findings in this study must be regarded as preliminary, and that various aspects of the calibration process and assumptions in particular need further work and refinement. Since the AIDS treatment costs are so high and since the system is unlikely to reach the steady state over reasonable planning period there are great dangers in imposing an artificial planning period of n years because one runs the risk of "pushing" important system behaviors beyond the period or of creating computational artifacts. While we concentrated on the economic cost, it will also be important to estimate the cost effectiveness of the multiple strategies. There is need to estimate the increased quality-adjusted life expectancy with the associated incremental cost per quality-adjusted year of life gained as compared with no particular intervention. There is also need to find out whether medical cost and life expectan! cy depend on the efficacy of the drugs and condoms. Finding the optimal timing of treatment and the most effective ways to reduce the risk of treatment failure is essential since in our model we assumed that anyone who can afford can be treated while WHO policy insists on all those whose CD4+ T cell count is less than $200mm^{-3}$. We also want to state that while we tried to include most costs of the epidemic, we did not include the cost of patients' time and some of the costs like, suffering, loss of friends and family members, which are intangible. Like what Paltiel *et al* [**11**] said, we also hope that research like this one will help to put quantifiable aspects of the epidemic into perspective.

References

1. G.Birkhoff and G.C. Rota , *Ordinary differential equations*, Ginn (1982).
2. J.S.Bollinger, R. Kerkhoven, G. Mutangadura, D. Mukurazita, *The Economic Impact of AIDS in Zimbabwe, The Futures Group International in collaboration with: Research Triangle Institute (RTI.)*, (1999)
3. D. Dickinson, E.M. Lungu and R. Cowen, *An African experience of Hydroxyurea containing regimes for HIV-1 positive patients*, The Lancet-Electronic Research Archive. www.thelancet.com/newlancet/eprint/16/index.html, (2000).
4. S. Gupta and R.M.Anderson, *Mathematical Models and the design of public health policy: HIV and antiviral therapy.* SIAM Review, *35*, (1993),1–16.
5. V. Hutson and K. Schmitt, *Permanence and the Dynamics of Biological Systems*, Math. Biosci., *111*, (1992),1–71.
6. J.P. LaSalle, *The Stability of Dynamical Systems*, CBMS-NSF Regional Conference Series in Applied Mathematics, *25*, SIAM: Philadephia, (1976).
7. L.S. Luboobi, *A Three Age-Groups Model for the HIV/AIDS Epidemic and Effects of Medical/Social Intervention*, (1993).
8. M.S.Moghadas , A.B. Gumel, R.G. Mcleod R.G and R. Gordon R, *Could condoms stop the AIDS epidemic?* Jour. Theor. Medic., *5*,(2003), 171–181.
9. Z. Mukandavire and W. Garira , *HIV/AIDS model for assessing the effects of prophylactic sterilizing vaccines, condoms and treatment with amelioration*, Jour. Biol. Syst., *14(3)*,(2006), 323–355.
10. F. Nyabadza, *A Mathematical Model for Combating HIV/AIDS in Southern Africa*, Journal of Biological Systems, *14*,(2006)
11. A.D. Paltiel, and E.H.Kaplan, *The Epidemiological and Economic Consequences of AIDS Clinical trials*, *14*, (1993).
12. P. van den Driessche and J. Watmough, *Reproduction numbers and sub-threshold endemic equilibrium for compartmental models of disease transmission*, Math. Biosci., *180*, (2002), 29–48.
13. J.R. Williams, and R.M. Anderson, *Mathematical models of the transmission dynamics of human immunodeficiency virus in England and Wales:mixing between different risk groups*, J. Roy. Stat. Soci., *157 part1*,(1996), 69–88.
14. UNAIDS report, *the global AIDS Epidemic*, Geneva (2002).
15. UNAIDS report, *the global AIDS Epidemic*, Geneva (2006).
16. *UNAIDS Practical Guidelines for Intensifying HIV Prevention*, (2007).

Department of Applied Mathematics, Modelling Biomedical Systems Research Group
E-mail address: sdmusekwa@nust.ac.zw
E-mail address: sdhmusekwa@gmail.com

National University of Science and Technology, Box AC 939 Ascot, Bulawayo, Zimbabwe

National University of Science and Technology, Box AC 939 Ascot, Bulawayo, Zimbabwe

DIMACS Series in Discrete Mathematics
and Theoretical Computer Science
Volume **75**, 2010

Mathematical Analysis of HIV Treatment Model With Variable Viral Load and Infection Stages

Oluwaseun Sharomi and Abba B. Gumel

ABSTRACT. A basic deterministic model for HIV transmission in a population, which accounts for viral load variability upon infection, is formulated and used to evaluate various ARV (anti-retroviral) drug treatment strategies. The strategies considered are to treat (i) every known infected individual (universal strategy), (ii) individuals with low viral load only, (iii) individuals with high viral load (including those with AIDS symptoms) only and (iv) people with clinical symptoms of AIDS only. In the absence of treatment, it is shown that the model has a globally-asymptotically stable (GAS) disease-free equilibrium (DFE) whenever a certain epidemiological threshold, known as the *basic reproduction number*, is less than unity. Using a non-linear Lyapunov function of Goh-Volterra type, it is further shown that the unique endemic equilibrium point (EEP) of the treatment-free model is GAS for a special case. The basic model with treatment also has a GAS DFE when the associated reproduction threshold ($\mathcal{R}_T$) is less than unity, and has a unique EEP when $\mathcal{R}_T > 1$. The basic treatment model is then extended to incorporate the staged-progression aspect of HIV disease. Numerical simulations of the extended model reveal that, for low treatment rate, the universal strategy gives the highest reduction in the total number of cases and AIDS-related mortality, whereas the AIDS-only treatment strategy gives the highest reduction in mortality if the treatment rates are high enough. For the other strategies, it is shown that the optimal choice of a treatment strategy is dependent on the value of σ (the fraction of HIV-infected individuals with high viral load upon initial infection).

1. Introduction

Ever since their introduction in the early 1990s [**38, 39**], antiretroviral drugs (ARVs), particularly the highly-active antiretroviral therapies (HAART), have had dramatic impact in curtailing the burden (morbidity and mortality) of the HIV pandemic in many countries where these drugs are accessible [**37**]. The use of such life-saving drugs, over long periods of time, reduces the viral loads in HIV-infected

1991 *Mathematics Subject Classification.* Primary 54C40, 14E20; Secondary 46E25, 20C20.
Key words and phrases. reproduction number, viral load, lyapunov functions.
One of the authors (ABG) acknowledges, with thanks, the support in part of the Natural Science and Engineering Research Council (NSERC) and Mathematics of Information Technology and Complex Systems (MITACS) of Canada. OS gratefully acknowledges the support of the Institute of Industrial Mathematical Sciences and the Department of Mathematics, University of Manitoba. The authors are grateful to the anonymous reviewers for their constructive comments.

individuals to non-detectable levels (typically characterized by HIV RNA of less than 50 copies/mm^3) [**24**]. In addition to making these individuals less infectious (owing to the positive correlation between viral load and HIV transmission [**17**]), HAART extends the life, and the quality of life, of infected individuals [**38**].

The type of strategy for implementing a HIV control program based on using ARVs is influenced by a number of factors ranging from biological, economics (availability of resources) and efficiency of the public health care system. Although the cost of ARVs has reduced significantly over the years, these drugs are still not widely available in many resource-poor nations. About 33 million people are now living with HIV, of whom more than 30 million live in low- and middle-income countries. The World Health Organization (WHO) [**44**] estimates that at least 9.7 million of these people are in need of ARVs. In nations where these drugs are readily available, while some have opted for universal (mass) treatment of all infected individuals (e.g., in Brazil [**29**]), other nations have adopted a more targeted approach, where only individuals with low CD4 count (generally below 200 cells/mm^3) are treated; individuals with such low CD4 count are essentially at the pre-AIDS or AIDS stage of HIV disease, and, therefore, have high viral loads. This late strategy is further justified by the results of the randomized clinical trials in [**5, 14, 16, 19**], which provide strong evidence of improved survival and reduced progression by treating symptomatic patients and patients with CD4 count of less than 200 cells/mm^3. Further, this strategy has the additional advantage of minimizing the potential impact of the evolution and spread of HAART-resistant HIV strain and also minimizing HAART-related side effects and toxicity.

It is worth emphasizing that the latter strategy (treating those with CD4 $<$ 200 cells/mm^3 or viral load above a certain threshold) forms part of the new HIV control guidelines in a number of countries, such as the USA [**9, 15**] and Canada [**15**]. Some developing nations, such as Botswana [**32**], also subscribe to the late (viral load-dependent) treatment strategy, perhaps due to reasons that may include economics. In summary, there are a number of ways HAART could be implemented to help combat the spread of HIV/AIDS in a community. These include targeting (i) all known infected individuals (universal strategy), (ii) infected individuals with low viral load, (iii) infected individuals with high viral load and clinical symptoms of AIDS and (iv) infected individuals with AIDS symptoms only. The key modelling question then is which of these strategies is most effective in minimizing HIV-related burden in a community?

A number of mathematical models, mostly of the form of deterministic or stochastic systems of non-linear differential equations, have been used, over the last few decades, to gain insights into the impact of antiretroviral therapies on the control of HIV spread in a population or *in vivo* [**1, 2, 17, 27, 38, 39, 43, 45**]. This paper complements, and extends, the aforementioned (and related) studies by designing, and rigorously analyzing, a new mathematical model which incorporates many of the known clinical features of HIV disease in the presence of ARVs. A basic HIV treatment model, which subdivides the infected population into those with low and high viral load upon initial infection (accounting for the differential infectivity property of HIV disease [**23**]), is considered first of all. In addition to incorporating the fact that HIV RNA vary in infected individuals (where individuals with larger viral loads during the chronic phase tend to develop AIDS more rapidly [**34**]), the model allows for HIV transmission by individuals with clinical symptoms of AIDS.

Although many HIV transmission models are built on the assumption that individuals in the AIDS stage do not transmit HIV, epidemiological evidence supports the hypothesis that AIDS patients are capable of, and do engage in, risky behavior such as having multiple sexual partners or inconsistent condom use [**28, 35, 36**]. Thus, it is plausible to incorporate the contribution of these individuals in further transmission of HIV. This phenomenon is also incorporated in [**10**].

The basic differential infectivity model is extended to account for the staged-progression aspect of HIV disease, where a HIV-infected individual is highly infectious during the pre-antibody phase (primary infection stage), maintaining low infectivity during the asymptomatic phase (secondary infection stage), and becoming highly infectious as s/he progresses toward AIDS (the AIDS stage) [**12, 21, 23, 30, 33, 38**]. The staged-progression model allows the assessment of the variation of infectiousness in a given individual over time, as well as the effects of treatment on HIV transmission as infected individuals pass through these different stages. The models are qualitatively analyzed and simulated to study the impact of various targeted treatment scenarios.

2. Basic Model

The development of the basic HIV transmission model is based on sub-dividing the total population at time t, denoted by $N(t)$, into a number of mutually-exclusive compartments namely, susceptible ($S(t)$), newly-infected individuals with low ($L(t)$), high ($H(t)$) viral load, infected individuals at the AIDS stage of infection ($A(t)$), treated individuals ($T(t)$) and individuals in whom treatment has failed ($F(t)$), so that

$$N(t) = S(t) + L(t) + H(t) + A(t) + T(t) + F(t).$$

The susceptible population is increased by the recruitment of individuals (assumed susceptible) into the population at a rate Π. These individuals acquire infection, following contact with infected individuals in the H, L, A, T and F classes, at a rate λ, where,

$$\lambda = \beta \frac{(L + \theta_H H + \theta_A A + \theta_T T + \theta_F F)}{N}.$$

The parameter β is the *effective contact rate*, while $\theta_H \geq 1$ is the relative risk of infectiousness of individuals with high viral load (in comparison to those with low viral load), $\theta_A \geq 1$ and $\theta_F \geq 1$ are similarly defined. The parameter $0 < \theta_T \leq 1$ accounts for the assumed reduced infectiousness of treated individuals.

To incorporate variability in viral load amongst infected individuals (differential infectivity), it is assumed that a proportion, $1-\sigma$, of the newly-infected individuals have low viral load upon diagnosis, and the remaining fraction (σ) have high viral load. Infected individuals in the low and high viral load classes progress to AIDS at rates α_L and α_H, respectively (where $\alpha_H > \alpha_L$ accounts for the fact that individuals with high viral load progress to AIDS faster than those with low viral load). It is worth stating that since the focus of the paper is to evaluate treatment strategies that target individuals with low or high viral load, transition to/from L to H is not incorporated; this is needed to help keep track of the two infection streams strictly (categorized in terms of low and high viral load). The parameters α_L and α_H account for the transition from the low and high viral load stages to AIDS, respectively. Individuals with low viral load are treated at a rate τ_1, whilst those with high viral load are treated at a rate τ_2. Similarly, individuals with symptoms of AIDS are treated at a rate τ_3.

Treated individuals fail treatment at a rate γ. Such failure arise due to various reasons, including non-compliance to the specified ARV regimen or development of resistance. In other words, individuals in the F class may have (and can transmit) a resistant strain (see, for instance, [**3, 4, 31**]), and are assumed to be in the final phase of the HIV disease. It is assumed that no alternative treatment exists for individuals in the F class, and these individuals suffer a disease-induced death at a rate η_F. For mathematical convenience, multiple HIV strains are not considered in this study. Further, natural mortality or removal occurs in all classes at a rate μ, and AIDS individuals suffer an additional disease-induced death at a rate δ (it is assumed that $\eta_F \geq \delta$, since individuals in the F class are not treated). The basic model is then given by the following system of non-linear differential equations (see Figure 1a for a flow diagram, and Table 2 for description of the variables and parameters of the model)

$$
\begin{aligned}
\frac{dS}{dt} &= \Pi - \beta\frac{(L+\theta_H H+\theta_A A+\theta_T T+\theta_F F)}{N}S - \mu S,\\
\frac{dL}{dt} &= (1-\sigma)\beta\frac{(L+\theta_H H+\theta_A A+\theta_T T+\theta_F F)}{N}S - (\mu+\alpha_L+\tau_1)L,\\
\frac{dH}{dt} &= \sigma\beta\frac{(L+\theta_H H+\theta_A A+\theta_T T+\theta_F F)}{N}S - (\mu+\alpha_H+\tau_2)H,\\
\frac{dA}{dt} &= \alpha_L L+\alpha_H H-(\mu+\tau_3+\delta)A,\\
\frac{dT}{dt} &= \tau_1 L+\tau_2 H+\tau_3 A-\mu T-\gamma T,\\
\frac{dF}{dt} &= \gamma T-\mu F-\eta_F F.
\end{aligned}
\tag{2.1}
$$

2.1. Basic Properties.

2.1.1. *Positivity and boundedness of solutions.* For the basic model (2.1) to be epidemiologically meaningful, it is important to prove that all its state variables are non-negative for all time. In other words, solutions of the model system (2.1) with positive initial data will remain positive for all time $t > 0$.

THEOREM 2.1. *Let the initial data* $S(0) > 0$, $L(0) > 0$, $H(0) > 0$, $A(0) > 0$, $T(0) > 0$, $F(0) > 0$. *Then the solutions* (S, L, H, A, T, F) *of the basic model* (2.1) *are positive for all* $t > 0$. *Furthermore,*

$$\limsup_{t\to\infty} N(t) \leq \frac{\Pi}{\mu}, \quad \text{with } N = S+L+H+A+T+F.$$

Proof. It follows from the first equation of the system (2.1) that

$$\frac{d}{dt}\left[S(t)\exp\left\{\int_0^t \lambda(u)du+\mu t\right\}\right] = \Pi\exp\left\{\int_0^t \lambda(u)du+\mu t\right\},$$

with,

$$\lambda(t) = \frac{\beta[L(t) + \theta_H H(t) + \theta_A A(t) + \theta_T T(t) + \theta_F F(t)]}{N(t)}.$$

Hence,

$$S(t_1)\exp\left\{\int_0^{t_1} \lambda(u)du + \mu t_1\right\} - S(0) = \int_0^{t_1} \Pi \exp\left\{\int_0^{x} \lambda(\nu)d\nu + \mu x\right\} dx,$$

so that,

$$\begin{aligned} S(t_1) &= S(0)\exp\left\{-\int_0^{t_1} \lambda(u)du + \mu t_1\right\} \\ &\quad + \exp\left\{-\int_0^{t_1} \lambda(u)du + \mu t_1\right\} \times \int_0^{t_1} \Pi \exp\left\{\int_0^{x} \lambda(\nu)d\nu + \mu x\right\} dx, \\ &> 0. \end{aligned}$$

Similarly, it can be shown that $L(t) > 0, H(t) > 0, A(t) > 0, T(t) > 0$ and $F(t) > 0$ for all time $t > 0$. For the second part of the proof, it should be noted that $0 < A(t) \leq N(t)$ and $0 < F(t) \leq N(t)$.

Adding all the equations in the differential equation system (2.1) gives

$$\frac{dN}{dt} = \Pi - \mu N(t) - \delta A(t) - \eta_F F(t). \tag{2.2}$$

It follows from (2.2) that,

$$\Pi - (\mu + \delta + \eta_F)N(t) \leq \frac{dN}{dt} < \Pi - \mu N(t).$$

Thus,

$$\frac{\Pi}{\mu + \delta + \eta_F} \leq \liminf_{t\to\infty} N(t) \leq \limsup_{t\to\infty} N(t) \leq \frac{\Pi}{\mu},$$

so that,

$$\limsup_{t\to\infty} N(t) \leq \frac{\Pi}{\mu},$$

as required. □

2.1.2. *Invariant regions.* Since all the parameters and state variables of the model (2.1) are non-negative for all $t \geq 0$, it follows from (2.2) that

$$\frac{dN}{dt} \leq \Pi - \mu N. \tag{2.3}$$

A standard comparison theorem [**26**] can be used to show that $N(t) \leq N(0)e^{-\mu t} + \frac{\Pi}{\mu}(1 - e^{-\mu t})$. In particular, $N(t) \leq \frac{\Pi}{\mu}$ if $N(0) \leq \frac{\Pi}{\mu}$. Consequently, the following biologically-feasible region

$$\mathcal{D}_1 = \left\{(S, L, H, A, T, F) \in \mathbb{R}^6_+ : S + L + H + A + T + F \leq \Pi/\mu\right\},$$

is positively-invariant (that is, all solutions of the model with initial conditions in $\mathcal{D}_1$ will remain in $\mathcal{D}_1$ for all $t \geq 0$). It is, therefore, sufficient to consider the solutions of the model in $\mathcal{D}_1$. In this region, the usual existence, uniqueness and continuation results hold for the system (2.1) (see also [**20**]).

3. Treatment-free Model

Before analyzing the model (2.1), the treatment-free model, obtained by setting $\tau_1 = \tau_2 = \tau_3 = \theta_T = \theta_F = T = F = 0$ in (2.1), is considered first of all. This (reduced) model is given by the following system of equations (see Figure 1b for a flow diagram)

$$
\begin{aligned}
\frac{dS}{dt} &= \Pi - \beta\frac{(L+\theta_H H+\theta_A A)}{N}S - \mu S,\\
\frac{dL}{dt} &= (1-\sigma)\beta\frac{(L+\theta_H H+\theta_A A)}{N}S - (\mu+\alpha_L)L,\\
\frac{dH}{dt} &= \sigma\beta\frac{(L+\theta_H H+\theta_A A)}{N}S - (\mu+\alpha_H)H,\\
\frac{dA}{dt} &= \alpha_L L + \alpha_H H - (\mu+\delta)A.
\end{aligned}
\tag{3.1}
$$

Using the approach in Section 2.1.2, it can be shown that the feasible region

$$\mathcal{D}_1^m = \left\{(S,L,H,A) \in \mathbb{R}_+^4 : S+L+H+A \leq \Pi/\mu\right\},$$

is positively-invariant for the treatment-free model (3.1). It is convenient to define:

$$\mathcal{D}_0^m = \{(S,L,H,A) \in \mathcal{D}_1^m : L = H = A = 0\}.$$

3.1. Local stability of disease-free equilibrium (DFE). The DFE of the treatment-free model (3.1), obtained by setting the right-hand sides of the model (3.1) to zero, is given by

$$e_0 = (S^*, L^*, H^*, A^*) = (\Pi/\mu, 0, 0, 0).$$

The linear stability of e_0 can be established using the next generation operator method in [**42**]. This entails writing the reduced model (3.1) in terms of the matrices F_1 and V_1, of new infections in each compartment and of transfer rates of individuals between compartments, respectively, given by (where $N^* = S^* + L^* + H^* + A^* = \Pi/\mu$)

$$F_1 = \begin{pmatrix} \beta(1-\sigma)\frac{S^*}{N^*} & \beta(1-\sigma)\theta_H\frac{S^*}{N^*} & \beta(1-\sigma)\theta_A\frac{S^*}{N^*} \\ \beta\sigma\frac{S^*}{N^*} & \beta\sigma\theta_H\frac{S^*}{N^*} & \beta\sigma\theta_A\frac{S^*}{N^*} \\ 0 & 0 & 0 \end{pmatrix},$$

$$V_1 = \begin{pmatrix} \mu+\alpha_L & 0 & 0 \\ 0 & \mu+\alpha_H & 0 \\ -\alpha_L & -\alpha_H & \mu+\delta \end{pmatrix}.$$

The *basic reproduction number*, denoted by $\mathcal{R}_0$, is then given by $\mathcal{R}_0 = \rho(F_1 V_1^{-1})$, where ρ denotes the spectral radius. It follows that (noting that, at the DFE, $N^* = S^*$)

$$\mathcal{R}_0 = \frac{(1-\sigma)(\mu+\delta+\theta_A\alpha_L)\beta}{(\mu+\alpha_L)(\mu+\delta)} + \frac{[(\mu+\delta)\theta_H+\theta_A\alpha_H]\beta\sigma}{(\mu+\alpha_H)(\mu+\delta)}. \tag{3.2}$$

The result below follows from Theorem 2 of [**42**].

LEMMA 3.1. *The DFE,* e_0*, of the treatment-free model* (3.1) *is locally-asymptotically stable (LAS) if* $\mathcal{R}_0 < 1$*, and unstable if* $\mathcal{R}_0 > 1$.

The threshold quantity $\mathcal{R}_0$ measures the average number of new cases generated by a single infected individual in a completely susceptible population. The epidemiological implication of Lemma 3.1 is that HIV can be eliminated from the community (when $\mathcal{R}_0 < 1$) if the initial sizes of the sub-populations of the model are in the basin of attraction of e_0. To ensure that eradication of the virus is independent of the initial size of the sub-populations, it is necessary to show that the DFE is globally-asymptotically stable (GAS). This is considered below.

3.2. Global stability of disease-free equilibrium.

THEOREM 3.2. *The DFE,* e_0*, of the treatment-free model* (3.1) *is GAS in* $\mathcal{D}_1^m$ *if* $\mathcal{R}_0 < 1$.

Proof.
The proof is based on using a comparison theorem. Notice, first of all, that the equations for the infected components of the treatment-free model (3.1) can be written in matrix-vector form as:

$$\begin{pmatrix} \frac{dL(t)}{dt} \\ \frac{dH(t)}{dt} \\ \frac{dA(t)}{dt} \end{pmatrix} = (F_1 - V_1)\begin{pmatrix} L(t) \\ H(t) \\ A(t) \end{pmatrix} - \left(1 - \frac{S}{N}\right) K \begin{pmatrix} L(t) \\ H(t) \\ A(t) \end{pmatrix}, \tag{3.3}$$

where the matrices F_1 and V_1 are as defined above, and K is a non-negative matrix given by

$$K = \begin{pmatrix} \beta(1-\sigma) & \beta(1-\sigma)\theta_H & \beta(1-\sigma)\theta_A \\ \beta\sigma & \beta\sigma\theta_H & \beta\sigma\theta_A \\ 0 & 0 & 0 \end{pmatrix}.$$

Since $S(t) \le N(t)$ (for all $t \ge 0$) in $\mathcal{D}_1^m$, it follows that

$$(3.4) \qquad \begin{pmatrix} \frac{dL(t)}{dt} \\ \frac{dH(t)}{dt} \\ \frac{dA(t)}{dt} \end{pmatrix} \le (F_1 - V_1) \begin{pmatrix} L(t) \\ H(t) \\ A(t) \end{pmatrix}.$$

Using the fact that the eigenvalues of the matrix $F_1 - V_1$ all have negative real parts (see local stability result in Section 3.1, where $\rho(F_1 V_1^{-1}) < 1$ if $\mathcal{R}_0 < 1$, which is equivalent to $F_1 - V_1$ having eigenvalues with negative real parts when $\mathcal{R}_0 < 1$.), it follows that the linearized differential inequality system (3.4) is stable whenever $\mathcal{R}_0 < 1$. It follows, by comparison theorem (see, for instance, [**26**], p. 31 and [**40**], Theorem B.1; Appendix B), that $(L(t), H(t), A(t)) \to (0, 0, 0)$ in the nonlinear system (3.1). Substituting $L = H = A = 0$ in the first equation of (3.1) gives $S(t) \to S^*$ as $t \to \infty$. Thus, $(S(t), L(t), H(t), A(t)) \to (S^*, 0, 0, 0)$ as $t \to \infty$ for $\mathcal{R}_0 < 1$, so that e_0 is GAS in $\mathcal{D}_1^m$ if $\mathcal{R}_0 < 1$.

□

Theorem 3.2 shows that HIV will be eliminated from the community if the threshold quantity, $\mathcal{R}_0$, can be brought to (and maintained at) a value less than unity.

3.3. Endemic equilibrium.

3.3.1. *Existence of endemic equilibrium.* Let $e_1 = (S^{**}, L^{**}, H^{**}, A^{**})$ denotes the endemic equilibrium of the model (3.1) (i.e., a steady-state solution with $L^{**} > 0$, $H^{**} > 0$, $A^{**} > 0$). Define

$$(3.5) \qquad G^{**} = \beta \frac{(L^{**} + \theta_H H^{**} + \theta_A A^{**})}{N^{**}}$$

as the *force of infection* at an endemic equilibrium of (3.1). Thus, at an endemic equilibrium, the equations in (3.1) can be expressed as:

(3.6)

$$S^{**} = \frac{\Pi}{\mu + G^{**}}, \quad L^{**} = \frac{(1-\sigma)G^{**}S^{**}}{\mu + \alpha_L}, \quad H^{**} = \frac{\sigma G^{**} S^{**}}{\mu + \alpha_H}, \quad A^{**} = \frac{\alpha_L L^{**} + \alpha_H H^{**}}{\mu + \delta}.$$

Using (3.6) in (3.5), and simplifying, gives the following unique non-zero solution for (3.5)

$$(3.7) \quad G^{**} = \frac{(\mu + \alpha_L)(\mu + \alpha_H)(\mu + \delta)(\mathcal{R}_0 - 1)}{(\mu + \alpha_H)\left[(1-\sigma)(\mu + \delta) + \alpha_L(1-\sigma)\right] + (\mu + \alpha_L)\left[\sigma(\mu + \delta) + \alpha_H \sigma\right]}.$$

The endemic equilibrium of (3.1) can then be obtained by substituting the expression for G^{**} from (3.7) into (3.6). It should be noted from (3.7) that $G^{**} > 0$ (so that, S^{**}, L^{**}, H^{**} and A^{**} are all positive) whenever $\mathcal{R}_0 > 1$. Thus, we have established the following result.

LEMMA 3.3. *The treatment-free model* (3.1) *has a unique positive (endemic) equilibrium if and only if* $\mathcal{R}_0 > 1$.

3.3.2. *Local stability of endemic equilibrium: special case.* The local stability of the unique endemic equilibrium of the treatment-free model (3.1) will now be considered for a special case, where the disease-induced mortality is negligible (i.e., $\delta = 0$). Setting $\delta = 0$ in the model (3.1) gives

$$\frac{dN}{dt} = \Pi - \mu N,$$

so that, $N \to \frac{\Pi}{\mu}$ as $t \to \infty$. Using $N = N^{**} = \frac{\Pi}{\mu}$ and $S = N^{**} - L - H - A$ in (3.1) gives the following system

$$\begin{aligned}
\frac{dL}{dt} &= (1-\sigma)\beta\frac{(L+\theta_H H+\theta_A A)}{N^{**}}(N^{**}-L-H-A) - k_1 L,\\
\frac{dH}{dt} &= \sigma\beta\frac{(L+\theta_H H+\theta_A A)}{N^{**}}(N^{**}-L-H-A) - k_2 H, \qquad (3.8)\\
\frac{dA}{dt} &= \alpha_L L + \alpha_H H - \mu A,
\end{aligned}$$

where, now,

$$k_1 = \mu + \alpha_L \quad \text{and} \quad k_2 = \mu + \alpha_H.$$

It is clear that the model (3.8) also has a unique endemic equilibrium, given by $e_2 = e_1|_{\delta=0}$, whenever the basic reproduction number

$$\mathcal{R}_0^m = \mathcal{R}_0|_{\delta=0} = \frac{(1-\sigma)(\mu+\theta_A\alpha_L)\beta}{(\mu+\alpha_L)\mu} + \frac{[\mu\theta_H+\theta_A\alpha_H]\beta\sigma}{(\mu+\alpha_H)\mu}$$

exceeds unity.

THEOREM 3.4. *The unique endemic equilibrium, e_2, of the model* (3.8), *is LAS whenever $\mathcal{R}_0^m > 1$.*

Proof. Consider the model (3.8) with $\mathcal{R}_0^m > 1$ (so that the endemic equilibrium e_2 exists). The method given in [**41**], which is based on using a Krasnoselskii sub-linearity trick (see also [**11, 22**]), will be used to prove Theorem 3.4. The method essentially entails proving that the linearized equation

$$\bar{Z}' = Df(e_2)\bar{Z} \qquad (3.9)$$

of the model (3.8), around the endemic equilibrium e_2, has no solutions of the form

$$\bar{Z}(t) = \bar{Z}_0 e^{\nu t} \qquad (3.10)$$

with $\bar{Z}_0 \in \mathbb{C}^3 \setminus \bar{0}$, $\nu \in \mathbb{C}$ and $\text{Re}(\nu) \geq 0$, where $\mathbb{C}$ denotes the complex numbers.

Let L^{**}, H^{**} and A^{**}, with $S^{**} = N^{**} - L^{**} - H^{**} - A^{**}$, denote the coordinates of the endemic equilibrium, e_2. Substituting a solution of the form (3.10) into the linearized system (3.9) around e_2 gives the following system of linear equations

$$\nu Z_1 = \left[\frac{(1-\sigma)\beta S^{**}}{N^{**}} - \frac{(1-\sigma)\beta(L^{**}+\theta_H H^{**}+\theta_A A^{**})}{N^{**}} - k_1\right] Z_1 + \left[\frac{(1-\sigma)\beta\theta_H S^{**}}{N^{**}} - \frac{(1-\sigma)\beta(L^{**}+\theta_H H^{**}+\theta_A A^{**})}{N^{**}}\right] Z_2 + \left[\frac{(1-\sigma)\beta\theta_A S^{**}}{N^{**}} - \frac{(1-\sigma)\beta(L^{**}+\theta_H H^{**}+\theta_A A^{**})}{N^{**}}\right] Z_3,$$

(3.11)
$$\nu Z_2 = \left[\frac{\sigma\beta S^{**}}{N^{**}} - \frac{\sigma\beta(L^{**}+\theta_H H^{**}+\theta_A A^{**})}{N^{**}}\right] Z_1 + \left[\frac{\sigma\beta\theta_H S^{**}}{N^{**}} - \frac{\sigma\beta(L^{**}+\theta_H H^{**}+\theta_A A^{**})}{N^{**}} - k_2\right] Z_2 + \left[\frac{\sigma\beta\theta_A S^{**}}{N^{**}} - \frac{\sigma\beta(L^{**}+\theta_H H^{**}+\theta_A A^{**})}{N^{**}}\right] Z_3,$$

$$\nu Z_3 = \alpha_L Z_1 + \alpha_H Z_2 - \mu Z_3.$$

Further algebraic manipulations give the following equivalent system:

$$Z_1\left\{1+\frac{1}{k_1}\left[\nu + \frac{(1-\sigma)\beta(L^{**}+\theta_H H^{**}+\theta_A A^{**})}{N^{**}}\right]\right\} = -\frac{\beta(1-\sigma)(L^{**}+\theta_H H^{**}+\theta_A A^{**})}{N^{**}k_1} Z_2 - \frac{\beta(1-\sigma)(L^{**}+\theta_H H^{**}+\theta_A A^{**})}{N^{**}k_1} Z_3 + \frac{\beta(1-\sigma)S^{**}}{N^{**}k_1} Z_1 + \frac{\beta\theta_H(1-\sigma)S^{**}}{N^{**}k_1} Z_2 + \frac{\beta\theta_A(1-\sigma)S^{**}}{N^{**}k_1} Z_3,$$

(3.12)
$$Z_2\left\{1+\frac{1}{k_2}\left[\nu + \frac{\sigma\beta(L^{**}+\theta_H H^{**}+\theta_A A^{**})}{N^{**}}\right]\right\} = -\frac{\sigma\beta(L^{**}+\theta_H H^{**}+\theta_A A^{**})}{N^{**}k_2} Z_1 - \frac{\sigma\beta(L^{**}+\theta_H H^{**}+\theta_A A^{**})}{N^{**}k_2} Z_3 + \frac{\sigma\beta S^{**}}{N^{**}k_2} Z_1 + \frac{\sigma\beta\theta_H S^{**}}{N^{**}k_2} Z_2 + \frac{\sigma\beta\theta_A S^{**}}{N^{**}k_2} Z_3,$$

$$Z_3\left(1+\frac{\nu}{\mu}\right) = \frac{\alpha_L}{\mu} Z_1 + \frac{\alpha_H}{\mu} Z_2.$$

Adding the three equations of (3.12), and then moving all the negative terms to their respective left-hand sides, gives

(3.13)
$$\sum_{i=1}^{3}[1+F_i(\nu)]Z_i = \sum_{i=1}^{3}(M\bar{Z})_i,$$

where,

$$F_1(\nu) = \frac{\nu}{k_1} + \frac{\beta(L^{**} + \theta_H H^{**} + \theta_A A^{**})}{N^{**}}\left(\frac{1-\sigma}{k_1} + \frac{\sigma}{k_2}\right),$$

$$F_2(\nu) = \frac{\nu}{k_2} + \frac{\beta(L^{**} + \theta_H H^{**} + \theta_A A^{**})}{N^{**}}\left(\frac{1-\sigma}{k_1} + \frac{\sigma}{k_2}\right), \tag{3.14}$$

$$F_3(\nu) = \frac{\nu}{\mu} + \frac{\beta(L^{**} + \theta_H H^{**} + \theta_A A^{**})}{N^{**}}\left(\frac{1-\sigma}{k_1} + \frac{\sigma}{k_2}\right),$$

with M defined by,

$$M = \begin{bmatrix} \frac{(1-\sigma)\beta S^{**}}{N^{**}k_1} & \frac{(1-\sigma)\beta\theta_H S^{**}}{N^{**}k_1} & \frac{(1-\sigma)\beta\theta_A S^{**}}{N^{**}k_1} \\ \frac{(1-\sigma)\beta S^{**}}{N^{**}k_2} & \frac{(1-\sigma)\beta\theta_H S^{**}}{N^{**}k_2} & \frac{(1-\sigma)\beta\theta_A S^{**}}{N^{**}k_2} \\ \frac{\alpha_L}{\mu} & \frac{\alpha_H}{\mu} & 0 \end{bmatrix}.$$

The notation $(M\bar{Z})_i$ (with $i = 1, 2, 3$) denotes the ith coordinate of the vector $(M\bar{Z})$. It should be noted that the matrix M has non-negative entries, and the equilibrium e_2 satisfies the relation:

$$e_2 = Me_2. \tag{3.15}$$

Since the coordinates of e_2 are positive, it follows that if $\bar{Z}$ is any solution of (3.13), then there exists a minimal positive real number s, depending on $\bar{Z}$, such that

$$|\bar{Z}| \leq se_2, \tag{3.16}$$

where $|\bar{Z}| = (|Z_1|, |Z_2|, |Z_3|)$ and $|\cdot|$ is the norm in $\mathbb{C}$.

Observe that s is also the minimal positive such that $|Z_1| + |Z_2| + |Z_3| \leq s(L^{**} + H^{**} + A^{**})$. Now, we want to show that $\mathrm{Re}(\nu) < 0$. Suppose the contrary (i.e., $\mathrm{Re}(\nu) \geq 0$). Thus, there are two cases to consider: $\nu = 0$ and $\nu \neq 0$. Suppose, first of all, that $\nu = 0$. It follows then that (3.11) is a homogenous linear system in the variables Z_i $(i = 1 \ldots 5)$. The determinant of this system corresponds to that of the Jacobian of system (3.8) evaluated at e_2, which is given by

$$\begin{aligned} \Delta &= -\frac{\beta(L^{**} + \theta_H H^{**} + \theta_A A^{**})k_1 k_2}{N^{**}} + \mu k_1 k_2 \left(\frac{\mathcal{R}_0^m S^{**}}{N^{**}} - 1\right), \\ &= -\frac{\beta(L^{**} + \theta_H H^{**} + \theta_A A^{**})k_1 k_2}{N^{**}}. \end{aligned} \tag{3.17}$$

It can be shown (from (3.17)) that $\frac{S^{**}}{N^{**}} = \frac{1}{\mathcal{R}_0^m}$. Thus, $\Delta < 0$. Consequently, the system (3.11) can only have the trivial solution $\bar{Z} = \bar{0}$ (which corresponds to the DFE, e_0). Hence, by the definition of $\bar{Z}$, this is a contradiction. Thus, $\nu \neq 0$.

For the case when $\nu \neq 0$, suppose that $\text{Re}(\nu) \geq 0$. Let $\mathcal{F}(\nu) = \min\{|1 + \mathcal{F}_i(\nu)|,\ i = 1\ldots 3\}$. It is easy to show that $|1 + \mathcal{F}_i(\nu)| > 1$, so that $\mathcal{F}(\nu) > 1$. Taking norms on both sides of the second equation of (3.13), and using the fact that the matrix M is non-negative, gives

$$\mathcal{F}(\nu)|\bar{Z}| \leq \left|\sum_{i=1}^{3}[1 + \mathcal{F}_i(\nu)]Z_i\right| = \left|\sum_{i=1}^{3}(M\bar{Z})_i\right| \leq \sum_{i=1}^{3}|(M\bar{Z})_i| = M|\bar{Z}|. \tag{3.18}$$

Using (3.16) and (3.18) gives

$$\mathcal{F}(\nu)|\bar{Z}| \leq M|\bar{Z}| \leq sMe_2 = se_2, \tag{3.19}$$

which implies that,

$$|\bar{Z}| \leq \frac{s}{\mathcal{F}(\nu)}e_2 < se_2, \tag{3.20}$$

contradicting the minimality of s. Therefore, $\text{Re}(\nu) \ngeq 0$ (so that $\text{Re}(\nu) < 0$, as required).

□

3.3.3. *Global stability of endemic equilibrium: special case.* Now we consider the special case of the reduced model (3.8) with $\sigma = 0$ (i.e., the case where all newly-infected individuals have low viral load upon primary infection). Using $\sigma = 0$ in (3.8), and setting $\beta_1 = \dfrac{\beta}{N^{**}}$, gives (it should be noted that for $\sigma = 0$, $H \to 0$ as $t \to \infty$):

$$\begin{aligned}
\frac{dS}{dt} &= \Pi - \beta_1(L + \theta_A A)S - \mu S,\\
\frac{dL}{dt} &= \beta_1(L + \theta_A A)S - k_1 L,\\
\frac{dA}{dt} &= \alpha_L L - \mu A.
\end{aligned} \tag{3.21}$$

For the model (3.21), the regions

$$\mathcal{D}_{1*}^m = \left\{(S, L, A) \in \mathbb{R}_+^3 : S + L + A \leq \Pi/\mu\right\} \text{ and } \mathcal{D}_{0*}^m = \{(S, L, A) \in \mathcal{D}_1^m : L = A = 0\},$$

are positively-invariant. Further, it is easy to see that the system (3.21) has a unique endemic equilibrium, given by $e_3 = e_2|_{\sigma=0}$, whenever the associated reproduction number

$$\mathcal{R}_1^m = \mathcal{R}_0^m|_{\sigma=0} = \frac{\beta(\mu + \theta_A\alpha_L)}{\mu(\mu + \alpha_L)},$$

exceeds unity.

THEOREM 3.5. *The unique endemic equilibrium, e_3, of the reduced treatment-free model (3.21) is GAS in $\mathcal{D}_{1*}^m \setminus \mathcal{D}_{0*}^m$, whenever $\mathcal{R}_1^m > 1$.*

Proof. Let $\mathcal{R}_1^m > 1$, so that the endemic equilibrium, e_3, of the model (3.21), exists. Consider the non-linear Lyapunov function,

$$\mathcal{F}_2 = S - S^{**} - S^{**}\ln\left(\frac{S}{S^{**}}\right) + L - L^{**} - L^{**}\ln\left(\frac{L}{L^{**}}\right) + \frac{\beta\theta_A S^{**}}{\mu}\left[A - A^{**} - A^{**}\ln\left(\frac{A}{A^{**}}\right)\right],$$

with Lyapunov derivative (where a dot represents differentiation with respect to t) given by

(3.22)
$$\dot{\mathcal{F}}_2 = \left(1 - \frac{S^{**}}{S}\right)\dot{S} + \left(1 - \frac{L^{**}}{L}\right)\dot{L} + \frac{\beta\theta_A S^{**}}{\mu}\left(1 - \frac{A^{**}}{A}\right)\dot{A},$$

$$= \left(1 - \frac{S^{**}}{S}\right)[\Pi - \beta_1(L + \theta_A A)S - \mu S] + \left(1 - \frac{L^{**}}{L}\right)[\beta_1(L + \theta_A A)S - k_1 L] + \frac{\beta\theta_A S^{**}}{\mu}\left(1 - \frac{A^{**}}{A}\right)(\alpha_L L - \mu A).$$

It is worth recalling that, at the endemic steady-state, the following equations hold:

$$\Pi = \beta_1 L^{**}S^{**} + \beta_1\theta_A A^{**}S^{**} + \mu S^{**},$$

(3.23)
$$k_1 L^{**} = \beta_1 L^{**}S^{**} + \beta_1\theta_A A^{**}S^{**}, \quad \mu A^{**} = \alpha_L L^{**}.$$

Substituting the relations in (3.23) into (3.22) gives

$$\begin{aligned}
\dot{\mathcal{F}}_2 &= \left(1 - \frac{S^{**}}{S}\right)(\beta_1 L^{**}S^{**} + \beta_1\theta_A A^{**}S^{**} + \mu S^{**} - \beta_1 LS - \beta_1\theta_A AS - \mu S) \\
&\quad + \left(1 - \frac{L^{**}}{L}\right)(\beta_1 LS + \beta_1\theta_A AS - k_1 L) + \frac{\beta\theta_A S^{**}}{\mu}\left(1 - \frac{A^{**}}{A}\right)(\alpha_L L - \mu A), \\
&= \beta_1 L^{**}S^{**} + \beta_1\theta_A A^{**}S^{**} + \mu S^{**} - \beta_1 LS - \beta_1\theta_A AS - \mu S \\
&\quad - \frac{S^{**}}{S}(\beta_1 L^{**}S^{**} + \beta_1\theta_A A^{**}S^{**} + \mu S^{**} - \beta_1 LS - \beta_1\theta_A AS - \mu S) \\
&\quad + \beta_1 LS + \beta_1\theta_A AS - k_1 L - \frac{L^{**}}{L}(\beta_1 LS + \beta_1\theta_A AS - k_1 L) \\
&\quad + \frac{\beta\theta_A S^{**}}{\mu}(\alpha_L L - \mu A) - \frac{\beta\theta_A S^{**}A^{**}}{\mu A}(\alpha_L L - \mu A),
\end{aligned}$$

$$
\begin{aligned}
&= \beta_1 L^{**}S^{**} + \beta_1\theta_A A^{**}S^{**} + \mu S^{**} - \beta_1 LS - \beta_1\theta_A AS - \mu S \\
&\quad -\frac{\beta_1 L^{**}S^{**2}}{S} - \frac{\beta_1\theta_A A^{**}S^{**2}}{S} - \frac{\mu S^{**2}}{S} + \beta_1 LS^{**} + \beta_1\theta_A AS^{**} + \mu S^{**} \\
&\quad +\beta_1 LS + \beta_1\theta_A AS - \beta_1 S^{**}L - \frac{\beta_1\theta_A A^{**}S^{**}L}{L^{**}} - \beta_1 SL^{**} - \frac{\beta_1\theta_A ASL^{**}}{L} + k_1 L^{**} \\
&\quad +\frac{\beta\theta_A S^{**}\alpha_L L}{\mu} - \beta\theta_A S^{**}A - \frac{\beta\theta_A S^{**}A^{**}\alpha_L L}{\mu A} + \beta\theta_A S^{**}A^{**}, \\
&= 2\mu S^{**} - \mu S - \frac{\mu S^{**2}}{S} + 2\beta_1 L^{**}S^{**} - \beta_1 SL^{**} - \frac{\beta_1 L^{**}S^{**2}}{S} \\
&\quad +3\beta_1\theta_A A^{**}S^{**} - \frac{\beta_1\theta_A A^{**}S^{**2}}{S} - \frac{\beta_1\theta_A S^{**}A^{**2}L}{AL^{**}} - \frac{\beta_1\theta_A ASL^{**}}{L}, \\
&= \mu S^{**}\left(2 - \frac{S}{S^{**}} - \frac{S^{**}}{S}\right) + \beta_1 L^{**}S^{**}\left(2 - \frac{S}{S^{**}} - \frac{S^{**}}{S}\right) \\
&\quad +\beta_1\theta_A A^{**}S^{**}\left(3 - \frac{S^{**}}{S} - \frac{A^{**}L}{AL^{**}} - \frac{ASL^{**}}{A^{**}S^{**}L}\right).
\end{aligned}
$$

Since the arithmetic mean exceeds the geometric mean, the following inequalities hold.

$$2 - \frac{S}{S^{**}} - \frac{S^{**}}{S} \leq 0 \text{ and } 3 - \frac{S^{**}}{S} - \frac{A^{**}L}{AL^{**}} - \frac{ASL^{**}}{A^{**}S^{**}L} \leq 0.$$

Thus, $\dot{\mathcal{F}}_2 \leq 0$ for $\mathcal{R}_1^m > 1$. Hence, $\mathcal{F}_2$ is a Lyapunov function of the system (3.21) on $\mathcal{D}_{1*}^m$. It follows, by LaSalle's Invariance Principle [**18**], that every solution to the equations of the model (3.21), and initial conditions in $\mathcal{D}_{1*}^m \setminus \mathcal{D}_{0*}^m$, approaches the associated unique endemic equilibrium, e_3, of the model (3.21), as $t \to \infty$ for $\mathcal{R}_1^m > 1$.

□

In summary, the treatment-free model (3.1) has:

i: a GAS DFE whenever $\mathcal{R}_0 < 1$ (Theorem 3.2);

ii: a unique EEP whenever $\mathcal{R}_0 > 1$ (Lemma 3.3);

iii: a GAS EEP whenever $\delta = \sigma = 0$ and $\mathcal{R}_0^m > 1$ (Theorem 3.5).

It is instructive, therefore, to determine whether the basic treatment model (2.1) has similar qualitative dynamics. This is explained in Section 4.

4. Analysis of Treatment Model

In this section, the basic treatment model, given by (2.1), will be analysed.

4.1. Local stability of the DFE. This model has a DFE given by

$$e_0^T = (S^*, L^*, H^*, A^*, T^*, F^*) = (\Pi/\mu, 0, 0, 0, 0, 0)\,.$$

Here, the associated next generation matrices F_2 and V_2 are, respectively, given by

$$F_2 = \begin{pmatrix} (1-\sigma)\beta & (1-\sigma)\beta\theta_H & (1-\sigma)\beta\theta_A & (1-\sigma)\beta\theta_T & (1-\sigma)\beta\theta_F \\ \sigma\beta & \sigma\beta\theta_H & \sigma\beta\theta_A & \sigma\beta\theta_T & \sigma\beta\theta_F \\ 0 & 0 & 0 & 0 & 0 \\ 0 & 0 & 0 & 0 & 0 \\ 0 & 0 & 0 & 0 & 0 \end{pmatrix},$$

and,

$$V_2 = \begin{pmatrix} P_1 & 0 & 0 & 0 & 0 \\ 0 & P_2 & 0 & 0 & 0 \\ -\alpha_L & -\alpha_H & P_3 & 0 & 0 \\ -\tau_1 & -\tau_2 & -\tau_3 & P_4 & 0 \\ 0 & 0 & 0 & -\gamma & P_5 \end{pmatrix},$$

where,

$$P_1 = \mu + \alpha_L + \tau_1, \; P_2 = \mu + \alpha_H + \tau_2, \; P_3 = \mu + \tau_3 + \delta, \; P_4 = \mu + \gamma, \; P_5 = \mu + \eta_F,$$

so that the associated *treatment reproduction number* is given by

$$\mathcal{R}_T = \rho(F_2 V_2^{-1}) = \frac{\beta\sigma A_1}{P_1P_2P_3P_4P_5} + \frac{\beta(1-\sigma)A_2}{P_1P_2P_3P_4P_5}, \tag{4.1}$$

with,

$$A_1 = P_1P_4P_5(\theta_H P_3 + \theta_A\alpha_H) + P_1(\theta_T P_5 + \theta_F\gamma)(P_3\tau_2 + \alpha_H\tau_3),$$

$$A_2 = P_2P_4P_5(P_3 + \theta_A\alpha_L) + P_2(\theta_T P_5 + \theta_F\gamma)(P_3\tau_1 + \alpha_L\tau_3).$$

The local asymptotic stability result of the DFE, e_0^T, follows from Theorem 2 of [**42**] (and is summarized below).

LEMMA 4.1. *The disease-free equilibrium, e_0^T, of the treatment model* (2.1), *is LAS if $\mathcal{R}_T < 1$, and unstable if $\mathcal{R}_T > 1$.*

4.2. Global stability of DFE.

THEOREM 4.2. *The disease-free equilibrium, e_0^T, of the treatment model* (2.1), *is GAS in $\mathcal{D}_1$ if $\mathcal{R}_T \leq 1$.*

Proof. Consider the Lyapunov function,

$$\mathcal{F} = f_1 L + f_2 H + f_3 A + f_4 T + f_5 F,$$

where,

$$\begin{aligned} f_1 &= P_2[P_4P_5(P_3 + \theta_A\alpha_L) + (\theta_T P_5 + \theta_F\gamma)(P_3\tau_1 + \alpha_L\tau_3)], \\ f_2 &= P_1[P_4P_5(\theta_H P_3 + \theta_A\alpha_H) + (\theta_T P_5 + \theta_F\gamma)(P_3\tau_2 + \alpha_H\tau_3)], \\ f_3 &= P_1P_2(\theta_A P_4P_5 + \theta_T\tau_3P_5 + \theta_F\gamma\tau_3), \\ f_4 &= P_1P_2P_3(\theta_T P_5 + \theta_F\gamma), \;\; f_5 = P_1P_2P_3P_4\theta_F. \end{aligned}$$

Let $G_T = \beta\dfrac{(L+\theta_H H+\theta_A A+\theta_T T+\theta_F Q)}{N}$. It follows that the Lyapunov derivative is given by

$$\begin{aligned}
\dot{\mathcal{F}} &= f_1\dot{L}+f_2\dot{H}+f_3\dot{A}+f_4\dot{T}+f_5\dot{F}\\
&= f_1[(1-\sigma)G_T S-P_1L]+f_2(\sigma G_T S-P_2H)+f_3(\alpha_L L+\alpha_H H-P_3A)\\
&\quad +f_4(\tau_1L+\tau_2H+\tau_3A-P_4T)+f_5(\gamma T-P_5F)\\
&= G_T(A_1+A_2)S-P_1P_2P_3P_4P_5(L+\theta_H H+\theta_A A+\theta_T T+\theta_F Q)\\
&= G_T(A_1+A_2)S-P_1P_2P_3P_4P_5\frac{G_T N}{\beta}\\
&= P_1P_2P_3P_4P_5\frac{G_T N}{\beta}\left[\frac{\beta(A_1+A_2)S}{P_1P_2P_3P_4P_5N}-1\right]\\
&\le P_1P_2P_3P_4P_5\frac{G_T N}{\beta}\left[\frac{\beta(A_1+A_2)}{P_1P_2P_3P_4P_5}-1\right] \qquad \text{since } S\le N \text{ in } \mathcal{D}_1\\
&= P_1P_2P_3P_4P_5(L+\theta_H H+\theta_A A+\theta_T T+\theta_F Q)(\mathcal{R}_T-1)\le 0 \quad \text{for } \mathcal{R}_T\le 1.
\end{aligned}$$

The proof is completed using similar argument as in the proof of Theorem 3.5. □

The epidemiological implication of Theorem 4.2 is that HIV will be eliminated from the community if the treatment program implemented can reduce (and maintain) the reproduction threshold, $\mathcal{R}_T$, to a value less than unity.

4.3. Existence of endemic equilibrium. As in the case of the treatment-free model (3.1), let

$$G^{**} = \beta\frac{(L^{**}+\theta_H H^{**}+\theta_A A^{**}+\theta_T T^{**}+\theta_F Q^{**})}{N^{**}}, \tag{4.2}$$

be the *force of infection* at an arbitrary endemic equilibrium of the treatment model (2.1), denoted by $e_1^T=(S^{**},L^{**},H^{**},A^{**},T^{**},F^{**})$. Thus, the equations in (2.1) can be expressed as:

$$\begin{aligned}
S^{**} &= \frac{\Pi}{\mu+G^{**}},\quad L^{**}=\frac{(1-\sigma)G^{**}S^{**}}{P_1},\quad H^{**}=\frac{\sigma G^{**}S^{**}}{P_2},\\
A^{**} &= \frac{\alpha_L L^{**}+\alpha_H H^{**}}{P_3},\quad T^{**}=\frac{\tau_1L^{**}+\tau_2H^{**}+\tau_3A^{**}}{P_4},\quad F^{**}=\frac{\gamma T^{**}}{P_5}.
\end{aligned}\tag{4.3}$$

Using (4.3) in (4.2), and simplifying, gives $G^{**}=0$ (corresponding to the DFE e_0^T; hence, not considered) and

$$G^{**} = \frac{P_1P_2P_3P_4P_5(\mathcal{R}_T-1)}{Z_1+Z_2}, \tag{4.4}$$

with,

$$Z_1 = [P_2P_5(P_3+\alpha_L)(P_4+\tau_T)+\gamma\tau_T P_2(P_3+\alpha_L)](1-\sigma),$$

$$Z_2 = [\gamma\tau_T P_1(P_3+\alpha_H)+P_1P_5(P_3+\alpha_H)(P_4+\tau_T)]\sigma.$$

Substituting the expression for G^{**} above into (4.3) gives the unique endemic equilibrium for the treatment model (2.1). It should be noted that, like in the treatment-free model, all components of the unique endemic equilibrium are positive whenever $\mathcal{R}_T > 1$. Thus, the following result has been established.

LEMMA 4.3. *The model* (2.1) *has a unique (positive) endemic equilibrium, given by* e_1^T, *whenever* $\mathcal{R}_T > 1$.

The approach in Section 3.3.2 can be used to show that the endemic equilibrium e_0^T is LAS whenever $\mathcal{R}_T|_{\delta=\eta_F=0} > 1$.

Overall, the differential infectivity treatment model (2.1) has similar qualitative dynamics as the treatment-free model (3.1), where, in each case, the associated disease-free equilibrium is globally-asymptotically stable when a certain threshold quantity reproduction number) is less than unity, and a unique endemic equilibrium exists when the threshold exceeds unity. It is worth noting that, unlike in HIV models that incorporate vaccination (see, for example, [**10**]), the treatment model does not undergo the phenomenon of backward bifurcation (where the disease-free equilibrium co-exists with a stable endemic equilibrium when the reproduction threshold is less than unity). This is because the DFE, e_0^T, is GAS in $\mathcal{D}_1$ whenever the reproduction threshold is less than unity.

5. Differential Infectivity Treatment Model With Staged Progression

One key biological feature of HIV disease is the fact that infected individuals display variations in infectiousness over time. In other word, infected individuals pass through various infection stages, where they are highly infectious during the pre-antibody phase, maintaining low infectivity during the asymptomatic phase, and becoming highly infectious as they progress toward clinical AIDS [**21, 23, 30, 33**]. The treatment model (2.1) is now extended to incorporate this property. For simplicity, three progression stages are assumed: L_1 and L_2 for two low viral load classes; and H_1 and H_2 for two high viral load classes. The AIDS class (A) is the last infection stage for both low and high viral load individuals.

Individuals in the L_1 stage progress to stage-2 (L_2) at a rate α_1; and those in L_2 progress to the AIDS stage at a rate α_2. Here, too, no transition from L_2 to H is allowed to enable us keep track of the two infection streams. It is assumed that individuals in low viral load classes (L_1, L_2) transmit infection at the same rate. Infected people in H_1 and H_2 classes are assumed to have (high) viral loads greater than a certain threshold but do not display clinical symptoms of AIDS yet. Individuals with low viral load are treated at a rate τ_1 whilst those with high viral load are treated at a rate τ_2.

Similarly, individuals in stage-1 of high viral load class (H_1) move to stage-2 (H_2) at an increased rate $\eta_1\alpha_1$, where $\eta_1 > 1$. Individuals in H_2 class progress to AIDS at a faster rate $\eta_2\alpha_2$ (with $\eta_2 > 1$) in comparison to those in the L_2 class. Treated individuals develop AIDS at a rate $\alpha_3 < \alpha_2$. Here, too, treated individuals fail treatment at a rate γ and suffer disease induced death, at a rate η_F. People in the AIDS stage are treated at a rate τ_3, and suffer a disease-induced death at a rate δ.

Putting all these together, the differential infectivity and staged-progression HIV treatment model (DISPT model) is given by (see Figure 1c for a flow diagram, and Table 3 for the description of the variables and parameters of the DISPT model)

$$
\begin{aligned}
\frac{dS}{dt} &= \Pi - \lambda S - \mu S,\\
\frac{dL_1}{dt} &= (1-\sigma)\lambda S - (\mu + \alpha_1 + \tau_1)L_1,\\
\frac{dL_2}{dt} &= \alpha_1 L_1 - (\mu + \alpha_2 + \tau_1)L_2,\\
\frac{dH_1}{dt} &= \sigma\lambda S - (\mu + \eta_1\alpha_1 + \tau_2)H_1,\\
\frac{dH_2}{dt} &= \eta_1\alpha_1 H_1 - (\mu + \eta_2\alpha_2 + \tau_2)H_2,\\
\frac{dA}{dt} &= \alpha_2 L_2 + \eta_2\alpha_2 H_2 - (\mu + \delta + \tau_3)A,\\
\frac{dT}{dt} &= \tau_1(L_1 + L_2) + \tau_2(H_1 + H_2) + \tau_3 A - (\mu + \gamma)T,\\
\frac{dF}{dt} &= \gamma T - (\mu + \eta_F)F,
\end{aligned}
\tag{5.1}
$$

where,

$$\lambda = \frac{\beta(L_1 + L_2 + \theta_1 H_1 + \theta_2 H_2 + \theta_3 A + \theta_4 T + \theta_5 F)}{N}.$$

For the DISPT model (5.1), the following biologically-feasible region is positively-invariant

$$\mathcal{D}_2 = \left\{(S, L_1, L_2, H_1, H_2, A, T, F) \in \mathbb{R}^8_+ : S + L_1 + L_2 + H_1 + H_2 + A + T + F \le \Pi/\mu\right\}.$$

5.1. Local stability of DFE. The DISPT model (5.1) has a DFE given by

$$\mathcal{E}_0 = (S^*, L_1^*, L_2^*, H_1^*, H_2^*, A^*, T^*, F^*) = (\Pi/\mu, 0, 0, 0, 0, 0, 0, 0).$$

Using the associated next generation matrices

$$F_3 = \begin{pmatrix} (1-\sigma)\beta & (1-\sigma)\beta & (1-\sigma)\beta\theta_1 & (1-\sigma)\beta\theta_2 & (1-\sigma)\beta\theta_3 & (1-\sigma)\beta\theta_4 & (1-\sigma)\beta\theta_5 \\ 0 & 0 & 0 & 0 & 0 & 0 & 0 \\ \sigma\beta & \sigma\beta & \sigma\beta\theta_1 & \sigma\beta\theta_2 & \sigma\beta\theta_3 & \sigma\beta\theta_4 & \sigma\beta\theta_5 \\ 0 & 0 & 0 & 0 & 0 & 0 & 0 \\ 0 & 0 & 0 & 0 & 0 & 0 & 0 \\ 0 & 0 & 0 & 0 & 0 & 0 & 0 \\ 0 & 0 & 0 & 0 & 0 & 0 & 0 \end{pmatrix},$$

and,

$$V_3 = \begin{pmatrix} B_1 & 0 & 0 & 0 & 0 & 0 & 0 \\ -\alpha_1 & B_2 & 0 & 0 & 0 & 0 & 0 \\ 0 & 0 & B_3 & 0 & 0 & 0 & 0 \\ 0 & 0 & -\eta_1\alpha_1 & B_4 & 0 & 0 & 0 \\ 0 & -\alpha_2 & 0 & -\eta_2\alpha_2 & B_5 & 0 & 0 \\ -\tau_1 & -\tau_1 & -\tau_2 & -\tau_2 & -\tau_3 & B_6 & 0 \\ 0 & 0 & 0 & 0 & 0 & -\gamma & B_7 \end{pmatrix},$$

with,

$$B_1 = \mu + \alpha_1 + \tau_1,\ B_2 = \mu + \alpha_2 + \tau_1,\ B_3 = \mu + \eta_1\alpha_1 + \tau_2,$$

$$B_4 = \mu + \eta_2\alpha_2 + \tau_2,\ B_5 = \mu + \delta + \tau_3,\ B_6 = \mu + \gamma,\ B_7 = \mu + \eta_F,$$

it follows that the associated *treatment reproduction number* is given by:

$$\mathcal{R}_{TS} = \rho(F_3V_3^{-1}) = \frac{\beta(1-\sigma)A_{11}}{B_1B_2B_5B_6B_7} + \frac{\beta\sigma A_{12}}{B_3B_4B_5B_6B_7},$$

where,

$$A_{11} = B_5(B_6B_7 + \theta_4B_7\tau_1 + \theta_5\gamma\tau_1)(B_2 + \alpha_1) + \alpha_2\alpha_1(\theta_3B_6B_7 + \theta_4B_7\tau_3 + \theta_5\gamma\tau_3),$$

$$A_{12} = B_6B_7[\theta_1B_4B_5 + \eta_1\alpha_1(\theta_2B_5 + \theta_3\eta_2\alpha_2)] + (\theta_4B_7 + \theta_5\gamma)[\tau_3\eta_2\alpha_2\eta_1\alpha_1 + \tau_2B_5(B_4 + \eta_1\alpha_1)].$$

Similarly, the following result is established

LEMMA 5.1. *The DFE, $\mathcal{E}_0$, of the DISPT model* (5.1), *is LAS if $\mathcal{R}_{TS} < 1$, and unstable if $\mathcal{R}_{TS} > 1$.*

5.2. Global stability of DFE.

THEOREM 5.2. *The DFE of the DISPT model* (5.1) *is GAS in $\mathcal{D}_2$ if $\mathcal{R}_{TS} \leq 1$.*

Proof. Consider the Lyapunov function given by,

$$\mathcal{F} = p_1L_1 + p_2L_2 + p_3H_1 + p_4H_2 + p_5A + p_6T + p_7F,$$

where,

$$
\begin{aligned}
p_1 &= B_3B_4\{B_5[B_6B_7 + \tau_1(\theta_4B_7 + \theta_5\gamma)](B_2 + \alpha_1) + \alpha_2\alpha_1[\theta_3B_6B_7 + \tau_3(\theta_4B_7 + \theta_5\gamma)]\},\\
p_2 &= B_1B_3B_4[B_6B_7(B_5 + \theta_3\alpha_2) + (\tau_1B_5 + \tau_3\alpha_2)(\theta_5\gamma + \theta_4B_7)],\\
p_3 &= B_1B_2\{B_6B_7[\theta_1B_4B_5 + \eta_1\alpha_1(\theta_2B_5 + \theta_3\eta_2\alpha_2)]\\
&\quad + (\theta_4B_7 + \theta_5\gamma)[\tau_3\eta_2\alpha_2\eta_1\alpha_1 + \tau_2B_5(B_4 + \eta_1\alpha_1)]\},\\
p_4 &= B_1B_2B_3[B_6B_7(\theta_2B_5 + \theta_3\eta_2\alpha_2) + (\theta_4B_7 + \theta_5\gamma)(\tau_2B_5 + \tau_3\eta_2\alpha_2)],\\
p_5 &= B_1B_2B_3B_4(\theta_3B_6B_7 + \theta_4\tau_3B_7 + \theta_5\gamma\tau_3),\\
p_6 &= B_1B_2B_3B_4B_5(\theta_4B_7 + \theta_5\gamma), \quad p_7 = \theta_5B_1B_2B_3B_4B_5B_6,
\end{aligned}
$$

with Lyapunov derivative given by,

$$
\begin{aligned}
\dot{\mathcal{F}} &= p_1\dot{L}_1 + p_2\dot{L}_2 + p_3\dot{H}_1 + p_4\dot{H}_2 + p_5\dot{A} + p_6\dot{T} + p_7\dot{F},\\
&= p_1((1-\sigma)\lambda S - B_1L_1) + p_2(\alpha_1L_1 - B_2L_2) + p_3(\sigma\lambda S - B_3H_1)\\
&\quad + p_4(\eta_1\alpha_1H_1 - B_4H_2) + p_5(\alpha_2L_2 + \eta_2\alpha_2H_2 - B_5A)\\
&\quad + p_6(\tau_1(L_1 + L_2) + \tau_2(H_1 + H_2) + \tau_3A - B_6T) + p_7(\gamma T - B_7F),\\
&= \lambda[B_3B_4(1-\sigma)A_{11} + B_1B_2\sigma A_{21}]S - B_1B_2B_3B_4B_5B_6B_7\frac{\lambda N}{\beta},\\
&= B_1B_2B_3B_4B_5B_6B_7\frac{\lambda N}{\beta}\left\{\frac{\beta[B_3B_4(1-\sigma)A_{11} + B_1B_2\sigma A_{21}]S}{B_1B_2B_3B_4B_5B_6B_7N} - 1\right\},\\
&\le B_1B_2B_3B_4B_5B_6B_7\frac{\lambda N}{\beta}\left\{\frac{\beta[B_3B_4(1-\sigma)A_{11} + B_1B_2\sigma A_{21}]}{B_1B_2B_3B_4B_5B_6B_7} - 1\right\},\\
&\quad \text{since } S \le N \text{ in } \mathcal{D}_2,\\
&= B_1B_2B_3B_4B_5B_6B_7\frac{\lambda N}{\beta}\left[\frac{\beta(1-\sigma)A_{11}}{B_1B_2B_5B_6B_7} + \frac{\beta\sigma A_{12}}{B_3B_4B_5B_6B_7} - 1\right],\\
&= B_1B_2B_3B_4B_5B_6B_7(L_1 + L_2 + \theta_1H_1 + \theta_2H_2 + \theta_3A + \theta_4T + \theta_5F)(\mathcal{R}_{TS} - 1)\\
&\le 0 \;\text{ for } \mathcal{R}_{TS} \le 1.
\end{aligned}
$$

The proof is completed using similar argument as in the proof of Theorem 3.5. □

5.3. Existence of Endemic Equilibrium. As in Section 4.3, let

$$
G^{**} = \beta\frac{(L_1^{**} + L_2^{**} + \theta_1H_1^{**} + \theta_2H_2^{**} + \theta_3A^{**} + \theta_4T^{**} + \theta_5F^{**})}{N^{**}}, \tag{5.2}
$$

be the force of infection at an endemic equilibrium of the DISPT model (5.1), denoted by

$$
\mathcal{E}_1 = (S^{**}, L_1^{**}, L_2^{**}, H_1^{**}, H_2^{**}, A^{**}, T^{**}, F^{**}).
$$

Thus, at $\mathcal{E}_1$, the equations in the DISPT model can be expressed as:

$$
\begin{aligned}
S^{**} &= \frac{\Pi}{\mu + G^{**}}, \quad L_1^{**} = \frac{(1-\sigma)G^{**}S^{**}}{B_1}, \quad L_2^{**} = \frac{\alpha_1L_1^{**}}{B_2},\\
H_1^{**} &= \frac{\sigma G^{**}S^{**}}{B_3}, \quad H_2^{**} = \frac{\eta_1\alpha_1H_1^{**}}{B_4}, \quad F^{**} = \frac{\gamma T^{**}}{B_7},\\
A^{**} &= \frac{\alpha_2L_2^{**} + \alpha_2\eta_2H_2^{**}}{B_5}, \quad T^{**} = \frac{\tau_1(L_1^{**} + L_2^{**}) + \tau_2(H_1^{**} + H_2^{**}) + \tau_3A^{**}}{B_6}.
\end{aligned}
\tag{5.3}
$$

Using (5.3) in (5.2), and simplifying, gives the following unique non-zero solution for (5.2)

$$G^{**} = \frac{B_1B_2B_3B_4B_5B_6B_7(\mathcal{R}_{TS}-1)}{B_8}, \tag{5.4}$$

where,

$$\begin{aligned} B_8 = {} & B_3B_4(1-\sigma) \\ & \cdot\{[\tau_3\alpha_2\alpha_1 + \tau_1B_5(\alpha_1+B_2)](B_7+\gamma) + B_6B_7[\alpha_2\alpha_1 + B_5(B_2+\alpha_1)]\} \\ & + \sigma B_1B_2\{B_5[B_6B_7 + \tau_2(B_7+\gamma)](B_4+\eta_1\alpha_1) + \alpha_2\alpha_1\eta_2\eta_1[B_6B_7 + \tau_3(B_7+\gamma)]\}. \end{aligned}$$

The positive endemic equilibrium of the DISPT model can then be obtained by substituting (5.4) into (5.3). It should be noted that $G^{**} > 0$ whenever $\mathcal{R}_{TS} > 1$. Thus, the following result is established.

LEMMA 5.3. *The DISPT model, given by* (5.1), *has a unique endemic equilibrium whenever* $\mathcal{R}_{TS} > 1$.

The approach in Section 3.3.2 can be used to establish the local stability of the unique endemic equilibrium of (5.1) (this is not reported here because of space limitation).

In summary, it can also be concluded that adding staged-progression to the differential infectivity treatment model (3.1) does not change its qualitative (equilibrium) dynamics (since, in each case, the associated DFE is GAS if the corresponding treatment reproduction number is less than unity; and a unique endemic equilibrium exists when this threshold exceeds unity). Overall, all three models considered in this study ((2.1), (3.1) and (5.1)) exhibit similar qualitative (equilibrium) dynamics.

6. Numerical Simulations

6.1. Assessment of Treatment Strategies. In this section, the DISPT model (5.1) will be used to assess the population-level impact of various treatment strategies. The following strategies are considered:

- **I:** Low viral load strategy ($\tau_1 \neq 0, \tau_2 = \tau_3 = 0$), where only individuals with low viral load are treated (i.e., those in L_1 and L_2 classes only);
- **II:** High viral load strategy ($\tau_1 = 0, \tau_2 \neq 0, \tau_3 \neq 0$), where only individuals with high viral load and clinical symptoms of AIDS are treated (i.e., those in H_1, H_2 and A classes only);
- **III:** AIDS-only strategy ($\tau_1 = \tau_2 = 0, \tau_3 \neq 0$), where only individuals with clinical symptoms of AIDS are treated (i.e., those in A class only);
- **IV:** Universal strategy ($\tau_1 \neq 0, \tau_2 \neq 0, \tau_3 \neq 0$), where all known infected individuals are treated (i.e., those in L_1, L_2, H_1, H_2 and A classes).

6.2. Discussions. Since the basic model (2.1) and the treatment model (3.1) are special cases of the DISPT model (5.1), numerical simulations will be carried out on the latter model using the parameters in Table 4 (unless otherwise stated). The model is now simulated to assess the impact of the various treatment strategies. Simulations are carried out at pre-treatment endemic equilibrium. Using the nominal values in Table 4, the values of the associated reproduction numbers are $\mathcal{R}_{TS} = 1.39$ and $\mathcal{R}_0 = 4.25$.

Using a relatively low treatment rate of $\tau_i = 0.5$ ($i = 1, 2, 3$) and various values of σ (the fraction of infected individuals with the high viral load upon infection), it is shown that the worst-case scenario, where no infected individual is treated ($\tau_1 = \tau_2 = \tau_3 = 0$), accounts for the highest number of cases, whereas the universal strategy ($\tau_1 = \tau_2 = \tau_3 = 0.5$) always gives the least number of cases (Figures 2A-E). As expected, the low viral load strategy is competitive when most of the new infections are in the low viral load category ($\sigma < 0.5$), and *vice versa* for the high viral load strategy ($\sigma \geq 0.5$). Nonetheless, it should be emphasized that, for this value of τ, the universal strategy is always the best strategy. Low treatment rate can be thought of as the case for which the supply of ARVs is limited; whereas high viral load models the case where ARVs are in abundant (or at least are in adequate) supply.

The impact of the various treatment strategies on mortality using different values of σ and low treatment rate ($\tau_i = 0.5$) is depicted in Figure 3. Here, the worst case scenario records the most number of fatalities, followed by the low viral load-only strategy. Although the high viral load and the AIDS-only strategies give reduced mortality, the universal strategy always records the least number of AIDS-related deaths. However, when the treatment rate is increased by 10-fold (from $\tau_i = 0.5$ to $\tau_i = 5$; $i = 1, 2, 3$), the AIDS-only strategy accounts for the least mortality (Figure 4). It is worth noting that for $\sigma = 0$ (i.e., all newly-infected individuals have low viral load), the AIDS-only strategy and the high viral load strategy coincide (Figure 4). This is because $H_1 \to 0$ and $H_2 \to 0$ as $t \to \infty$. Similarly, when $\sigma = 1$ (i.e., all newly-infected individuals are in the high viral load class, H_1), the low viral load strategy coincides with the worst case scenario of not treating anyone at all, whereas the high viral load strategy coincides with the universal strategy. Unlike in the simulations for the number of cases (Figure 2), there is no instance where the low viral load-only strategy is better than the high viral load-only or AIDS-only strategy in terms of deaths averted.

Figure 5 depicts the number of new cases averted using the various treatment strategies for $\tau_i = 0.5$ ($i = 1, 2, 3$). It is evident from this figure that the universal strategy prevents more cumulative new cases than any of the other strategies. Further, this figure shows the impact of σ on the cumulative number of new cases averted. For low values of σ (i.e., $\sigma \leq 0.5$), the low viral load-only strategy is more effective than the high viral load-only and AIDS-only strategies (Figures 5A-C). Similarly, if $\sigma \geq 0.5$, the high viral load-only strategy is more effective than the low viral load-only and AIDS-only strategies (Figures 5A-C). It is also evident that the AIDS-only strategy averts fewer number of new cases compared to the other strategies for various values of σ (Figure 5C). The corresponding plots for the case when the treatment rate is increased by 10-fold are depicted in Figure 6. It is clear that these plots are qualitatively-consistent with those in Figure 5 (so that the same conclusions hold).

In conclusion, these simulations show that the universal strategy is the best in terms of preventing new cases and mortality, regardless of which of the two treatment rates are used ($\tau_i = 0.5$ or $\tau_i = 5$; $i = 1, 2, 3$). In the case when there is limited supply of resources, the choice of an optimal treatment strategy depends on the value of σ.

7. Conclusions

A basic HIV transmission model, which stratifies the infected population in terms of their viral load, is designed and rigorously analysed to gain insights into its dynamical features. The model was shown to have a globally-asymptotically stable DFE whenever the associated reproduction threshold is less than unity and a unique endemic equilibrium when the threshold exceeds unity. In the absence of treatment, the basic model is shown to have a globally-asymptotically stable endemic equilibrium for a special case.

The differential infectivity treatment model is then extended to incorporate the staged-progression property of HIV disease. Here, too, the extended model is shown to have a globally-asymptotically stable DFE when its associated reproduction threshold is less than unity, and a unique endemic equilibrium when the threshold is greater than unity. The extended model is then used to evaluate various treatment strategies, namely

- **a:** treating individuals with low viral load only;
- **b:** treating individuals with high viral load and symptoms of AIDS;
- **c:** treating those with clinical symptoms of AIDS only;
- **d:** universal treatment (of all infected people).

Using a set of parameter values (some taken from the literature) and pre-treatment endemic initial data, the model gives the following results (for two sets of treatment rates):

- **i:** The universal strategy gives the highest reduction in the cumulative number of new cases, while the AIDS-only strategy gives the lowest reduction of cumulative number of new cases;
- **ii:** For low treatment rates (e.g., $\tau_i = 0.5$), the universal strategy averts more AIDS-related mortality than any of the remaining strategies;
- **iii:** For high treatment rates (e.g., $\tau_i = 5$), the AID-only strategy averts more AIDS-related mortality than any of the remaining strategies;
- **iv:** For low values of σ (i.e., $\sigma < 0.5$), the low viral load-only strategy is more effective in reducing new cases than the high viral load-only and AIDS-only strategies;
- **v:** For high values of σ (i.e., $\sigma \geq 0.5$), the high viral load-only strategy is more effective than the low viral load-only and AIDS-only strategies;
- **vi:** The AIDS-only strategy averts fewer cumulative new cases compared to the other strategies for various values of σ;
- **vii:** In terms of reduction of new cases, the strategies are listed in descending order of significance as follows:
  - **a:** for $\sigma < 0.5$, the order of significance is: universal, low viral load-only, high viral load-only and then AIDS-only strategy.
  - **b:** for $\sigma \geq 0.5$, the order of significance is: universal, high viral load-only, AIDS-only and then low viral load-only strategy.

Overall, this study shows that optimum reductions in new cases of HIV can be achieved using the universal strategy rather than any of the other targeted strategies. Further, the universal strategy accounts for the largest reductions in AIDS-related mortality if the treatment rate is low. For high treatment rates, the AIDS-only strategy averts more deaths. Since a universal strategy is probably not always feasible (for economic reasons) or preferred (for biological reasons), this study shows that, for a modest value of σ ($\sigma \geq 0.5$), a targeted high viral load strategy can be quite competitive in reducing HIV burden.

Although these results suggest promising prospects of using affordable ARV strategies to combat the spread of HIV in various settings (including resource-poor nations), it should be emphasized that the numerical simulation results obtained are dependent on the choice of parameter values used. In other words, the effect of possible uncertainties in the values of the associated parameters should be taken into account when interpreting the simulation results. This study would be extended to address the aforementioned uncertainties (as more data becomes available) and the effect of the emergence and transmission of ARV-resistant mutants.

Table 1: Glossary

Abbreviation	Meaning
LAS	Locally-asymptotically stable
GAS	Globally-asymptotically stable
DFE	Disease-free equilibrium
EEP	Endemic equilibrium point
AIDS	Acquired immune deficiency syndrome
HIV	Human immuno-deficiency virus
ARVs	Anti-retroviral drugs
HAART	Highly-active anti-retroviral therapy
SP	Staged-progression
DI	Differential infectivity
DISPT	Differential infectivity and staged-progression with treatment

Table 2: Description of variables and parameters for the basic model (2.1) *and the treatment-free model* (3.1)

Variable Parameter	**Description**
$S(t)$	susceptible individuals
$L(t)$	infected individuals with low viral load
$H(t)$	infected individuals with high viral load
$A(t)$	infected individuals showing clinical symptoms of AIDS
$T(t)$	treated infected individuals
$F(t)$	individuals in whom treatment fails
Π	recruitment rate into the sexually-active population
β	effective contact rate
μ	natural death rate
δ	disease-induced mortality rate for individuals in the AIDS stage
η_F	disease-induced mortality rate for individuals who failed treatment
θ_H	relative risk of infectiousness of high viral load individuals
θ_A	relative risk of infectiousness of AIDS individuals
θ_T	relative risk of infectiousness of treated individuals
θ_F	relative risk of infectiousness of individuals who failed treatment
τ_1, τ_2, τ_3	treatment rates for individuals in L, H and A classes, respectively
α_L	progression rate to AIDS of individuals with low viral load
α_H	progression rate to AIDS of individuals with high viral load
γ	rate at which treated individuals fail treatment
σ	fraction of newly-infected individuals with high viral load

Table 3: Description of variables and parameters for the DISPT model (5.1)

Variable Parameter	**Description**
$S(t)$	susceptible individuals
$L_1(t)$	infected individuals with low viral load stage 1
$L_2(t)$	infected individuals with low viral load stage 2
$H_1(t)$	infected individuals with high viral load stage 1
$H_2(t)$	infected individuals with high viral load stage 2
$A(t)$	infected individuals showing clinical symptoms of AIDS
$T(t)$	treated infected individuals
$F(t)$	individuals in whom treatment fails
Π	recruitment rate into the sexually-active population
β	effective contact rate
μ	natural death rate
δ	disease-induced mortality rate for individuals in the AIDS stage
η_F	disease-induced mortality rate for individuals who failed treatment
θ_1, θ_2	relative risk of infectiousness of high viral load individuals (H_1 and H_2)
θ_3	relative risk of infectiousness of AIDS individuals
θ_4	relative risk of infectiousness of treated individuals
θ_5	relative risk of infectiousness of individuals in whom treatment fails
α_1	progression rate from L_1 to L_2 class
α_2	progression rate to AIDS of individuals from L_2 class
γ	rate at which treated individuals fail treatment
η_1, η_2	modification parameters
σ	fraction of newly-infected individuals with high viral load
τ_1, τ_2, τ_3	treatment rates for individuals in L_1, L_2, H_1, H_2 and A classes, respectively

Table 4: Parameter Values

Parameter	**Nominal Value**	**References**
Π	1000 year^{-1}	assumed
β	0.4 year^{-1}	[**10**]
$\frac{1}{\mu}$	30 years	[**13**]
δ	0.2 year^{-1}	[**13**]
η_F	1.2δ year^{-1}	assumed
θ_1	1.5	assumed
θ_2	1.5	assumed
θ_3	1.5	assumed
θ_4	0.15	assumed
θ_5	1.5	assumed
α_1	1/15 year^{-1}	[**13, 23**]
α_2	1/10 year^{-1}	[**13, 23**]
τ_1	$[0.5, 5]$ year^{-1}	assumed
τ_2	$[0.5, 5]$ year^{-1}	assumed
τ_3	$[0.5, 5]$ year^{-1}	assumed
γ	0.01	assumed
η_1	1.1	assumed
η_2	1.2	assumed
σ	$[0, 1]$	assumed

References

[1] Baggaley, R.F., N.M. Ferguson and G.P. Garnett (2005). The epidemiological impact of antiretroviral use predicted by mathematical models: a review. *Emerging Themes in Epidemiology.* **2**:9 (doi:10.1186/1742-7622-2-9).

[2] Blower, S.M., Gershengorn, H.B. and R.M. Grant (2000). A tale of two futures: HIV and antiretroviral therapy in san Francisco. *Science.* **287**: 650-654.

[3] Blower, S.M., Aschenbach, A.N., Gershengorn, H.B and J.O. Kahin (2001). Predicting the unpredictable: transmission of drug resistant HIV. *Nature Medicine.* **7**(9): 1016-1020.

[4] Blower, S.M. and P. Volberding (2002). What can modeling tell us about the threat of antiviral drug resistance? *Current Options in Infectious Diseases.* **15**: 609-614.

[5] Cameron, D.W., Heath-Chiozzi, M., Danner, S., Cohen, C., Kravcik, S., Maurath, C., Sun, E., Henry, D., Rode, R., Potthoff, A. and Leonard, J. (1998). Randomised placebo-controlled trial of ritonavir in advanced HIV-1 disease. The Advanced HIV Disease Ritonavir Study Group. *Lancet.* **351**(9102): 536-537.

[6] Carr, J. (1981). Applications Centre Manifold Theory, Springer-Verlag, New York.

[7] Castillo-Chavez, C. and B. Song (2004). Dynamical models of tuberculosis and their applications. *Mathematical Biosci. and Engrg.* **1**(2): 361-404.

[8] Castillo-Chavez, C., Feng, Z. and Huang Wenzhang (2002). On the computation of $\mathcal{R}_0$ and its role on global stability. Mathematical Approaches for Emerging and Reemerging Infectious Diseases: An Introduction. The IMA Volumes in Mathematics and its Applications. Volume 125, pp. 229-250, Springer, New York. Castillo-Chavez, C. with S. Blower, P. van den Driessche, D. Kirschner and A.-A. Yakubu (Eds.)

[9] Department of Health and Human Services (DHHS) and National Guidelines Clearing house (2006). Guidelines for the use of antiretroviral agents in HIV-1-infected adults and adolescents. `http://www.guideline.gov/summary/summary.aspx?ss=15&doc_id=12195&nbr=6292`. Accessed November 6, 2008.

[10] Elbasha, E.H. and A. B. Gumel (2006). Theoretical Assessment of Public Health Impact of Imperfect Prophylactic HIV−1 Vaccines with Therapeutic Benefits. *Bull.Math. Biol.* **68**: 577-614.

[11] Esteva, L and C. Vargas (2000). Influence of vertical and mechanical transmission on the dynamics of dengue disease. *Math. Biosci.* 167: 51-64.

[12] Fauci, A.S., Pantaleo, G., Stanley, S. and D. Weissman. (1996). Immunopathogenic mechanisms of HIV infection. *Ann. Intern. Med.* **124**: 654-663.

[13] Gumel, A.B., Connell C. McCluskey and P. van den Driessche (2006). Mathematical analysis of a staged-progression HIV model with imperfect vaccine. *Bull. Math. Biol.* **68**(8): 2105-2128.

[14] Garcia, F., de Lazzari, E., Plana, M., Castrom P., Mestre, G., Nomdedeu, M., Fumero, E., Martinez, E., Mallolas, J., Blanco, J.L., Miro, J.M., Pumarola, T., Gallart, T. and Gatell, J.M. (2004). Long-term CD4+ T-cell response to highly active antiretroviral therapy according to baseline CD4+ T-cell count. *J Acquir Immune Defic Syndr.* **36**(2):702-713.

[15] Group of the Office of AIDS Research Advisory Council (2006). Guidelines for the Use of Antiretroviral Agents in HIV-1 Infected Adults and Adolescents.

[16] Gulick, R.M., Mellors, J.W., Havlir, D., Eron, J.J., Gonzalez, C., McMahon, D, Richman, D.D., Valentine, F.T., Jonas, L., Meibohm, A., Emini, E.A. and Chodakewitz, J.A. (1997). Treatment with indinavir, zidovudine, and lamivudine in adults with human immunodeficiency virus infection and prior antiretroviral therapy. *N Engl J Med.* **337**(11): 779-781.

[17] Gray, R.H., Li, X., Wawer, M.J., Gange, S.J., Serwadda, D. Sewankambo, N.K., Moore, R., Wabwire-Mangen, F., Lutalo, T. and T.C. Quinn (2003). Stochastic simulation of the impact of antiretroviral therapy and HIV vaccines on HIV trasmission; Rakai, Uganda. *AIDS.* **17**(13): 1941-1951.

[18] Hale, J.K. (1969). Ordinary differential equations. John Wiley and Sons, New York.

[19] Hammer, S.M., Squires, K.E., Hughes, M.D., Grimes, J.M., Demeter, L.M., Currier, J.S., Eron, J.J. Jr., Feinberg, J.E., Balfour, H.H. Jr., Deyton, L.R., Chodakewitz, J.A. and Fischl, M.A. (1997). A controlled trial of two nucleoside analogues plus indinavir in persons with human immunodeficiency virus infection and CD4 cell counts of 200 per cubic millimeter or less. AIDS Clinical Trials Group 320 Study Team. *N. Engl. J. Med.* **337**(11): 725-733.

[20] Hethcote, H. W (2000). The Mathematics of infectious diseases. *SIAM Review.* **42**(4): 599-653.

[21] Hethcote, H. W. and J. Van Ark (1992). Modeling HIV transmission and AIDS in the United States. Lecture Notes in Biomathematics **95**. New York: Springer-Verlag.

[22] Hethcote, H.W and H.R. Thieme (1985). Stability of the endemic equilibrium in epidemic models with subpopulations. *Math. Biosci.* **75**: 205-227.

[23] Hyman, J. M., J. Li and E.A. Stanley (1999). The differential infectivity and staged progression models for the transmission of HIV. *Math. Biosci.* **208**: 227−249.

[24] Jones, L.E. and A.S. Perelson (2005). Opportunistic infection as a cause of transient viremia in chronically infected HIV patients under treatment with HAART. *Bulletin of Maths. Bio.* **67**: 1227-1251.

[25] Kgosimore, M and E.M. Lungu (2004). The effects of vaccination and treatment on the spread of HIV/AIDS. *Journal of Biological Systems.* **12**(4): 399-417

[26] Lakshmikantham, V., S. Leela and A.A. Martynyuk (1989). Stability Analysis of Nonlinear Systems. Marcel Dekker, Inc., New York and Basel.

[27] Law, M.G., Prestage, G., Grulich, A., Van de Ven P and S. Kippax (2001). Modelling the effect of combination antiretroviral treatments on HIV incidence. *AIDS.* **15**(10): 1287-1294.

[28] Lee, D. et al. (2004). Breakthrough infections during phase 1 and 2 prime-boost HIV-1 vaccine trials with canarypox vectors (ALVAC) and booster dose of recombinant gp120 or gp160. *J. Infect. Dis.*. **190:** 903-907.

[29] Lopez, L.F., Coutinho, F.A.B., Burattini, M.N. and E. Massad. (2006). A schematic age-structured compartment model of the impact of antiretroviral therapy on HIV incidence and prevalence. *Mathematics and Computers in Simulation.* **71**: 131-148.

[30] Longini, I., W. Clark and R. Byers (1989). Statistical analysis of the stages of HIV infections using a Markov model. *Stat. Med.* **8**: 831−843.

[31] Martin, A.N. and R.M. May (2000). Virus dynamics: Mathematical principles of immunology and virology. Oxford University Press.

[32] MASA - The national antiretroviral Therapy programme of Botswana. Ministry of Health, Republic of Botswana.

[33] McCluskey, C. (2003). A model of HIV/AIDS with staged progression and amelioration. *Math. Biosci.* **181**: 1−16.

[34] Mellors, J., A. Munoz , J. Giorgi, J. Margolick, C. Tassoni, *et al.* (1997). Plasma viral load and CD4+ lymphocytes as prognostic markers of HIV-1 infection. *Ann. Intern. Med.* **126**: 946−954.

[35] Nicolosi, A., M. Musicco, A. Saracco and A. Lazzarin (1994). Risk factors for woman-to-man sexual transmission of the human immunodeficieny virus. *J. Acquir. Immune. Defic. Syndr.* **7**: 296-300.

[36] O'Brien, T., M. Busch, E. Donegan, J. Ward, L. Wong, et al. (1994). Heterosexual transmission of human immunodeficieny virus type 1 from transfusion recipents to their sex partners. *J. Acquir. Immune. Defic. Syndr.* **7**: 704-710.

[37] Palella, F.J. (Jr), Delaney, K.M., Moorman, A.C., Loveless, N.O., Fuher, J., Saten, G.A., Achman, D.J. and S.D. Homberg (1998). Declining morbidity and mortality among patients with advanced human immunodeficiency virus infection. HIV outpatients study investigators. *N.Engl.J.Med.* **338**(13): 853-860.

[38] Perelson, A.S and P.W. Nelson (1999). Mathematical Analysis of HIV-1 Dynamics in *vivo.* *SIAM Review.* **41**(1): 3-44.

[39] Perelson, A.S., Essunger, P., Cao, Y., Vesanej, M,, Hurley, A., Saksela, K., Markowitz, M. and D.D. Ho. (1997). Decay characteristics of HIV-1-infected compartments during combination therapy, *Nature.* **387**: 188-191.

[40] Smith, H.L. and P. Waltman (1995). The Theory of the Chemostat. Cambridge University Press.

[41] Thieme, H.R. (1985). in: Capasso, V., Grosso, E. and S.L. Paveri-Fontana (Eds.), Local Stability in Epidemic Models for Heterogenous Populations, in: Lecture Notes in Biomathematics, Springer. **57**: 185-189.

[42] van den Driessche, P. and Watmough, J. (2002). Reproduction numbers and sub-threshold endemic equilibria for compartmental models of disease transmission. *Mathematical Biosciences.* **180**: 29–48.

[43] Velasco-Hernandez, J.X., Gershengorn, H.B. and S.M. Blower. (2002). Could widespread use of combination antiretroviral therapy eradicate HIV epidemics? *Lancet Infect Dis.* **2**: 487-493.

[44] World Health Organization (2003). Scaling up antiretroviral therapy in resource-limited settings: treatment guidelines for a public health approach. `http://www.who.int/entity/hiv/pub/prev_care/en/arvrevision2003en.pdf` Accessed November 6, 2008.

[45] Xiridou, M., Geskus, R., De Wit, J., and M. Kretzschmar (2004). Primary HIV infection as a source of HIV transmission within steady and casual partnerships among homosexual men. *AIDS.* **18**: 1311-1320.

Department of Mathematics, University of Manitoba, Winnipeg, Manitoba, R3T 2N2, Canada.
E-mail address: umsharom@cc.umanitoba.ca

Department of Mathematics, University of Manitoba, Winnipeg, Manitoba, R3T 2N2, Canada.
E-mail address: gumelab@cc.umanitoba.ca

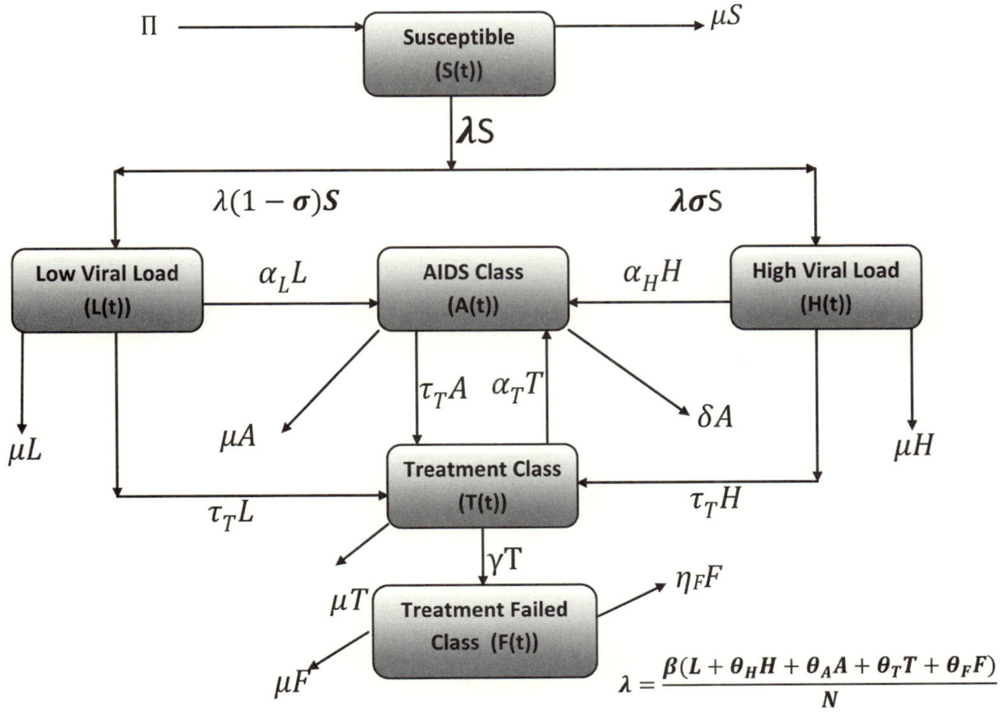

FIGURE 1A. Flow diagram for the basic treatment model (2.1)

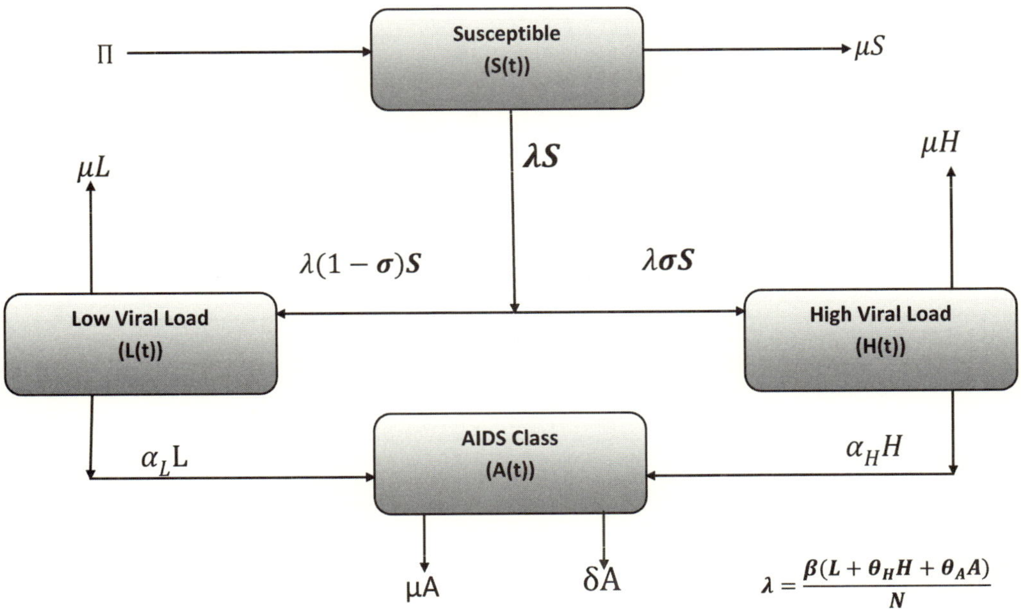

FIGURE 1B. Flow diagram for the treatment-free model (3.1)

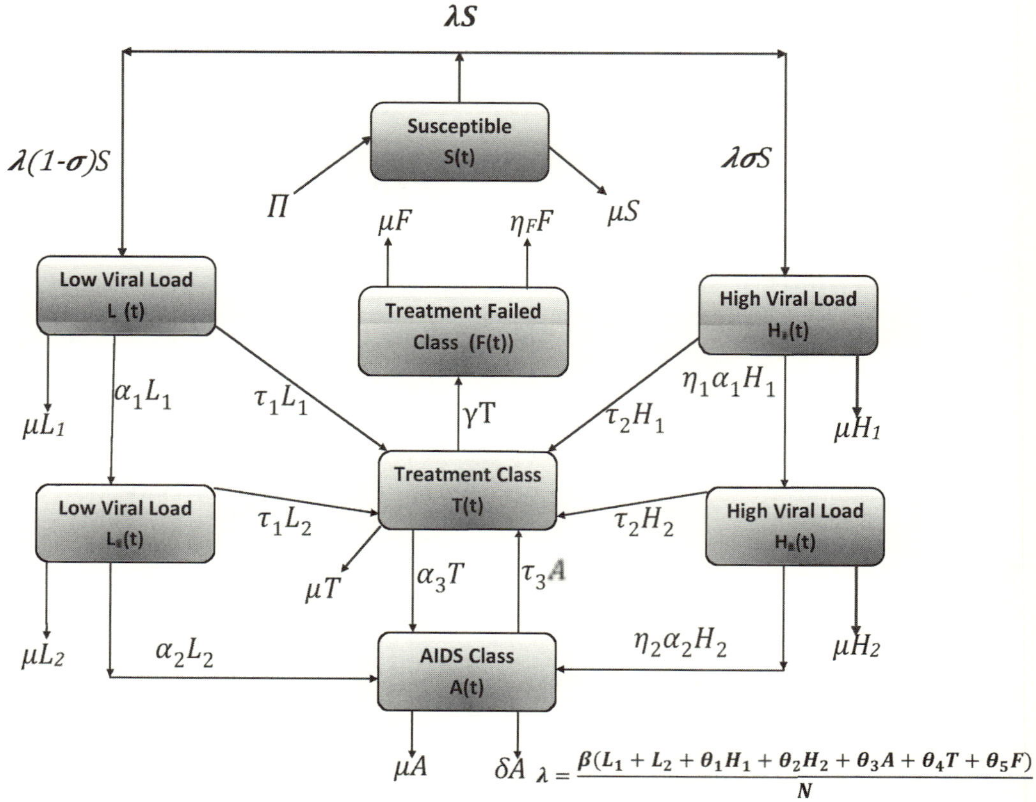

FIGURE 1C. Flow diagram for the DISPT model (5.1)

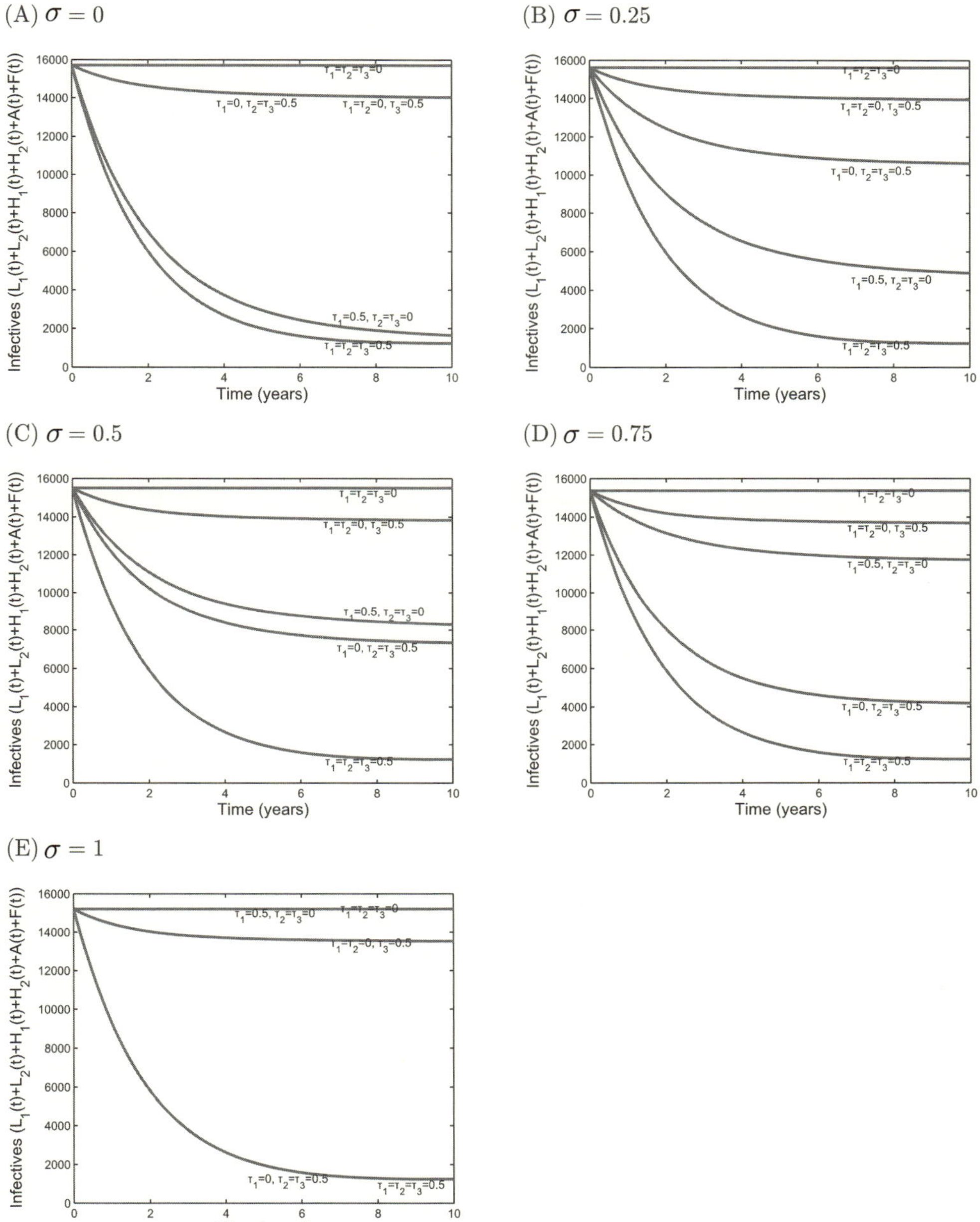

FIGURE 2. Plots of total number of cases as a function of time using various values of σ and low treatment rate. All other parameters as in Table 4.

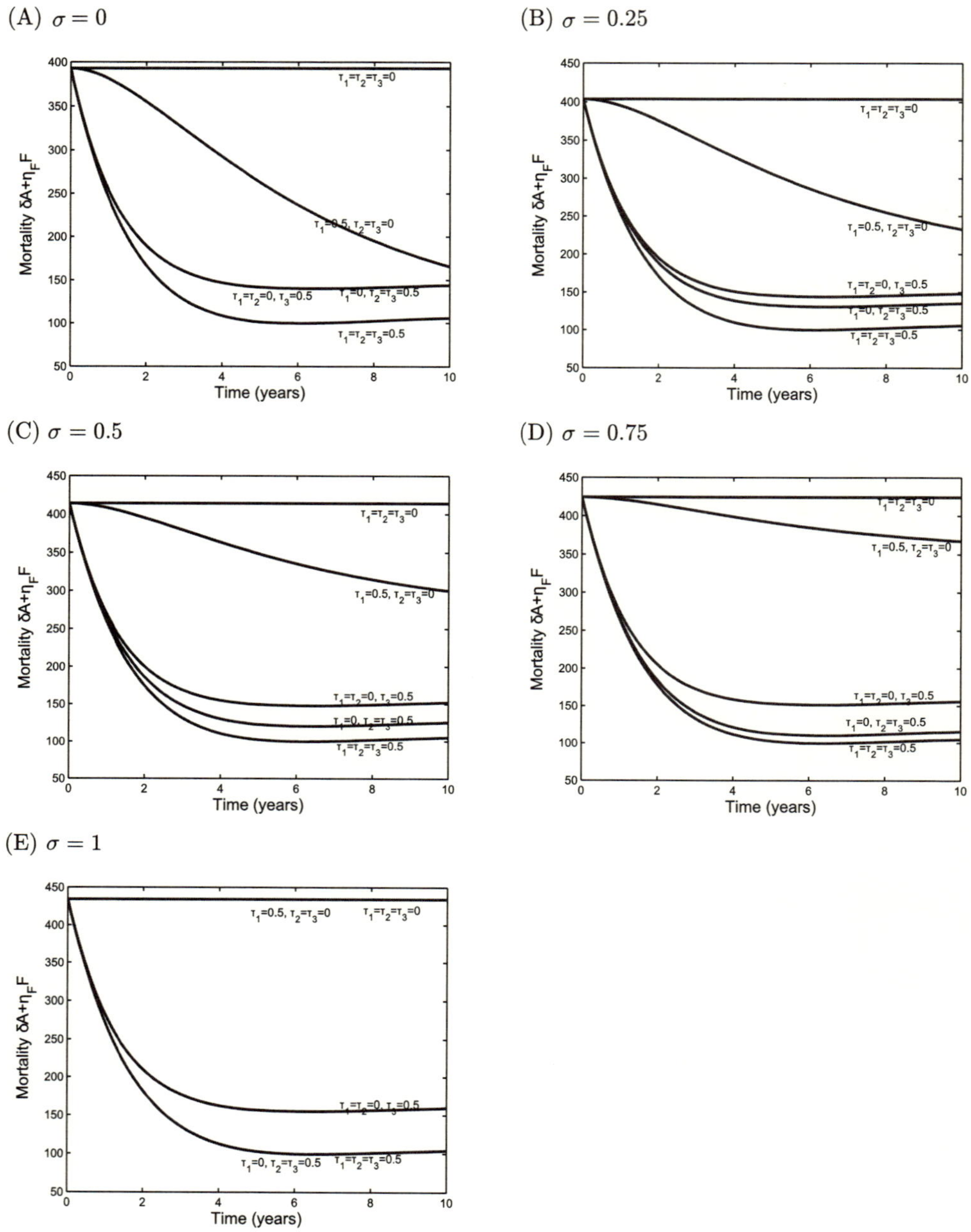

FIGURE 3. Plots of total mortality as a function of time for various values of σ and low treatment rate. All other parameters as in Table 4.

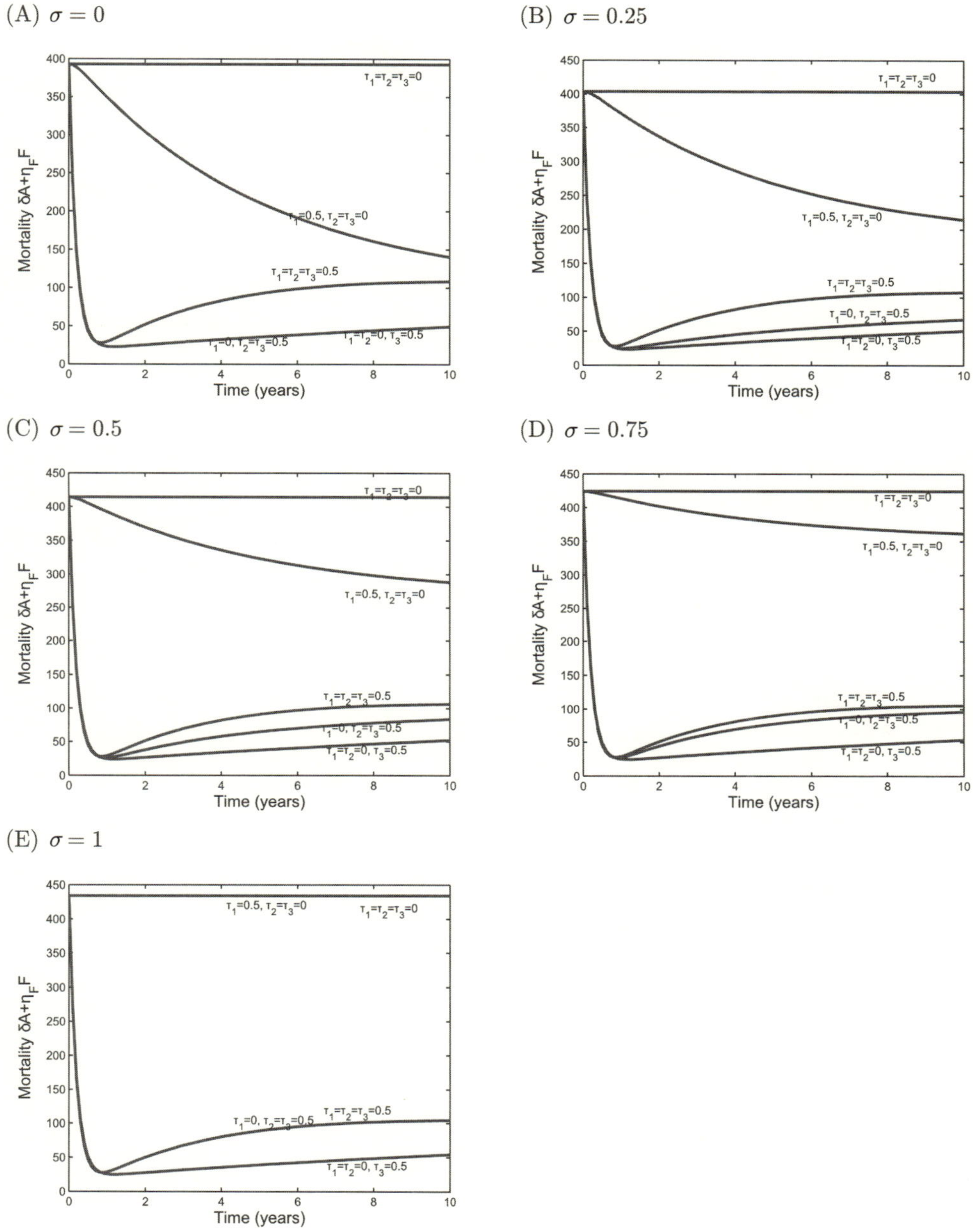

FIGURE 4. Plots of total mortality as a function of time for various values of σ and high treatment rate. All other parameters as in Table 4.

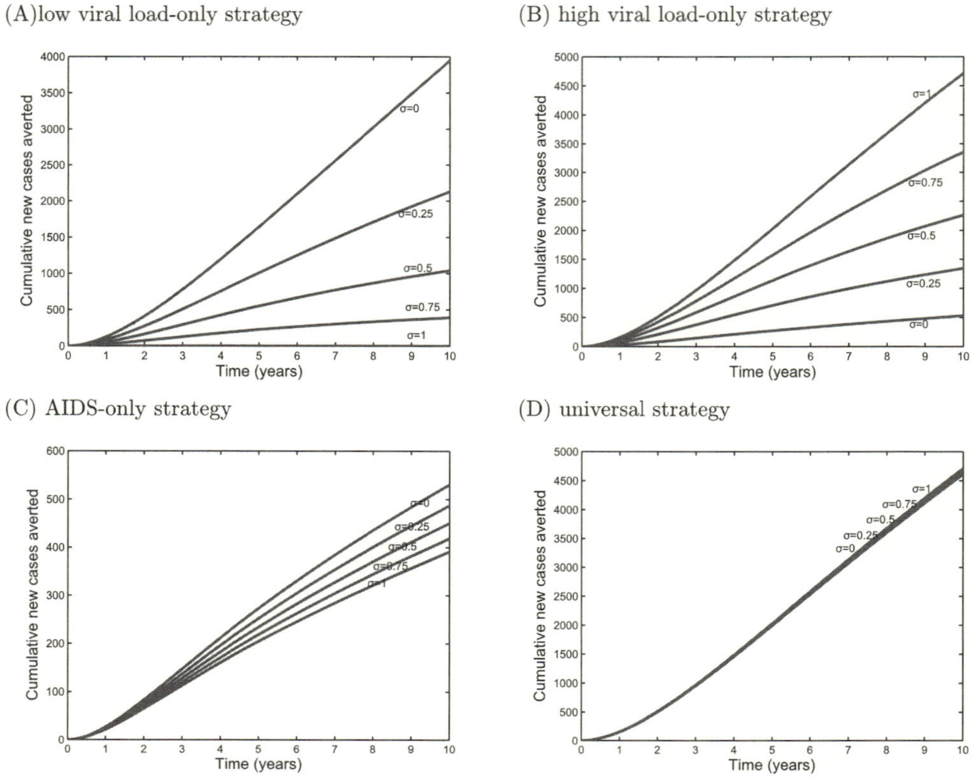

FIGURE 5. Cumulative new cases averted using various strategies and low treatment rate. (A) $\tau_1 = 0.5, \tau_2 = \tau_3 = 0$, (B) $\tau_1 = 0, \tau_2 = \tau_3 = 0.5$, (C) $\tau_1 = \tau_2 = 0, \tau_3 = 0.5$, (D) $\tau_1 = \tau_2 = \tau_3 = 0.5$. All other parameters as in Table 4.

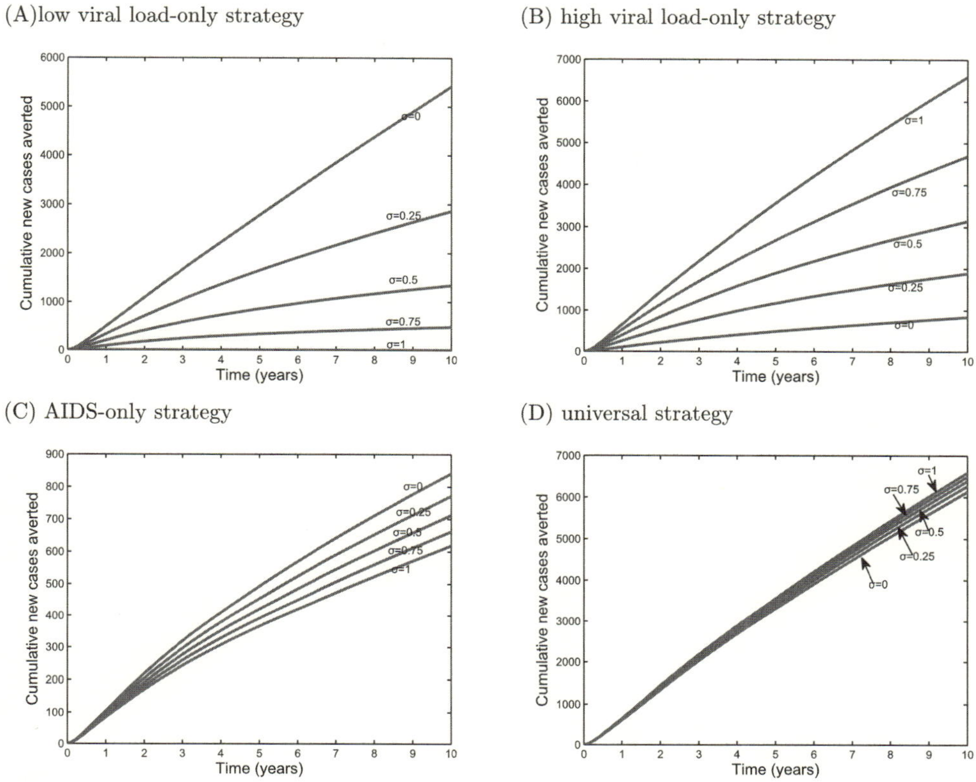

FIGURE 6. Cumulative new cases averted using various strategies and high treatment rate. (A) $\tau_1 = 5, \tau_2 = \tau_3 = 0$, (B) $\tau_1 = 0, \tau_2 = \tau_3 = 5$, (C) $\tau_1 = \tau_2 = 0, \tau_3 = 5$, (D) $\tau_1 = \tau_2 = \tau_3 = 5$. All other parameters as in Table 4.

DIMACS Series in Discrete Mathematics
and Theoretical Computer Science
Volume **75**, 2010

Greedy Algorithms in Economic Epidemiology

Fred S. Roberts

ABSTRACT. Economic issues are central to the control of disease because of the limited funds available for public health everywhere in the world, even in the wealthiest nations. These economic issues are closely related to issues of individual human behavior, as well as to fundamental disease processes and their relation to the environment. While mathematical formulation of epidemiological processes is an old discipline, combining such formulations with economic, behavioral, and environmental formalisms is relatively new, and has come to define the field of "Economic Epidemiology." Many problems in Economic Epidemiology can be formulated as optimization problems. The simplest approach to solving such a problem is often a greedy algorithm, one that always chooses the best available (cheapest, highest rated, ...) alternative at each step. We review some classical operations research problems arising in Economic Epidemiology for which the greedy algorithm in fact gives an optimal solution, and others for which it can be guaranteed to be reasonably close. We then present two examples from our own work. Examples will be chosen from: assigning workers to health care tasks; choosing medical supplies to maximize value and minimize cost; locating a health care facility so as to minimize the travel times of users; and reopening flooded roads to allow the passage of emergency vehicles. Other examples will include optimal strategies for vaccination given a limited supply; and optimal strategies for sequencing medical tests or public health interventions in order to minimize costs and maximize success.

1. Introduction

Economic issues are central to the control of disease because of the limited funds available for public health everywhere in the world, even in the wealthiest nations. These economic issues are closely related to issues of individual human behavior, as well as to fundamental disease processes and their relation to the environment. While mathematical formulation of epidemiological processes is an old

---

2010 *Mathematics Subject Classification.* Primary: 92C60 Medical epidemiology, 05C90 Graph theory applications, 05C05 Trees, 90B80 Discrete location and assignment, 91B99 Economics .

The author gratefully acknowledges the support of the National Science Foundation under grant numbers INT-0629714, INT-0629720, EIA-0205116, and DMS-0829652 to Rutgers University.

discipline, combining such formulations with economic, behavioral, and environmental formalisms is relatively new, and has come to define the field of "Economic Epidemiology."

Economic Epidemiology deals with the interplay among economics, individual and group human behavior, and disease ecology, and depends heavily on mathematical formulations of this interplay.[1] Among other things the field seeks optimal strategies and policy to improve our understanding of the spread of infectious agents and of ways to control that spread [**5, 6, 7, 61**]. In recent years, many mathematical models have been developed to compare alternative public health intervention strategies. However, these models commonly disregard varying individual responses to disease outbreaks and the economic contexts in which public health policies and individual responses to them must be evaluated. To evaluate health interventions and potential public policies, models of disease spread must incorporate behaviors of individuals and groups and economic scenarios, and we must develop methods that individuals and public institutions can utilize in response to or preparation for disease events. Some recent surveys of economic epidemiology are [**43, 76**]. Some workshops on Economic Epidemiology contain useful introductions to the field. See [**25, 26**]).

Many problems in Economic Epidemiology can be formulated as optimization problems:

- Find a solution that maximizes or minimizes some value such as lives saved.
- Find the optimal location for a clinic or hospital.
- Find the optimal assignment of health care workers to jobs.
- Optimize investment in health care supplies.
- Minimize the total cost of a series of interventions or medical tests.
- Control an outbreak with as small an investment in vaccines as possible.

Such optimization problems naturally invite inclusion of economic variables. They are also readily modified to include ways of measuring behavioral variables, for example through inclusion of individual or societal utility functions and measures of risk averseness. The challenge here is how to measure utility, risk, and more subtle factors such as peer pressure, motivation, etc. For a discussion of measurement of relevant epidemiological and behavioral variables, see [**66, 67, 68, 69**]. Some ideas of how to measure behavioral variables that can be brought into optimization models are discussed in [**55**], which summarizes a DIMACS workshop aimed at modeling social responses to bioterrorism involving infectious agents.

Often, the simplest approach to an optimization problem is a ***greedy algorithm***: Choose the best (cheapest, highest-rated, ...) available alternative at each step. In general, greedy algorithms will find locally optimal solutions, but not globally optimal ones. We give examples from Economic Epidemiology, some where a greedy solution achieves a global optimum and others where it doesn't, but where we can either make modifications or get a bound on how far from optimal we are. We quickly review some classical operations research problems arising in Economic Epidemiology for which the greedy algorithm in fact gives an optimal solution and others for which it can be guaranteed to be reasonably close. We then present two longer examples from our own work. Examples will be chosen from: assigning

[1]Thanks to Abba Gumel and Ramanan Laxminararayan for introducing me to the topic of Economic Epidemiology and for the ideas in this paragraph.

TABLE 1. Workers and Jobs they Are Qualified For

Worker W_i	W_1	W_2	W_3	W_4	W_5	W_6
Jobs Qualified For	J_2, J_3, J_5,	J_2, J_3	J_2, J_3	J_2, J_3	J_1, J_5	J_3
Cost of Using W_i	90	50	80	60	60	100

workers to health care tasks; choosing medical supplies to maximize value and minimize cost; locating a health care facility so as to minimize the travel times of users; and reopening flooded roads to allow the passage of emergency vehicles. The more detailed examples concern optimal strategies for vaccination given a limited supply; and optimal strategies for sequencing medical tests or public health interventions in order to minimize costs and maximize success.

2. Assigning Health Care Workers to Jobs

Suppose we have n health care workers $W_1, W_2, \ldots, W_n$ and m health care jobs $J_1, J_2, \ldots, J_m$ to be filled. We know which workers are qualified to do which jobs and the cost of using each worker. Our goal is to assign workers to jobs they are qualified for, each to at most one job, filling as many jobs as possible, and among all ways of filling as many jobs as possible, find the way to do it with minimum total cost. This is known in Operations Research as the ***Minimum Cost Assignment Problem***. (For a discussion of this problem, see for example [**9**].)

The following is a greedy algorithm for this problem. (See [**9**].) Create a set C of workers chosen. Choose first for C the least expensive worker and assign the worker to any acceptable job. (Choose arbitrarily throughout all the steps if there are ties.) At each stage, add the next least expensive worker to C if there is an acceptable (feasible) assignment using all the workers in the new C obtained by adding this worker. (This might require reassigning jobs from an earlier assignment of workers previously in C.) If a next least expensive worker cannot be added to C, go to the next least expensive one in the list. Continue until you have gone through all the workers. (This is a greedy algorithm because at each step we are choosing the least expensive worker.)

To illustrate this algorithm, consider the data of Table 1. With this data, the algorithm proceeds as follows.

- Step 1: Pick W_2 for C and assign it to, say, J_2.
- Step 2: Pick W_4 for C and use the assignment $W_2 - J_2, W_4 - J_3$. Now, $C = \{W_2, W_4\}$.
- Step 3: Pick W_5 and use the assignment $W_2 - J_2, W_4 - J_3, W_5 - J_5$. Now, $C = \{W_2, W_4, W_5\}$.
- Step 4: Pick W_3. Note that W_2, W_3, W_4 can only be assigned to J_2 and J_3, so there is no way to add W_3 to the set C.
- Step 5: Pick W_1. This can only be assigned to J_2, J_3, or J_5, all of which are already in the assignment. However, we could switch W_5 to J_1 and then assign W_1 to J_5, so we add W_1 to C. C is now $\{W_1, W_2, W_4, W_5\}$.
- Step 6: Pick W_6. Since one of W_2, W_4 has to be assigned to J_3, there is no way to make an assignment for W_6. Thus, we end with $C = \{W_1, W_2, W_4, W_5\}$ and only jobs J_1, J_2, J_3, J_5 are covered.

This solution turns out to be optimal. It is not hard to show that the greedy algorithm always gives an optimal solution to the Minimum Cost Assignment Problem. (See [**9**] for a discussion of why this works.)

3. Investing in Health Care Options

Suppose we are faced with a selection of health care options in which to invest. Option i has an estimated cost c_i and an estimated value v_i. We might be considering alternative health care facilities; alternative supplies for a clinic; alternative research programs; alternative interventions; etc. The problem is to determine which ones to invest in so that the total cost is within budget and the total value is as large as possible.

This is an example of a ***Knapsack Problem***. We have a fixed size knapsack, a number of items we can take, each of a certain size and value, and we want to choose items for the knapsack so as to maximize their value but not exceed the capacity of the knapsack. In general, knapsack problems are difficult to solve computationally: They are NP-complete. The problem we have posed can be stated as follows:

$$\text{Maximize } \sum v_i x_i$$
$$\text{Subject to } \sum c_i x_i \leq B,$$

where x_i = number of items i chosen. There are several variants of the problem. For example, if we allow at most one of each item, then we have the restriction $x_i = 0$ or 1. If the number of items i we can take is bounded for each i, we speak of a ***Bounded Knapsack Problem*** and have the restriction $x_i \in \{0, 1, \ldots, b_i\}$. If we allow an arbitrary number of copies of each item, then we speak of the ***Unbounded Knapsack Problem*** and x_i can be any integer. We shall discuss the latter problem here.

A greedy algorithm for the Unbounded Knapsack Problem is due to George Dantzig [**24**]. Sort items in decreasing order of value per unit cost: v_i/c_i. Pick as many copies of the first item as possible until no more are possible or until one more would violate the budget constraint $\sum c_i x_i \leq B$. Continue in the same way with the second item, then the third, etc. (This is a greedy algorithm since at each step we pick the most valuable item available to us that does not violate the constraint.) To illustrate, consider the data in Table 2. The options in the case of AIDS prevention could be things like: (1) Condom Distribution; (2) Educational Posters; (3) Distribution of Clean Needles; (4) Testing Programs; (5) Funded Research; etc. With this data, the algorithm proceeds as follows.

- Item 1 has the highest ratio v_i/c_i, i.e., 10. We can pick two copies of item 1, with a total cost of 70+70 = 140.
- Item 3 has the next highest ratio v_i/c_i, i.e., 9. We can pick one copy of item 3. The total cost of our knapsak is now 140+35 = 175.
- Next, we pick three copies of item 5, and our knapsack cost is 175+24 = 199.
- Next, we consider item 4, but it is too costly to add to the knapsack.
- Finally, we pick one copy of item 2, and our knapsack cost is 199+5 = 204.

For the Unbounded Knapsack Problem, the greedy algorithm does not always attain the optimal value. For example, consider the data of Table 3. Then the

TABLE 2. Value and Cost of Alternative Health Care Investments

Option i	1	2	3	4	5
Value v_i	700	15	315	35	64
Cost c_i	70	5	35	7	8
Available Budget $B = 205$					

TABLE 3. Value and Cost of Alternative Health Care Investments

Option i	1	2	3
Value v_i	50	52	1
Cost c_i	10	11	1
Available Budget $B = 99$			

greedy algorithm has us pick nine copies of item 1 plus nine copies of item 3, at a total value of 459, while picking nine copies of item 2 gives us a higher value, 468. In fact, the greedy algorithm can lead to solutions that are not close to the optimal value. However, if A is the maximum total value $\sum v_i x_i$ achievable, then the greedy algorithm always achieves a total value of at least $A/2$ [**79**]. Is this a satisfactory outcome? It depends upon the application and the tradeoff between the need to make a speedy decision and the ability to wait and do a complicated calculation. For instance, in a natural disaster such as a hurricane or earthquake, or a rapidly escalating newly-emerging disease outbreak, we might need to make rapid decisions. A case in point is a bioterrorist attack. After it is discovered, e.g., when a plume might still be in the air, we might only have several hours or even minutes to make quick decisions in response. However, if we have the time to do a more time-consuming calculation, we might do better than the relatively speedy greedy algorithm. For the Bounded Knapsack Problem, the algorithm can lead to a solution that is quite a bit further from the optimal. In fact, consider the case where there are two items, with $v_1 = 2, c_1 = 1, v_2 = v, c_2 = v$. If the budget B is v and at most one copy of each item can be chosen, the greedy algorithm chooses item 1 for a total value of 2, whereas choosing item 2 gives a total value of v. Thus, the ratio between the value of the greedy solution and that of the optimal solution can be arbitrarily close to 0.

Representative examples of greedy algorithms for general knapsack problems can be found in [**1, 62, 63, 74**]. Some references on greedy algorithms for the Unbounded Knapsack Problem are [**38, 42, 49, 53, 54**].

4. Locating Health Care Facilities

Suppose that we have a number of users of a planned set of health care facilities. Where do we put the facilities and how do we assign a user to a facility? Suppose we always associate a user to the facility she can get to with minimum cost (choosing arbitrarily in case of ties). There are two costs associated with a choice of locations for the facilities. One is the cost f_i of locating (building, opening, maintaining) a facility at location i. This is either a one-time, fixed cost, or a continuing cost, or a combination of the two. Another cost is the cost c_{ij} of assigning a user at location j to a facility at location i, which is the distance between i and j (or in some applications the distance multiplied by the importance of the user at j

or the demand for facility use at j). We wish to minimize the sum of these two costs, summed over all facilities that are located and over all j corresponding to users. Note that we allow more than one facility and there is a tradeoff between the increased cost if we have more facilities and the corresponding reduced cost of getting users to them.

Given a set S of facilities, let F be the sum of costs f_i over all facilities in S and C be the sum of distances c_{ij} over all users j, where i is the (a) closest facility to j. We seek to find S so that $F + C$ is as small as possible. Of course, if there is a one-time fixed cost for locating facilities and a minimal cost for maintaining them, this could be dominated by the continuing costs of getting users to facilities, and the costs f_i could be disregarded entirely. However, in other cases, the facility location costs are quite high and continuing regularly. There are many variants of the facility location problem. (For reference, see for example [**28**].) This version is called the ***Uncapacitated Facility Location Problem*** - uncapacitated since we have no limit on the number of facilities.

In many cases in the literature, the potential facility locations and the users are located along the edges or at the nodes of a network, with edges having "weights" corresponding to distance between nodes or some other measure of cost of going between the nodes. Charikar and Guha [**18**] consider the case where both facility locations and users are only at nodes of such a network. They use a greedy algorithm to first find a preliminary solution S. To find this, order the nodes of the network in order of increasing cost of locating a facility at the node (choosing arbitrarily in case of ties). Choose p so that if S is the set of the first p facilities, then the cost $F + C$ associated with S is as small as possible. (Note of course that adding facilities would increase F, but decrease (or not increase) C.) (This involves a greedy algorithm because one chooses at each stage the node where the cost of building a facility is as small as possible. This is then greedy in a second sense of choosing how many nodes to include so as to minimize a combination of costs, though this latter choice is not repeated at each step in the way we have defined greedy algorithm.)

To illustrate this part of the algorithm, consider the network of Figure 1. In this, the number on the edge $\{x, y\}$ represents the distance $d(x, y)$ between the nodes x and y if traveling along that edge, while if u and v are not joined by an edge, $d(u, v)$ is the length of a shortest path between u and v in the network. In our example, all distances are taken to be 1. Thus, the distance $d(b, f)$ between b and f is 2 (take the cycle from b to a to f). The costs of locating the facilities are given in the figure next to each node. Suppose that we have three users, located at b, c, f as indicated by circles in the figure. Ordering nodes in order of increasing cost gives the order f, d, b, e, a, c. First take $S = \{f\}$. Then the costs associated with S are $F =$ cost of $f = 0.5$, $C = d(f, f) + d(b, f) + d(c, f) = 0 + 2 + 3 = 5$, so $F + C = 5.5$. Next, take $S = \{f, d\}$. Here, $F =$ cost of f + cost of $d = 0.5 + 1 = 1.5, C = d(f, f) + d(b, f) + d(c, d) = 0 + 2 + 1 = 3, F + C = 4.5$. The third step is to take $S = \{f, d, b\}$. This gives a cost of $F = 4.5$ and $C = 1$, so $F + C = 5.5$. All subsequent sets S have $F > 4.5$, so $F + C > 4.5$. We conclude by the greedy algorithm that the preliminary solution is $S = \{f, d\}$.

The algorithm continues as follows. At each step, we try to improve the cost of the current solution S, starting with the preliminary solution. Choose a node k at random. (It may be one already in S.) Choose a subset T of facilities in S to remove from S. If a user at node j is closer to k than to the facility i in S she is

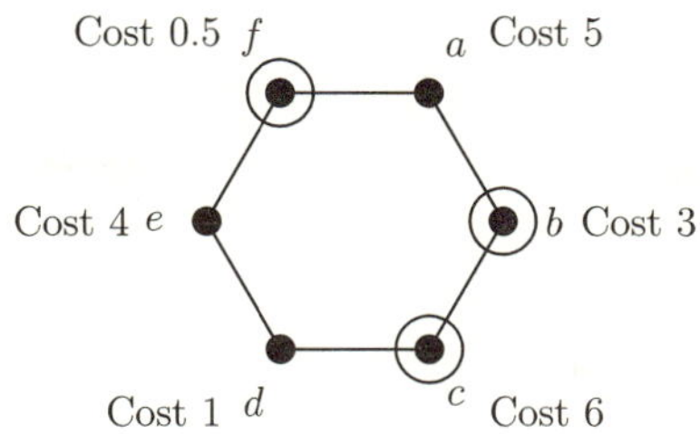

FIGURE 1. Users are located at circled nodes of this network, distances are indicated along edges, and costs of locating facilities are indicated next to nodes where facilities would be located.

assigned to, change her assignment to k and add k to S. If a user at node j was assigned to a facility that was removed from S, i.e., a facility in T, assign her to k and add k to S. Call the resulting set of facilities S^+. For the chosen k, over all possible sets T, find one to remove from S so that S^+ minimizes the total cost $F+C$ of the revised assignment. If the new set of facilities that results has a smaller total cost $F+C$ than that associated with S, use it for the new S. Otherwise, stay with the previous S.

Charikar and Guha [**18**] show that, given ϵ, the algorithm is guaranteed to achieve a cost $F+C$ that is at most $2F^*+3C^*+\epsilon(F^*+C^*)$ in at most $O(nlog(n/\epsilon))$ steps, where F^* and C^* are costs associated with an arbitrary optimal solution.

Note that the way Charikar and Guha define S^+, it is possible that in some steps, node j is not assigned to its closest facility in S^+. We could be tempted to change the definition of S^+ to include a step that would reassign a user at node j to its closest facility i in S^+ and then removing from S^+ all nodes not used for facilities. However, this method does not attain any better bound on the outcome value of $F+C$ and takes longer because we have to find closest facilities.

Representative publications on the Uncapacitated Facility Location Problem, including some with greedy algorithm approaches, are [**16, 34, 39, 40**].

5. Rerouting Emergency Vehicles in Case of Floods

When there is a flood or other natural disaster that results in roads being closed, we need to find fast ways to reroute emergency vehicles such as ambulances. We might want to reroute emergency rescue vehicles to avoid rising flood waters while minimizing delay in provision of medical attention and still getting afflicted people to available hospital facilities. A well-known and widely studied Operations Research problem that arises in this context is the ***Minimum Spanning Tree Problem*** [**70**]. Given a graph or network with positive real numbers as weights on the edges, a ***spanning tree*** is a tree using the edges of the graph and containing all of the nodes. It is ***minimum*** if the sum of the numbers on the edges used is as small as possible. Minimum spanning trees arise in many applications. The emergency vehicle routing problem can be looked at as follows: Given a road network, find usable roads that allow you to go from any node to any other node, minimizing the lengths of the roads used. This is exactly the problem of finding a minimum spanning tree.

A well-known and efficient greedy algorithm for solving the Minimum Spanning Tree problem is Kruskal's algorithm [**47**]: List the edges of the graph in order of

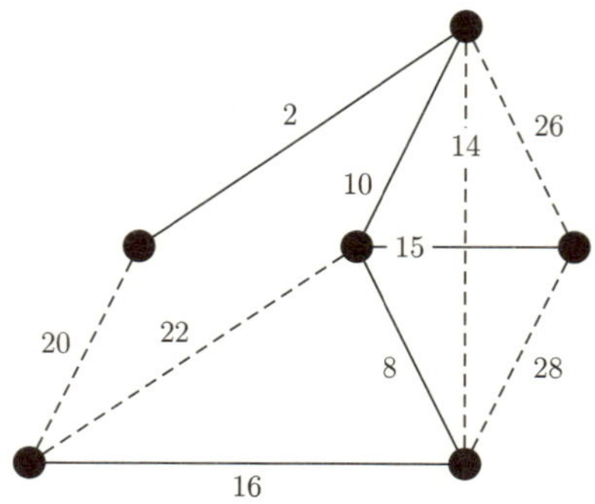

FIGURE 2. The solid edges define a minimum spanning tree.

increasing weight (choosing arbitrarily in case of ties). Going through the edges in this order, for each edge, greedily include it if it does not form a cycle with edges already chosen. Stop when no more edges can be included. (The algorithm is greedy because at each step we choose the least weight alternative that does not violate the constraint about cycles.)

A simple example illustating this algorithm is defined by the network shown in Figure 2. The lowest weight edge is that with weight 2 and the next lowest is that with weight 8. Both are included. The next lowest has weight 10 and it is also included. However, the weight 14 edge, which is next, forms a triangle with the edges of weights 8 and 10, so it is not included. We next include the edge of weight 15 and then the edge of weight 16. The remaining edges all form cycles with edges previously included. The resulting edges form the chosen spanning tree, which is illustrated with the solid lines in the figure. It is well known that Kruskal's algorithm always gives an optimal solution to the Mininum Spanning Tree problem [**22, 47, 70**].

6. Vaccination Strategies for Control of a Highly Infectious Disease Spreading through a Social Network

Many diseases spread through social networks by going from infected people to those with whom they are in contact. We can represent the contacts in a social network in a graph: The nodes are people and an edge between two people indicates contact. In such a social network, nodes are in different states at different times. In one very simple case, suppose there are only two states, susceptible (0) and infected (1). Suppose that $s_i(t)$ gives the state of node i at time t and that times are discrete, i.e., that $t = 0, 1, 2, \ldots$. In the simple case of a highly infectious disease, let us assume that an individual changes state from susceptible to infected at time $t+1$ if at least one of its neighbors are in the infected state at time t and that an individual never leaves the infected state. (More generally, we can study the variant of this model where an individual changes state from susceptible to infected at time $t+1$ if at least k of its neighbors are in the infected state at time t. This model has been studied in [**27**], who call it an ***irreversible k-threshold process.*** See also [**11, 46**].)

In this simple situation, we can investigate vaccination strategies. Let us say you have a limited amount of vaccine available each time period, say v doses. Whom should you vaccinate? More precisely: What vaccination strategy minimizes number of people ultimately infected if a disease breaks out with one infection? Here, we assume that a vaccinated node cannot move into the infected state. This problem in the context of the model above is sometimes known as the ***Firefighter Problem***. The latter problem arises when we have a forest and a fire (epidemic) starts at one tree. At each time period, some trees are burning (infected) and once they start burning, they don't stop. At every time period, we can place v firefighters (think of vaccinating) at unburned nodes. Then the fire spreads to neighboring trees that are not yet burning (susceptible) and not protected by a firefighter (vaccinated node). A rather large literature has grown up about this problem. For some references, see [**27, 36**]. Some of the questions that have been asked in connection with the firefighter problem include:

- Can the fire be contained?
- How many time steps are required before the fire is contained?
- How many firefighters per time step are necessary?
- What fraction of all nodes will be saved (burnt)?
- Does where the fire breaks out matter?
- What if the fire starts at more than one node?
- How does containment work for different graph topologies?
- How can we construct graph topologies to minimize damage?
- What is the complexity of different formalizations of this problem in the computer science sense?

Let $MVS(G, u)$ be the maximum number of nodes that can be saved in graph G if a fire starts at node u and there is one firefighter per time period. MacGillivray and Wang [**50**] asked whether at least p nodes can be saved, i.e., whether there a vaccination strategy such that $MVS(G, u) \geq p$? They showed that this problem is NP-complete.

The firefighter problem has been studied for a variety of particular types of graphs. To give one example, consider the case of an infinite d-dimensional square grid L_d. Here, nodes are located at points $(i, j, \ldots)$ in d-space with integer coordinates $i, j, \ldots$ and two nodes are neighbors if they differ by 1 on one component. Assume that the fire starts at one node. If $d = 1$, then we have nodes on a line and it is trivial to control a fire in two steps with three burned nodes if the number of firefighters v per time step is 1. If $d = 2$, it is impossible to control the fire (epidemic) with $v = 1$. But $v = 2$ suffices and with this case of two firefighters per time step, the fire (epidemic) can be controlled in eight steps with 18 burned trees (infected individuals). To illustrate the latter, consider Figure 3. Each node has an (x, y) coordinate starting with $x = 0$ on the left-most vertical line and with $y = 0$ on the bottom horizontal line. Suppose a fire starts at node (2,2). Here, nodes on fire are shown with black circles, nodes with firefighters with white circles.

- Step 1. Place two firefighters, at nodes (1,2) and (2,1).
- Step 2. The fire spreads to nodes (2,3) and (3,2). We now place firefighters at (1,3) and (2,4).
- Step 3. The fire spreads to (3,1), (3,3), and (4,2) and we place firefighters at (3,0) and (4,1).
- Step 4. The fire now spreads to (3,4), (4,3), and (5,2) and we place firefighters at (5,1) and (6,2).
- Step 5. The fire spreads to (3,5), (4,4), and (5,3) and firefighters are put at (2,5) and (3,6).

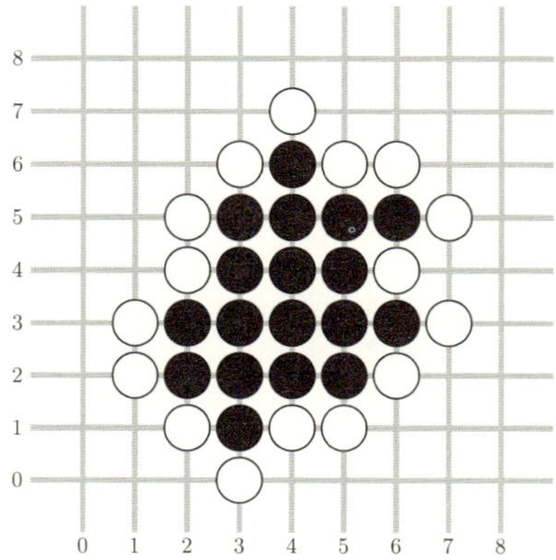

FIGURE 3. Spread of a fire on the grid when we have two firefighters available each time period. Burnt nodes are in black circles, firefighters are placed on nodes with white circles.

- Step 6. The fire spreads to (4,5), (5,4), (6,3) and we place firefighters at (6,4) and (7,3).
- Step 7. The fire spreads to (4,6) and (5,5) and firefighters are placed at (4,7) and (5,6).
- Step 8. The fire spreads to (6,5) and firefighters are placed at (6,6) and (7,5), thus controlling the fire.

We now consider the case $d \geq 3$. A graph is called ***r-regular*** if every node has exactly r neighbors. Wang and Moeller [**77**] observed that in such a graph, $r-1$ firefighters per time step are always sufficient to contain any fire outbreak (at a single node). In L_d, every node has degree $2d$. Thus, when $d \geq 3, 2d-1$ firefighters per time step are sufficient to contain any outbreak starting at a single node. Hartke [**36**] showed that $2d-2$ firefighters per time step are not enough to contain an outbreak of this kind in L_d. Thus, $2d-1$ firefighters per time step is the minimum number required to contain an outbreak in L_d and containment can be attained in two time steps.

If a fire can start at more than one node, then the following are some interesting results about outbreaks in L_d. If $d = 2$, Fogarty [**30**] showed that two firefighters per time step are sufficient to contain any outbreak at a finite number of nodes. If $d \geq 3$, Hartke [**36**] showed that for any positive integer f, f firefighters per time step is not sufficient to contain all finite outbreaks in L_d. In other words, for $d \geq 3$ and any positive integer f, there is an outbreak such that f firefighters per time step cannot contain the outbreak.

Ng and Raff [**59**] have studied L_d and modified the assumption that f is the same for each time period. Let $f(t)$ be the number firefighters available at time t. Ng and Raff assume that $f(t)$ is periodic with period p_f. This could happen for example if firefighters (doses of vaccine) arrive in batches. Then if

$$N_f = f(1) + f(2) + \quad + f(p_f),$$

$R_f = N_f/p_f$ is the average number firefighters available per time period. Ng and Raff showed that if $d = 2$ and f is periodic with period $p_f \geq 1$ and $R_f > 1.5$, then an outbreak at any number of nodes can be contained at a finite number of nodes.

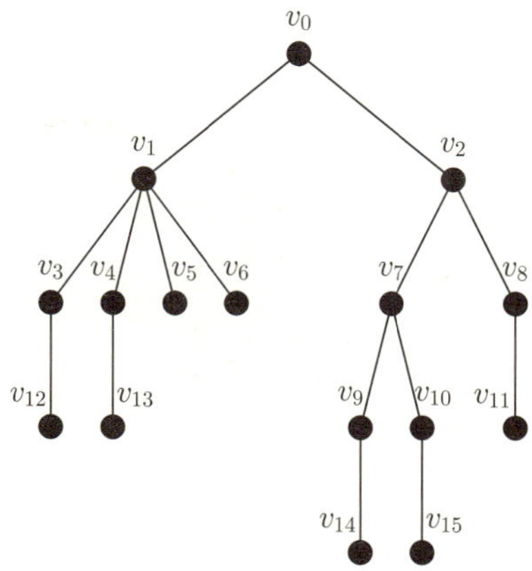

FIGURE 4. The greedy algorithm does not obtain the optimal firefighting solution for this tree.

The firefighter problem has also been studied on graphs that are trees. Consider a rooted tree with a fire starting at the root and suppose that $v = 1$. In a rooted tree, every edge goes down from a node to its immediate "children" one level below it. We define the ***weight*** of node x to be the number of descendants of x in the rooted tree, where a descendant of x is a node obtained from x by following a path that goes from x to a child y of x to a child z of $y \ldots$. In such a tree, once a firefighter is placed at a node, it and all of its descendants are "saved" and cannot be burned. A greedy algorithm for deploying firefighters in a rooted tree is the following: At each time step, place a firefighter at a node x that has not been saved or burned, such that the weight of x is maximized (choosing arbitrarily in case of ties). (This algorithm is greedy since at each step it looks to place a firefighter so as to maximize the number of nodes that can be saved at that stage of the procedure.) Consider for example the tree of Figure 4. Suppose a fire starts at node v_0. Clearly the weight is maximized by using immediate descendants, i.e., children, of v_0, and of these, v_2 has higher weight (7) than v_1 (6). Thus, we put a firefighter at node v_2. In the next time period, the fire spreads to v_1. Note that in the next stage, we can limit ourselves to descendants of v_1 since all descendants of v_2 are saved. We now look at the children of v_1 and put a firefighter on one of them. Two of them maximize weight, i.e., v_3 and v_4, so we put a firefigher on one of them, say v_3. The fire now spreads to the remaining children of v_1, i.e., v_4, v_5, v_6. Finally, we place a firefighter on one of the children of v_4, v_5, v_6, namely v_{13}. In the end, we have saved 11 nodes.

It is not hard to show that the greedy algorithm does not obtain the maximum number of saved nodes, i.e., $M(G, u)$, where u is the root. Indeed, suppose at the first step we put a firefighter at v_1 instead of v_2. The fire now spreads to v_2 and we put the next firefighter at v_7, with the fire spreading to v_8. Finally, we put a firefigher at v_{11}. In this way, we save 13 nodes.

Hartnell and Li [**37**] showed that for any tree G with one fire starting at the root u and one firefighter to be deployed per time step, the greedy algorithm always saves more than one half of $M(G, u)$ nodes, i.e., more than one half of the number of nodes that the best possible algorithm saves. Is this a satisfactory accomplishment?

It could be if time is of the essence, we have a fast-moving epidemic or bioterrorist attack, and we need to develop and implement an efficient algorithm very quickly.

7. Algorithms for Sequential Public Health or Medical Decision Making

Suppose that a patient presents with certain symptoms. Which test do we do first? On the basis of the outcome of the first test, which test do we do next? Tests are expensive. So are false positive and false negative results. In this situation, "cost" is a combination of cost of testing and cost of false results. We might ask: In what order should we do tests in order to minimize total "cost"?

An analogous problem is the following. We have several potential interventions for a public health crisis. Assume funds limit us to one intervention at a time. Which intervention do we invest in first? On the basis of the outcome of the first intervention, which do we launch next? Interventions are expensive. So are false positive and false negative assessments of the outcome of our interventions. "Cost" is a combination of cost of the intervention and cost of false results. In what order should we launch the interventions in order to minimize total "cost"?

Similar "sequential diagnosis" problems arise in many areas: communication networks (testing connectivity, paging cellular customers, sequencing tasks, etc.), manufacturing (testing machines, fault diagnosis, routing customer service calls, etc.), artificial intelligence and computer science (optimal derivation strategies in knowledge bases, best-value satisficing search, coding decision tables, etc.), inspecting containers in ports, etc. An illustrative list of references for such applications includes [**14, 15, 17, 21, 23, 29, 33, 41, 44, 45, 48, 60, 64, 65, 72, 73, 78, 80**]. Sequential diagnosis/decision making is an old subject, but one that has become increasingly important with the need for new models and algorithms as the traditional methods for making decisions sequentially do not scale.

The following approach builds on the approach to sequential diagnosis in inspection of containers at ports, originally presented by Stroud and Saeger [**75**]. In particular, we describe a method that was developed in a series of papers on container inspection: [**2, 10, 51, 52**].

Consider the medical testing problem. A physician is looking to determine if a patient has disease x. The doctor has a variety of tests to choose from (complete blood count, endoscopy, MRI, stress test, etc.). In the end, the patient is to be classified into one of several categories. Simple case: $0 =$ "doesn't have the disease," $1 =$ "does have the disease." A testing scheme specifies which test is to be made based on previous observations.

In the case of public health interventions, say we are looking to determine if an epidemic can be controlled. We have a variety of interventions to choose from (close schools if absenteeism is above 15%, close airports, invest in prophylactics, vaccinate health care workers, etc.). In the end, the epidemic is to be classified into one of several categories, in the simplest case "$0 =$ controllable," "$1 =$ not controllable." An intervention scheme specifies which intervention is to be made based on assessments of previous interventions. We shall present our discussion in the language of the medical testing problem, though an analogous discussion cojuld apply to the public health intervention problem.

The 0's and 1's suggest binary digits (bits). A ***bit string*** is a sequence of bits, e.g., 0001, 1101. A ***Boolean function*** on n variables is a function that assigns to each bit string of length n a 0 or a 1. Patients have ***attributes*** related to the disease being tested for, each in a number of states. (Sample attributes could be white blood cell count, PSA, creatinin clearance, fever greater than 40 degrees Centigrade, severe cough, severe fatigue). In the simplest case, attributes are in state 0 or 1 (absent or present). Then a patient corresponds to a bit string like 011001 and classification is a decision function F that assigns each bit string to a category. If there are two categories, 0 and 1 ("has disease" or "doesn't have disease"), the decision function F is a Boolean function. This is the case to be discussed here.

There are 2^{2^n} Boolean functions of n variables. This number grows rapidly and it quickly becomes infeasible to look at all possible Boolean functions when considering a testing problem. The problem is then: Given a patient, test her attributes until we know enough to calculate the value of F. A testing scheme tells us in which order to test the attributes to minimize cost. Even this simplified problem is hard computationally. Simplifications include the assumption that F is known. Another is that attributes are independent. Other complications that might arise would be if there were precedence relations in the attributes (e.g., we can't test attribute a_4 before testing attribute a_6). Moreover, the cost of testing for an attribute may depend on attributes tested before, or F may depend on variables that cannot be directly tested or for which tests are too costly. Such problems are hard computationally. There are many possible Boolean functions F. Even if F is fixed, the problem of finding a good (least cost) testing scheme is NP-complete. Several classes of Boolean functions F allow for efficient testing schemes: k-out-of-n systems [**8, 31, 32, 35, 72**], certain series-parallel systems [**4, 13, 57, 71**], read-once systems [**3, 58**], "regular systems" [**12**], and Horn systems [**78**].

We can represent Boolean functions by using binary rooted (directed) trees. All directed edges (arcs) head from a node to either a left or right child. Nodes with no outgoing arcs (no children) are called ***leaves***. When a Boolean function is based on testing for attributes, we can represent it as a binary rooted tree called a ***binary decision tree (BDT)*** where leaf nodes correspond to categories 0 or 1 and other nodes correspond to tests. We take a right arc from a test node if the test indicates that the attribute it is testing for is present, and a left arc otherwise. Consider for example the BDT shown in Figure 5. We reach category 1 from the root by going from a_0 left to a_1, then right to a_2, and then right to 1 or by going from a_0 right to a_2 and then right to 1. Hence, a patient is classified in category 1 iff she has attributes a_1 and a_2 and not a_0 or attributes a_0 and a_2 and possibly a_1. The corresponding Boolean function is given by $F(111) = F(101) = F(011) = 1, F(abc) = 0$ otherwise.

Note that two different BDTs can correspond to the same Boolean function. The BDT of Figure 6 corresponds to the same Boolean function as the BDT of Figure 5. Since the second BDT has fewer test nodes than the first, if all test nodes in a BDT are equally likely to be visited, then the BDT with fewer test nodes would be preferable, at least in the simple case where all tests cost the same and all tests are equally likely to lead to false positives or false negatives. Even in the simple case where the "cost" of a BDT is measured by the number of test nodes, the problem of finding the least cost BDT for a given fixed Boolean function is hard. Doing it by enumerating all possible BDTs is already impractical when there are only four kinds of tests, i.e., we have a Boolean function of $n = 4$ variables. In practice, we don't know what Boolean function to use and seek one that is least

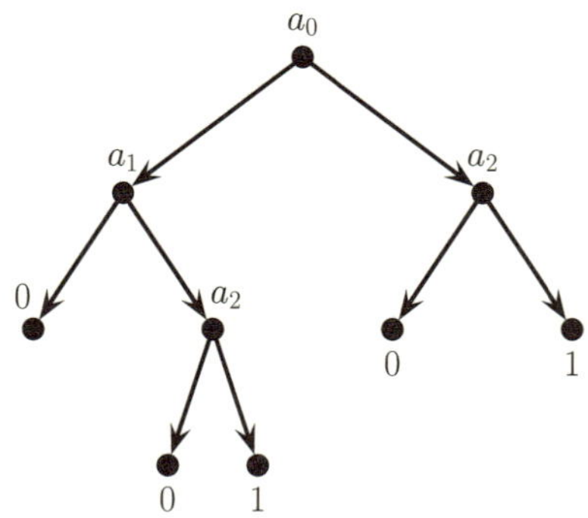

FIGURE 5. A binary decision tree for sequential testing.

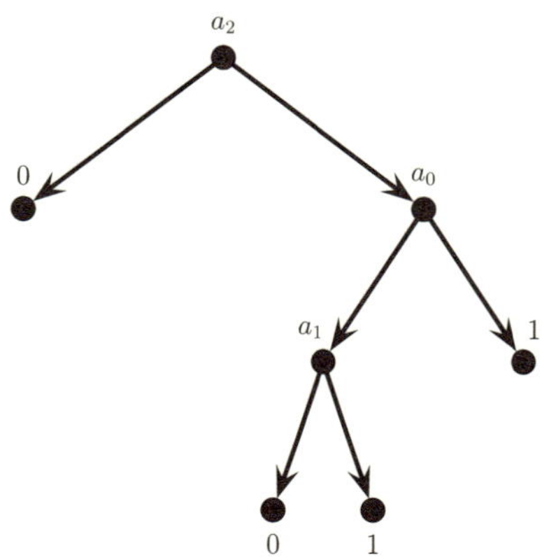

FIGURE 6. A binary decision tree corresponding to the same Boolean function as the BDT of Figure 5.

costly in some sense. Then one approach is to limit the problem to special types of Boolean functions, lest it get totally out of hand.

This is the idea developed by Stroud and Saeger [**75**]. They enumerated all "complete, monotone" Boolean functions and calculated the least expensive corresponding BDTs. Their method is practical for $n \leq 4$ but not for $n = 5$. Given two bit strings $x_1x_2 \dots x_n, y_1y_2 \dots y_n$, suppose that $x_i \geq y_i$ for all i implies that $F(x_1x_2 \dots x_n) \geq F(y_1y_2 \dots y_n)$. Then we say that F is ***monotone***. Here 111 has highest probability of being in category 1. A Boolean function F of n variables is ***incomplete*** if F can be calculated by finding at most $n-1$ variables and knowing the value of the input string on those variables, and F is ***complete*** otherwise.

Stroud and Saeger found the least cost tree by enumerating all BDTs corresponding to a given complete, monotone Boolean function and repeating this for all complete, monotone Boolean functions. The problem is that there are too many complete, monotone Boolean functions. When $n = 2$, there are 6 monotone Boolean functions, only 2 of them are complete, monotone, and there are 4 BDTs for calculating these 2 complete, monotone Boolean functions. When $n = 3$, there are 9 complete, monotone Boolean functions and 60 distinct BDTs for calculating them. When $n = 4$, there are 114 complete, monotone Boolean functions and 11,808 distinct BDTs for calculating them. (Compare 1,079,779,602 BDTs for all Boolean functions.) When $n = 5$, there are 6,894 complete, monotone Boolean functions and 263,515,920 corresponding BDTs. (Even worse: compare $5x10^{18}$ BDTs corresponding to all Boolean functions.) We need alternative approaches; enumeration is not feasible!

So far, we have considered only one possibility: that one BDT is cheaper than another if it has fewer nodes. This is oversimplified. There are more complex costs involved than number of tests in a tree. The Stroud-Saeger method can still be applied here. Performing a test has a number of costs. There is a ***unit cost*** of performing the test, a ***fixed cost*** of purchasing the equipment to make the test, and a ***delay cost*** from waiting to take the test and waiting for the results. Much of the work so far has disregarded fixed and delay costs and has been aimed at minimizing unit costs (though Stroud and Saeger have done some work with queueing models to take into account delay costs). Even if we just consider unit costs, the answer may be complicated; it depends on how many (or which) nodes of the decision tree are actually visited during an "average" procedure toward diagnosis. This will depend on the costs of doing a test for a given attribute and on a "distribution" of the disease in the population from which individuals to be tested are chosen. Moreover, it can also depend on the probability of test errors, i.e., the probability that a test for attribute a_i gives a false positive result (saying a_i is present when it is not) or a false negative (saying a_i is not present when it is). If we are given the probability of an error for each kind of test (and assume that this probability is independent of the time that the test is given) and given the a priori probability that a patient has the disease, we can calculate the "expected" cost of utilization of the tree, which we denote by C_{util}. Under these assumptions, we can also calculate the probability P_{FP} that a given BDT leads to a false positive outcome, or the probability P_{FN} that it leads to a false negative outcome in the classification scheme, i.e., the probability that the patient is classified as having the disease when she doesn't or not having it when she does. A challenge is to put costs on these false positive and false negative classifications, C_{FP}, C_{FN} respectively. Both of these costs are hard to measure. In the former case, if it means beginning a series of treatments, it could be expensive, not to mention having a psychological cost to patient. In the latter case, it would mean that the patient would go untreated. In our work [**2, 10, 51, 52**], following Stroud and Saeger, we have used the cost function

$$C_{Tot} = C_{FP} \times P_{FP} + C_{FN} \times P_{FN} + C_{util}$$

.

To repeat: P_{FP}, P_{FN} are calculated from the tree and C_{util} is calculated from the tree, the costs of the tests for the attributes, the a priori probability of disease, and the probabilities of test errors. The values of C_{FP}, C_{FN} are inputs. Note: a model for developing probability of errors in individual tests for attributes, that depends on thresholds, is also developed by Stroud and Saeger [**75**] and by Madigan, Mittal and Roberts [**51, 52**].

Sometimes adding more possibilities results in being able to do more efficient searches. Madigan, Mittal and Roberts expanded the space of trees from those corresponding to Stroud and Saeger's complete, monotonic Boolean Functions to "complete and monotonic" BDTs. There are some advantages to this: Unlike Boolean functions, BDTs may not have to consider all test inputs to give a final decision. Moreover, we might allow more potentially useful trees to participate in the analysis. In [**51, 52**], a binary tree is called ***monotonic*** if all the left leaves are class "0" and all the right leaves are class "1." A binary tree is called ***complete*** if every type of test occurs at least once in the tree and, at any non-leaf node in the tree, its left and right sub-trees are not identical. We consider the space of ***CM Trees***, trees that are complete and monotonic. This is a much richer space than the space of BDTs corresponding to complete, monotone Boolean functions. If $n = 3$, there 60 BDTs from complete, monotone Boolean functions, but 114 CM trees. If $n = 4$, it is 11,808 for the former, 66,600 for the latter.

Madigan, Mittal, and Roberts define a way of moving in CM Tree Space from one tree to a neighboring one. This follows ideas in the literature from Chipman, George, and McCulloch [**20**] and Miglio and Soffritti [**56**], who provide a comparison of various definitions of neighborhood and proximity between trees, and from Chipman, George, and McCulloch [**19**], who describe methods to traverse the tree space. Specifically, Madigan, Mittal and Roberts define four operations that take a CM tree into a "neighboring" CM tree. We ***split*** a CM tree when we pick a leaf node and replace it with a test node that is not already present in that branch, and then insert arcs from that test node to 0 and to 1. We perform a ***swap*** on a CM tree if we pick a non-leaf node in the tree and swap it with its parent node such that the new tree is still monotonic and complete and no test node occurs more than once in any branch. In the operation ***merge***, we pick a parent node of two leaf nodes and make it a leaf node by collapsing the two leaf nodes below it, or pick a parent node with one leaf node, collapse both the parent node and its one leaf node, and shift the sub-tree up in the tree by one level. Finally, we perform the operation ***replace*** on a CM tree when we pick a test node occurring more than once in the tree and replace it with any other test node such that no test node occurs more than once in any branch. Madigan, Mittal and Roberts showed that any tree in CM tree space can be reached from any other tree by using these neighborhood operations repetitively. These neighborhood operations are the basis of algorithms for searching through CM Tree Space.

The basic idea of Madigan, Mittal, and Roberts is to use a greedy search algorithm. In this algorithm, we randomly start at any tree in CM tree space, find its neighboring trees using the above operations, move to the neighbor with the lowest cost, and iterate until we find a minimum. The problem with this algorithm is that CM Tree Space is highly multi-modal (with more than one local minimum) and it is easy to get stuck at a local minimum. This led Madigan, Mittal, and Roberts to implement a stochastic search algorithm coupled with the method known as simulated annealing to find the best tree. This is a variant of the greedy algorithm. The algorithm is stochastic: It selects a neighboring tree according to a probability distribution over neighboring trees. The simulated annealing aspect involves a so-called "temperature" t, initiated to one and lowered in discrete unequal steps after every h hops so that as the temperature decreases, the probability of moving to the least expensive tree in the neighborhood increases. This greedy search algorithm allowed calculations with n up to 5 types of tests, leading to BDTs with cost very close to (and in many cases equal to) the minimum and finding them significantly faster than existing methods of searching through BDTs obtained from complete, monotonic Boolean functions.

8. Concluding Comments

Allocation of scarce resources, health care or otherwise, has been a topic of mathematical analysis for a long time. In the case of health care, we might try to define "optimality" and seek "optimal" allocation strategies, or near-optimal strategies. In the context of infectious disease prevention, there is the potential to focus our efforts to optimize different, more complex outcomes: the fewest cumulative number of infections, the fewest cumulative number of deaths, the cumulative cost of infection control, the indirect societal impacts caused by an outbreak of disease, the average utility of an outcome to individuals in the population, etc. For many of these, the simplest algorithmic approach is sometimes a greedy one. As we have seen: Sometimes it pays to be greedy.

References

1. Akay, Y., Li, H.,and Xu, S., "Greedy algorithm for the general multidimensional knapsack problem," *Annals of Operations Research*, **150** (2007), 17-29.
2. Anand, S., Madigan, D. Mammone, R., Pathak, S., and Roberts, F., "Experimental analysis of sequential decision making algorithms for port of entry inspection procedures, in S. Mehrotra, D. Zeng, H. Chen, B. Thuraisingham, and F-X Wang (eds.), *Intelligence and Security Informatics, Proceedings of ISI-2006*, Lecture Notes in Computer Science #3975, Springer-Verlag, New York, 2006, 319-330.
3. Angluin, D., Hellerstein, L., and Karpinski, M., "Learning read-once formulas with queries," *Journal of the Association for Computing Machinery*, **40** (1993), 185-210.
4. Arseneau, L., *Optimal Testing Strategies for s,t-Series Parallel Systems*, Master's Thesis, Combinatorics and Optimization, University of Waterloo, 1996.
5. Barrett, S., "Eradication versus control: the economics of global infectious disease policies, *Bull. World Health Organ.*, **82** (2004), 683-688.
6. Bauch, C.T., "Imitation dynamics predict vaccinating behaviour," *Proc. Biol. Sci.*, **272** (2005), 1669-1675.
7. Bauch, C.T., and Earn, D.J., "Vaccination and the theory of games, *Proc. Natl. Acad. Sci. USA*, **101** (2004), 13391-13394.
8. Ben-Dov, Y., "Optimal testing procedures for special structures of coherent systems," *Management Science*, **27** (1981), 1410-1420.
9. Bogart, K.P., *Introductory Combinatorics*, Pitman Publishing, Marshfield, MA, 1983.
10. Boros, E., Elsayed, E., Kantor, P. Roberts, F., and Xie, M., "Optimization problems for port-of-entry detection systems," in H. Chen and C.C. Yang eds.O, *Intelligence and Security Informatics: Techniques and Applications*, Springer, 2008, 319-335.
11. Boros, E., and Gurvich, V., "On complexity of algorithms for modeling disease transmission and optimal vaccination strategy," RUTCOR Research Report 16-2007, Rutgers University, 2007.
12. Boros, E., and Ünlüyurt, T., "Diagnosing double regular systems," *Annals of Mathematics and Artificial Intelligence*, **26** (1999), 171-191.
13. Boros, E., and Ünlüyurt, T., "Sequential testing of series-parallel systems of small depth," in M. Laguna and J. L. Gonzáles Velarde (eds.), *OR Computing Tools for the New Millennium* (Proc. Conference of the INFORMS Computing Society, Cancun, Mexico, January 5-7, 2000), 2000, 39-74.
14. Brule, J.D., Johnson, R.A., and Kletsky, E.J., "Diagnosis of equipment failures," *IRE Transactions on Reliability and Quality Control*, **RQC-9** (1960), 23-34.
15. Butterworth, R., "Some reliability fault testing models," *Operations Research*, **20** (1972), 335-343.
16. Byrka, J., "An optimal bifactor approximation algorithm for the metric uncapacitated facility location problem," in *International Workshop on Approximation Algorithms for Combinatorial Optimization Problems (APPROX)*, 2007.
17. Chang, C.L., and Slage, J.R., "An admissible and optimal algorithm for searching and-or graphs," *Artificial Intelligence*, **2** (1971), 117-128.

18. Charikar, M., and Guha, S., "Improved combinatorial algorithms for facility location problems," *SIAM Journal on Computing*, **34** (2005), 803-824.
19. Chipman, H.A., George, E.I., and McCulloch, R.E., "Bayesian CART model search, *Journal of the American Statistical Association*, **93** (1998), 935-960.
20. Chipman, H.A., George, E.I., and McCulloch, R.E., "Extracting representative tree models from a forest," working paper 98-07, Department of Statistics and Actuarial Science, University of Waterloo, 1998.
21. Chiu, S.Y., Cox, L.A., and Sun, X., "Least-cost failure diagnosis in uncertain reliability systems," *Reliability Engineering and System Safety*, **54** (1996), 203–216.
22. Cormen, T.H., Leiserson, C.E., Rivest, R.L., and Stein, C., *Introduction to Algorithms*, Second Edition, MIT Press and McGraw-Hill, 2001.
23. Cox, L.A., Jr., and Qiu, Y., "Optimal inspection and repair of renewable coherent systems with independent components and constant failure rates," *Naval Research Logistics*, **41** (1994), 771-788.
24. Dantzig, G.B., "Discrete-variable extremum problems," *Operations Research*, **5** (1957), 266-288.
25. DIMACS, DIMACS Workshop on Economic Epidemiology, 2005, http://dimacs.rutgers.edu/Workshops/EconEpid/.
26. DIMACS, DIMACS/MBI/MITACS Workshop on Economic Epidemiology, July-August 2009, http://dimacs.rutgers.edu/Workshops/WSEconEpi/.
27. Dreyer, P.A., and Roberts, F.S., "Irreversible k-threshold processes: Graph-theoretical threshold models of the spread of disease and of opinion," *Discrete Applied Mathematics*, **157** (2009), 1615-1627.
28. Drezner, Z, and Hamacher, H.W., *Facility Location: Applications and Theory*, Springer, 2004.
29. Duffuaa, S.O., and Raouf, A., "An optimal sequence in multicharacteristics inspection," *Journal of Optimization Theory and Applications*, **67** (1990), 79-87.
30. Fogarty, P., *Catching the Fire on Grids*, Masters Thesis, University of Vermont, 2003.
31. Garey, M.R., "Simple binary identification problems," *IEEE Transactions on Computers*, **21** (1972), 588-590.
32. Garey, M.R., "Optimal task sequencing with precedence constraints," *Discrete Mathematics*, **4** (1973), 37-56.
33. Geiger, D., and Barnett, J.A., "Optimal satisficing tree searches," in *AAAI91*, Morgan Kaufmann, Anaheim, CA, 1991, 441-445.
34. Guha, S., and Khuller, S., "Greedy strikes back: Improved algorithms for facility location," *Journal of Algorithms,* **31** (1999), 228-248.
35. Halpern, J.Y., "Fault testing for a k-out-of-n system," *Operations Research*, **22** (1974), 1267-1271.
36. Hartke, S.G., *Graph-theoretic Models of Spread and Competition*, Ph.D. Thesis, Rutgers University, 2004.
37. Hartnell, B., and Li, Q., "Firefighting on trees: How bad is the greedy algorithm?", *Congressus Numerantium*, **145** (2000) 1-192.
38. Hu, T.C., and Lenard, M.L., " Optimality of a heuristic solution for a class of knapsack problems." *Oper. Res.*, **24** (1976), 193-196.
39. Jain, K., Mahdian, M., Markakis, E., Saberi, A., and Vazirani, V., "A greedy facility location algorithm analyzed using dual-fitting with factor-revealing LP," *Journal of the ACM*, **50** (2003), 795-824.
40. Jain, K., Mahdian, M, and Saberi, A. , "A new greedy approach for facility location problem," *Proceedings of the Symposium on Theory of Computing*, 2002.
41. Kadane, J.B., "Quiz show problems," *Journal of Mathematical Analysis and Applications*, **27** (1969), 609-623.
42. Kellerer, H., Pferschy, U., and Pisinger, D., *Knapsack Problems,* Springer, New York, 2004.
43. Klein, E., Laxminarayan, R., Smith, D.L., and Gilligan, C.A., "Economic incentives and mathematical models of diseases, *Environment and Development Economics*, **12** (2007), 707-732.
44. Kowalski, R., "Search strategies for theorem proving," in B. Meltzer and D. Mitchie (eds.) *Machine Intelligence*, **5**, Edinburgh University Press. Edinburgh, 1969, 181-201.

45. Kowalski, R., "And-or graphs, theorem proving graphs and bi-directional search," in B. Meltzer and D. Mitchie (eds.) *Machine Intelligence*, **7**, Edinburgh University Press, Edinburgh, 1972, 167-194.
46. Kynčl, J., Lidický, B. and Vyskočil, T., "Irreversible 2-conversion set is NP-complete," preprint, Institute for Theoretical Computer Science, Charles University, 2009.
47. Kruskal, J.B., "On the shortest spanning subtree of a graph and the traveling salesman problem," *Proceedings of the American Mathematical Society*, **7** (1956), 4850.
48. Lauritzen, S.L. and Nilsson, D., "Representing and solving decision problems with limited information," *Management Science*, **47** (2001), 1238-1251.
49. Lueker, G.S., "Two NP-complete problems in nonnegative integer programming," Report No. 178, Computer Science Laboratory, Princeton University, 1975.
50. MacGillivray, G., and Wang, P., "On the firefighter problem," *Journal of Combinatorial Mathematics and Combinatorial Computing*, **47** (2003) 83-96.
51. Madigan, D., Mittal, S., and Roberts, F.S., "Efficient sequential decision-making algorithms for container inspection operations," preprint, DIMACS, Rutgers University, 2009.
52. Madigan, D., Mittal, S., and Roberts, F.S., "Sequential decision making algorithms for port of entry inspection: Overcoming computational challenges, in G. Muresan, T. Altiok, B. Melamed, and D. Zeng (eds.), *Proceedings of IEEE International Conference on Intelligence and Security Informatics (ISI-2007)*, IEEE Press, Piscataway, NJ, 2007, 1-7.
53. Magazine, M., Nemhauser, G.L., and Trotter, L.E., Jr., "When the greedy solution solves a class of knapsack problems, " *Oper. Res.*, **23** (1975), 207-217.
54. Martello, S., and Toth, P., *Knapsack Problems: Algorithms and Computer Implementations*, Wiley, England, 1990.
55. McKenzie, E., and Roberts, F.S., "Modeling social responses to bioterrorism involving infectious agents," Technical Report, DIMACS Center, Rutgers University, Piscataway, NJ, July 24, 2003. (Available at http://dimacs.rutgers.edu/Workshops/Modeling/.)
56. Miglio, R., and Soffritti, G., "The comparison between classification trees through proximity measures," *Computational Statistics and Data Analysis*, **45** (2004), 577-593.
57. Monma, C.L., and Sidney, J.B., "Optimal sequencing via modular decomposition: Characterization of sequencing functions," *Mathematics of Operations Research*, **4** (1979), 215-224.
58. Mundici, D., "Functions computed by monotone boolean formulas with no repeated variables," *Theoretical Computer Science*, **66** (1989), 113-114.
59. Ng, K.L., and Raff, P., "A generalization of the firefighter problem on $Z \times Z$," *Discrete Applied Mathematics*, **156** (2008), 730-745.
60. Nilsson, N.J., *Problem-solving Methods in Artificial Intelligence*, McGraw-Hill, New York, 1971.
61. Perry, B.D., and Young, A.S., "The past and future roles of epidemiology and economics in the control of tick-borne diseases of livestock in Africa: The case of theileriosis," *Preventive Veterinary Medicine*, **25** (1995), 107-120.
62. Pisinger, D., "A minimal algorithm for the 0-1 knapsack problem," *Operations Research*, **45** (1997), 758-767.
63. Pisinger, D., "Where are the hard knapsack problems?", *Computers & Operations Research*, **32** (2005), 2271-2284.
64. Pohl, I., "Bi-directional search," in B. Meltzer and D. Mitchie (eds.) *Machine Intelligence*, **6**, Edinburgh University Press, Edinburgh, 1971, 127-140.
65. Reinwald, L.T., and Soland, R.M., "Conversion of limited-entry decision tables to optimal computer programs I: Minimum average processing time," *Journal of the Association for Computing Machinery*, **13** (1966), 339-358.
66. Roberts, F.S., *Measurement Theory, with Applications to Decisionmaking, Utility, and the Social Sciences*, Addison-Wesley, Reading, MA, 1979. Reprinted, Cambridge University Press, Cambridge, UK, 2009.
67. Roberts, F.S., "Meaningfulness of conclusions from combinatorial optimization," *Discr. Appl. Math.* **29** (1990), 221-241.
68. Roberts, F.S., "Limitations on conclusions using scales of measurement," in S.M. Pollock, M.H. Rothkopf, and A. Barnett (eds.), *Operations Research and the Public Sector*, Vol. 6 in *Handbooks in Operations Research and Management Science*, North-Holland, Amsterdam, 1994, 621-671.

69. Roberts, F.S., "Meaningful and meaningless statements in epidemiology and public health," preprint, DIMACS, Rutgers University, 2009, submitted for publication.
70. Roberts, F.S., and Tesman, B., *Applied Combinatorics*, 2nd ed., Chapman & Hall/CRC, 2009.
71. Salloum, S., and Breuer, M.A., "An optimum testing algorithm for some symmetric coherent systems," *Journal of Mathematical Analysis and Applications*, **101** (1984), 170–194.
72. Simon, H.A., and Kadane, J.B., "Optimal problem-solving search: All-or-none solutions," *Artificial Intelligence*, **6** (1975), 235-247.
73. Smith, D.E., "Controlling backward inference," *Artificial Intelligence*, **39** (1989), 145-208.
74. Sriram, J., "KS-Solve: Local search for the knapsack problem," http://www.cs.dartmouth.edu/ afra/courses/cs44/winter09/project/report/sriram-report.eps, March 14, 2009,
75. Stroud, P.D, and Saeger, K.J., "Enumeration of increasing Boolean expressions and alternative digraph implementations for diagnostic applications," *Proceedings Volume IV, Computer, Communication and Control Technologies* 2003, 328-333.
76. Tanaka, M.M., Kumm, J., and Feldman, M.W., "Coevolution of pathogens and cultural practices: A new look at behavioral heterogeneity in epidemics," *Theoretical Population Biology*, **62** (2002), 111-119.
77. Wang, P., and Moeller, S.A., "Fire control on graphs," *Journal of Combinatorial Mathematics and Combinatorial Computing*, **41** (2002) 19-34.
78. Wang, J., and Vande Vate, J., "Question asking strategies for Horn clause systems," *AMAI*, **1** (1990), 359-370.
79. http://en.wikipedia.org/wiki/Knapsack_problem#Greedy_approximation_algorithm, September 14, 2009.
80. Yener, A., and Rose, C., "Highly mobile users and paging: Optimal polling strategies," *IEEE Transactions on Vehicular Technology*, **47** (1998), 1251-1257.

DIMACS Center, Rutgers University, Piscataway NJ 08854 USA
E-mail address: froberts@dimacs.rutgers.edu

Titles in This Series

75 **Abba B. Gumel and Suzanne Lenhart, Editors,** Modeling Paradigms and Analysis of Disease Transmission Models

74 **Camil Demetrescu, Andrew V. Goldberg, and David S. Johnson, Editors,** The Shortest Path Problem: Ninth DIMACS Implementation Challenge

73 **Paul H. Siegel, Emina Soljanin, Adriaan J. van Wijngaarden, and Bane Vasić, Editors,** Advances in Information Recording

72 **Regina Y. Liu, Robert Serfling, and Diane Souvaine, Editors,** Data Depth: Robust Multivariate Analysis, Computational Geometry and Applications

71 **Zhilan Feng, Ulf Dieckmann, and Simon Levin, Editors,** Disease Evolution: Models, Concepts, and Data Analyses

70 **James Abello and Graham Cormode, Editors,** Discrete Methods in Epidemiology

69 **Siemion Fajtlowicz, Patrick W. Fowler, Pierre Hansen, Melvin F. Janowitz, and Fred S. Roberts, Editors,** Graphs and Discovery

68 **A. Ashikhmin and A. Barg, Editors,** Algebraic Coding Theory and Information Theory

67 **Ravi Janardan, Michiel Smid, and Debasish Dutta, Editors,** Geometric and Algorithmic Aspects of Computer-Aided Design and Manufacturing

66 **Piyush Gupta, Gerhard Kramer, and Adriaan J. van Wijngaarden, Editors,** Advances in Network Information Theory

65 **Santosh S. Vempala,** The Random Projection Method

64 **Melvyn B. Nathanson, Editor,** Unusual Applications of Number Theory

63 **J. Nešetřil and P. Winkler, Editors,** Graphs, Morphisms and Statistical Physics

62 **Gerard J. Foschini and Sergio Verdú, Editors,** Multiantenna Channels: Capacity, Coding and Signal Processing

61 **M. F. Janowitz, F.-J. Lapointe, F. R. McMorris, B. Mirkin, and F. S. Roberts, Editors,** Bioconsensus

60 **Saugata Basu and Laureano Gonzalez-Vega, Editors,** Algorithmic and Quantitative Real Algebraic Geometry

59 **Michael H. Goldwasser, David S. Johnson, and Catherine C. McGeoch, Editors,** Data Structures, Near Neighbor Searches, and Methodology: Fifth and Sixth DIMACS Implementation Challenges

58 **Simon Thomas, Editor,** Set Theory: The Hajnal Conference

57 **Eugene C. Freuder and Richard J. Wallace, Editors,** Constraint Programming and Large Scale Discrete Optimization

56 **Alexander Barg and Simon Litsyn, Editors,** Codes and Association Schemes

55 **Ding-Zhu Du, Panos M. Pardalos, and Jie Wang, Editors,** Discrete Mathematical Problems with Medical Applications

54 **Erik Winfree and David K. Gifford, Editors,** DNA Based Computers V

53 **Nathaniel Dean, D. Frank Hsu, and R. Ravi, Editors,** Robust Communication Networks: Interconnection and Survivability

52 **Sanguthevar Rajasekaran, Panos Pardalos, and D. Frank Hsu, Editors,** Mobile Networks and Computing

51 **Pierre Hansen, Patrick Fowler, and Maolin Zheng, Editors,** Discrete Mathematical Chemistry

50 **James M. Abello and Jeffrey Scott Vitter, Editors,** External Memory Algorithms

49 **Ronald L. Graham, Jan Kratochvíl, Jaroslav Nešetřil, and Fred S. Roberts, Editors,** Contemporary Trends in Discrete Mathematics

48 **Harvey Rubin and David Harlan Wood, Editors,** DNA Based Computers III

47 **Martin Farach-Colton, Fred S. Roberts, Martin Vingron, and Michael Waterman, Editors,** Mathematical Support for Molecular Biology

46 **Peng-Jun Wan, Ding-Zhu Du, and Panos M. Pardalos, Editors,** Multichannel Optical Networks: Theory and Practice

45 **Marios Mavronicolas, Michael Merritt, and Nir Shavit, Editors,** Networks in Distributed Computing

44 **Laura F. Landweber and Eric B. Baum, Editors,** DNA Based Computers II

43 **Panos Pardalos, Sanguthevar Rajasekaran, and José Rolim, Editors,** Randomization Methods in Algorithm Design

42 **Ding-Zhu Du and Frank K. Hwang, Editors,** Advances in Switching Networks

41 **David Aldous and James Propp, Editors,** Microsurveys in Discrete Probability

40 **Panos M. Pardalos and Dingzhu Du, Editors,** Network Design: Connectivity and Facilities Location

39 **Paul W. Beame and Samuel R Buss, Editors,** Proof Complexity and Feasible Arithmetics

38 **Rebecca N. Wright and Peter G. Neumann, Editors,** Network Threats

37 **Boris Mirkin, F. R. McMorris, Fred S. Roberts, and Andrey Rzhetsky, Editors,** Mathematical Hierarchies and Biology

36 **Joseph G. Rosenstein, Deborah S. Franzblau, and Fred S. Roberts, Editors,** Discrete Mathematics in the Schools

35 **Dingzhu Du, Jun Gu, and Panos M. Pardalos, Editors,** Satisfiability Problem: Theory and Applications

34 **Nathaniel Dean, Editor,** African Americans in Mathematics

33 **Ravi B. Boppana and James F. Lynch, Editors,** Logic and Random Structures

32 **Jean-Charles Grégoire, Gerard J. Holzmann, and Doron A. Peled, Editors,** The SPIN Verification System

31 **Neil Immerman and Phokion G. Kolaitis, Editors,** Descriptive Complexity and Finite Models

30 **Sandeep N. Bhatt, Editor,** Parallel Algorithms: Third DIMACS Implementation Challenge

29 **Doron A. Peled, Vaughan R. Pratt, and Gerard J. Holzmann, Editors,** Partial Order Methods in Verification

28 **Larry Finkelstein and William M. Kantor, Editors,** Groups and Computation II

27 **Richard J. Lipton and Eric B. Baum, Editors,** DNA Based Computers

26 **David S. Johnson and Michael A. Trick, Editors,** Cliques, Coloring, and Satisfiability: Second DIMACS Implementation Challenge

25 **Gilbert Baumslag, David Epstein, Robert Gilman, Hamish Short, and Charles Sims, Editors,** Geometric and Computational Perspectives on Infinite Groups

24 **Louis J. Billera, Curtis Greene, Rodica Simion, and Richard P. Stanley, Editors,** Formal Power Series and Algebraic Combinatorics/Séries Formelles et Combinatoire Algébrique, 1994

23 **Panos M. Pardalos, David I. Shalloway, and Guoliang Xue, Editors,** Global Minimization of Nonconvex Energy Functions: Molecular Conformation and Protein Folding

22 **Panos M. Pardalos, Mauricio G. C. Resende, and K. G. Ramakrishnan, Editors,** Parallel Processing of Discrete Optimization Problems

21 **D. Frank Hsu, Arnold L. Rosenberg, and Dominique Sotteau, Editors,** Interconnection Networks and Mapping and Scheduling Parallel Computations

20 **William Cook, László Lovász, and Paul Seymour, Editors,** Combinatorial Optimization

19 **Ingemar J. Cox, Pierre Hansen, and Bela Julesz, Editors,** Partitioning Data Sets

18 **Guy E. Blelloch, K. Mani Chandy, and Suresh Jagannathan, Editors,** Specification of Parallel Algorithms